Headache

Series Editor

Paolo Martelletti
Roma, Italy

The purpose of this Series, endorsed by the European Headache Federation (EHF), is to describe in detail all aspects of headache disorders that are of importance in primary care and the hospital setting, including pathophysiology, diagnosis, management, comorbidities, and issues in particular patient groups. A key feature of the Series is its multidisciplinary approach, and it will have wide appeal to internists, rheumatologists, neurologists, pain doctors, general practitioners, primary care givers, and pediatricians. Readers will find that the Series assists not only in understanding, recognizing, and treating the primary headache disorders, but also in identifying the potentially dangerous underlying causes of secondary headache disorders and avoiding mismanagement and overuse of medications for acute headache, which are major risk factors for disease aggravation. Each volume is designed to meet the needs of both more experienced professionals and medical students, residents, and trainees.

More information about this series at http://www.springer.com/series/11801

Massimo Leone • Arne May

Editors

Cluster Headache and other Trigeminal Autonomic Cephalgias

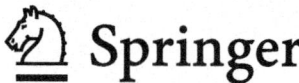 Springer

Editors
Massimo Leone
Department of Neurology
Neuroalgology Unit
The Foundation of the Carlo Besta
Neurological Institute, IRCCS
Milano
Italy

Arne May
Department of Systems Neuroscience
University of Hamburg
Hamburg
Germany

ISSN 2197-652X   ISSN 2197-6538   (electronic)
Headache
ISBN 978-3-030-12437-3   ISBN 978-3-030-12438-0   (eBook)
https://doi.org/10.1007/978-3-030-12438-0

This Springer imprint is published by the registered company Springer Nature Switzerland AG
The registered company address is: Gewerbestrasse 11, 6330 Cham, Switzerland

Foreword

Cluster headache has always been the object of researchers' desire for understanding. I must confess that I too have succumbed to its dark fascination and applied myself for more than 15 years to the visionary study of its neuroimmunological mechanisms, well before the era of monoclonal antibodies started.

This new volume of the Headache Series, endorsed by the European Headache Federation, carefully scans all the corners of laboratory and clinical research on cluster headache and offers a complete pathophysiological picture. Although it is so typical to be unmistakable, it often escapes the untrained eye in everyday practice; these diagnostic delays remain completely unacceptable, especially because they can be extremely serious or fatal. Although very dated, prevention therapies of cluster headache are not always correctly applied everywhere and in a timely manner, often missing the appropriate cardiovascular evaluations.

Always keeping an eye to the past, the present of these patients is more promising, due to a better awareness of this crucial illness and better educational activities.

The near future seems to promise a new pharmacological class, but we still need to make better use of the available therapeutic armaments.

This volume, edited by two giants of the sector, Arne May and Massimo Leone, offers to expert readers new food for thought, to young physicians basics know-how to properly recognize and treat cluster headache, and to students a safe and solid point of integration of what they often do not find adequately detailed in their textbooks—all cleverly presented by a *parterre de roi* list of authors.

Rome, Italy   Paolo Martelletti

Foreword

In the last decade, scientific attention on cluster headache and related syndromes has much increased. For a rather rare disease as cluster headache, this is a good news. On the other side, it has emerged the need to have a reappraisal of the knowledge on the worst primary headache, i.e. cluster headache, as well as on related disorders. In this book, clinical data and research findings are well mixed so that it can be intelligible to the vast majority of physicians and neurologists not expert in the headache field.

I have met several cluster headache patients who have remained for many years without a proper diagnosis, hence, poorly treated. Cluster headache produces high disability during the cluster periods and even more when it has a chronic course. How to reduce all this sufferance? Carefully listening to these patients will easily guide to properly diagnose the disease. Empathy with patients is crucial to develop good research and improve science.

Some peculiar characteristics of cluster headache as the strict unilaterality of the pain and the circadian and circannual recurrence of the attacks are convincing evidence that this is a disease of the brain. Along the 1980s, a number of neuroendocrinological studies showed alterations pointing to a hypothalamic involvement in cluster headache.

In the late 1990s, the seminal neuroimaging studies by Arne May, Peter Goadsby and colleagues opened a window on the brain of cluster headache patients, confirming that the area of the posterior hypothalamus is involved in the pathophysiology of the disease. Their observation led our group in Milan to introduce for the first time the stimulation of that brain area to relieve otherwise intractable chronic cluster headache. So far, stimulation of this brain area has been used in various centres to relieve otherwise intractable cluster headaches as well as other trigeminal autonomic cephalgias. This opens up avenues to better understand the role of certain brain areas in the pathophysiology of these headache forms (and maybe beyond that).

Before the 1988 headache classification, cluster headache was considered a migraine variant in the "vascular headaches" chapter. Lee Kudrow's book in 1980 and Ottar Sjaastad's book in 1992 have much contributed to spread knowledge on the disease and to give scientific dignity to such a devastating disorder. This book follows the line traced by those books and represents a "continuum" bridging the past, present and future. It can help the new generations of clinicians and researchers in this field.

Young neurologists and doctors will much benefit to have such a book in their library.

Milan, Italy   Gennaro Bussone

Contents

Chapter 1
Cluster Headache and Related Syndromes in History and Literature

Gian Camillo Manzoni and Paola Torelli

Unlike migraine, for which there are multiple and clear indications about its knowledge since ancient times, cluster headache (CH) has been recognized only fairly recently.

The history of CH can be divided in three time periods: the first, since the mid-seventeenth century to the first part of the nineteenth century, was characterized by occasional reports of individual patients suffering from headache forms with clinical aspects suggestive of CH; the second, during the first half of the twentieth century, saw the first reports on case series with CH under the most varied names; and the third, in the second half of the twentieth century, was marked by the accurate clinical description of CH and the identification of some of its subtypes (Table 1.1).

1.1 Mid-seventeenth Century to the First Part of the Nineteenth Century

Based on a review of the studies on CH history conducted so far, the first, albeit incomplete, description can be attributed to Nicolaas Pieterszoon Tulp, a Dutch physician born in Amsterdam in 1593 who was portrayed in the famous canvas by Rembrandt *The Anatomy Lesson*. In his 1641 treatise *Observationum medicarum libri tres* [1], Tulp discussed some cases of headache and about one of them wrote: "[...] (Isaak van Halmaal) in the beginning of the summer season, was afflicted with

G. C. Manzoni (✉)
Poliambulatorio Dalla Rosa Prati, Centro Diagnostico Europeo, Parma, Italy
e-mail: giancamillo.manzoni@unipr.it

P. Torelli
Dipartimento di Medicina e Chirurgia, Centro Cefalee, Università di Parma, Parma, Italy

© Springer Nature Switzerland AG 2020
M. Leone, A. May (eds.), *Cluster Headache and other Trigeminal Autonomic Cephalgias*, Headache, https://doi.org/10.1007/978-3-030-12438-0_1

Table 1.1 Historic periods in the development of knowledge of cluster headache

First period (mid-seventeenth century to the first part of the nineteenth century)		
Nicolaas Pieterszoon Tulp	Amsterdam	1641
Thomas Willis	Oxford	1672
Abraham de la Pryme	South Yorkshire	1702
Gerhard van Swieten	Vienna	1745
Johann Christoph Ulrich Oppermann	Regensburg	1747
Johann Müller	Frankfurt	1813
Second period (first half of the twentieth century)		
Robert Bing	Basel	1913
Wifred Harris	London	1926
Bayard Taylor Horton	Rochester	1939
Third period (second half of the twentieth century)		
Lee Kudrow	USA	(1933–)
Karl Ekbom jr	Sweden	(1935–)
Ottar Sjaastad	Norway	(1928–)

a very severe headache, occurring and disappearing daily on fixed hours, with such an intensity that he often assured me that he could not bear the pain anymore or he would succumb shortly. For rarely it lasted longer than two hours. And the rest of the day there was no fever, nor indisposition of the urine, nor any infirmity of the pulse. But this recurring pain lasted until the fourteenth day". The extremely severe pain and the attacks lasting 2 h and recurring every day at fixed hours for 2 weeks are highly suggestive of CH. However, in his description Tulp says nothing about the location of pain and the presence of any accompanying symptoms.

The typical temporal pattern of CH, with active periods (cluster periods) alternating with other, even longer periods without attacks (periods of remission), was precisely defined by Thomas Willis, a professor of philosophy at Oxford University in 1672 when in *De anima brutorum* [2] he described headache periods regularly recurring at fixed intervals: "Usually the attacks of seemingly suppressed headache recur around the solstices and equinoxes [...] but the majority, provided with subordinate periods, habitually molests at fixed hours within every cycle of 24 hours".

In 1702, the British antiques dealer Abraham de la Pryme described the headache of one of his brother's servants and attributed its cause to hydrophobia, because 3 weeks before onset, the man had come into contact with some dogs with rabies [3]. In fact, the headache he described was actually more similar to CH [4]: "[...] my brother's servant, a most strong laborious man, began to be troubled with an exceeding acute pain in the head, sometimes once, sometimes twice a day, so very vehement that he was forced to hold his head with both his hands to hinder it from riving in two, which fits commonly held him about an hour at a time; [...] and his eyes behold every thing of a fiery red colour. Thus was he tormented for a whole week together, but being of a strong constitution, and returning to his labour in every interval, he sweat and wrought it off, without any physic". There is no clear indication of the location of pain, but the description of the physical appearance of the patient is interesting, because it anticipates much more recent observations in this regard [5, 6]. According to Arkink [4], this would be the first CH description ever in English, because Willis [2], as well as Tulp [1], had used Latin.

In 1745, in his *Commentaria in Hermanni Boerhaave aphorismos de cognoscendis et curandis morbis* written in Latin [5], Gerhard van Swieten, a disciple of Herman Boerhaave who founded the Vienna Medical School and served also as the personal physician of Austrian empress Maria Theresa, described a headache attack that, according to Isler [6], had all the features modern neurologists consider necessary for a diagnosis of CH [7]: "A healthy, robust men of middle age was, each day, at the same hour troubled by pain above the orbit of the left eye, where the nerve leaves the bony frontal opening; after a short time the left eye began to redden and tears to flow; then he felt as his eye was protruding from its orbit with so much pain that he became mad. After a few hours all this evil ceased and nothing in the eye appeared at all changed".

Two years later, Johann Christoph Ulrich Oppermann in his *Dissertatio medica inauguralis de hemicrania horologica* [8] reported the case of a 35-year-old woman who since age 29 had suffered from daily attacks lasting about 15 min and recurring every hour, both at night and during the day, with such regularity that she could tell time more precisely than the clock tower in the town square. Oppermann's hemicrania horologica bears close similarities to the chronic paroxysmal hemicrania that Sjaastad and Dale were able to describe only two centuries later [9].

In 1813, 56-year-old Johann Müller, general practitioner in Frankfurt, provided a detailed description of the headache that had afflicted him from age 20 to age 54 [10]: "[…] April 28, 1777 at 8 o'clock in the morning (I felt) in correspondence of the right orbit, at the level of the eyebrow, in a region that could be covered by a threepenny piece, a particular sensation of heaviness, localized in depth, that increased from minute to minute and was becoming a more and more intense pain, until it became unbearable. The pain was dull, lancinating, bothering, throbbing, as if a blacksmith was beating on his anvil; the eye had become so sensitive that it could not tolerate light, red, spasmodically contracted and full of tears; the temporal vessels were pulsing stronger than ever […] I could not find relief in any position, until the pain became so severe that I rolled on the floor. […] The attack occurred at exactly 8 o'clock every morning for seven consecutive days. […] Fortunately it then resolved; I have been suffering for 34 years from this form of disease, that afflicts me each year in fairly irregular periods". This is a very interesting description, especially because it points out two features that are typical of CH: the patient's peculiar behaviour during attacks and the periodic temporal pattern of the headache.

In the following years of the nineteenth century, eminent researchers like von Moellendorff [11], Eulenburg [12], and Charcot [13] all reported migrainous conditions characterized by attacks with signs and symptoms that were more typical of CH than of migraine, but no significant progress was made in the study of CH.

Table 1.2 Possible names of
cluster headache before 1952

Sphenopalatine neuralgia	Sluder [14]
Erythroprosopalgia	Bing [15]
Migrainous neuralgia	Harris [16]
Erythromelalgia	Bing [17]
Nasal neuralgia	Charlin [18]
Vidian neuralgia	Vail [19]
Ciliary neuralgia	Harris [20]
Histaminic cephalgia	Horton [21]
Greater superficial petrosal neuralgia	Gardner et al. [22]

Table 1.2 Possible names of cluster headache before 1952

1.2 First Half of the Twentieth Century

This was a crucial period for CH history, owing to two different sets of events.

The first was the descriptions, by several authors, of headache forms that seemed to have much in common with CH but were given the most diverse names [14–22] (Table 1.2).

The second was the progress made in the knowledge of CH thanks to the work by Robert Bing in Basel, Wilfred Harris in London, and Bayard Taylor Horton in Rochester. A testimony to Bing's contribution to CH history is the eponym "Bing-Horton syndrome", which is not uncommon in current medical German usage [6]. Harris provided very accurate descriptions of CH, which he named migrainous neuralgia, from as early as 1926 [16] and he was probably the first to report on the efficacy of ergotamine in blocking the attacks [23]. But it is especially to Horton that we owe a clinical definition of CH and its recognition as a separate clinical entity, thanks to his description of very large case series [21].

1.3 Second Half of the Twentieth Century

This period began in 1952 with the publication by Kunkle et al. [24] of the paper *Recurrent brief headaches in* "cluster" *pattern*, which resulted in the final naming now universally accepted and used for CH.

Retracing the history of a disease, it could seem strange that we mention a period, the second half of the twentieth century, that is still very close. However, for CH this was a period that was marked by a huge number of clinical, therapeutic, and pathogenetic studies conducted by different researchers in various countries, which have made it possible to shed light on several aspects of this peculiar and interesting form of primary headache. More importantly, this was a period that saw the work of three scientists who can already be said to have made the history of CH: Lee Kudrow from California, Karl Ekbom Jr from Sweden, and Ottar Sjaastad from Norway. Using a simple and clear writing style to illustrate the case series of CH patients that he followed with intelligent attention, Kudrow was able to disseminate knowledge of this disorder and to propose that the brain is the main responsible of CH pathophysiology [25]. A committed, accurate, and scrupulous researcher as Karl Ekbom gave a very detailed and precise description of CH [26]. Finally, thanks to his perspicacity and ingenious creativity, Sjaastad managed to identify three important CH subtypes: paroxysmal hemicrania [9], short-lasting unilateral neuralgiform headache with conjunctival injection and tearing (SUNCT) [27], and hemicrania continua [28], all of which today are officially recognized and listed in the international classification of headache disorders [7].

References

1. Koehler PJ. Prevalence of headache in Tulp's Observationes Meddicae (1641) with a description of cluster headache. Cephalalgia. 1993;13:318–20.
2. Willis T. De Anima Brutorum, quae hominis vitalis ac sensitive est, exercitationes duae. Pars 2,C.II:303. Oxford: Theatro Sheldoniano; 1672.
3. De la Pryme A. Extracts of two letters from the reverend Mr Abraham de la Pryme, F.R.S. to the publisher, concerning subterraneous trees, bitings of mad dogs, etc. Philos Trans. 1702;23:1073–7.
4. Arkink EB, van Buchem MA, Haan J, Ferrari MD, Kruit MC. An early 18th-century case description of cluster headache. Cephalalgia. 2010;30:1392–5.
5. Van Swieten G. Commentaria in Hermanni Boerhaave Aphorismos de cognoscendis et curandis morbis, vol. II. Lugduni Batavorum (Leiden): Apud Johannem et Hermanum Verbeek; 1745.
6. Isler H. Episodic cluster headache from a textbook of 1745: van Switen's classic description. Cephalalgia. 1993;13:172–4.
7. Headache Classification Committee of the International Headache Society (IHS). The international classification of headache disorders, 3rd edition. Cephalalgia. 2018;38:1–211.
8. Oppermann JCU. Dissertatio Medica Inauguralis de Hemicrania Horologica … Halle (Magdeburg): Typis Joannis Christiani Hilligeri; 1747.
9. Sjaastad O, Dale I. Evidence for a new (?) treatable headache entity. Headache. 1974;14:105–8.
10. Mueller J. Praktische Bemerkungen ueber di Kur des Halbseitigen Kopfwehes oder des sogenannten Migraine mit beigefuegten diaetetischen Vorschriften fuer Nervenkranke und Hypochondristen. Frankfurt am Mein: H Broenner; 1813.
11. Moellendorff W. Ueber Hemikranie. In: Archiv fuer pathologische anatomie un fuer klinische medizin, vol. 41. Berlin: Springer; 1867. p. 385–95.
12. Eulenburg A. Lehrbuch des functionellen Nervenkrankheiten auf physiologischen Basis. Berlin: A Hirschwald; 1871.
13. Charcot JM, Bouchard CJ, Brissaud E. Traité de Medécine, vol. VI. Paris: G Masson éditeur; 1894.
14. Sluder G. The syndrome of sphenopalatine neurosis. Am J Med Sci. 1910;140:868–78.
15. Bing R. Lehrbuch des Nervenkrankheiten. Berlin: Urban & Schwarzenberg; 1913.
16. Harris W. Neuritis and neuralgia. London: Oxford University Press; 1926.
17. Bing R. Ueber traumatische Erythromelalgie und Erythroprosopalgie. Nervenarzt. 1930;3:506–12.
18. Charlin C. Le syndrome du nerf nasal. Ann Oculist (Paris). 1931;168:808.
19. Vail V. Vidian neuralgia. Ann Otol Rhinol. 1932;41:837–56.
20. Harris W. Ciliary (migrainous) neuralgia and its treatment. Br Med J. 1936;1:457–60.
21. Horton BT. Histaminic cephalgia. Lancet. 1952;72(2):92–8.

22. Gardner WJ, Stowell A, Dutlinger R. Resection of the greater superficial petrosal nerve in the treatment of unilateral headache. J Neurosurg. 1947;4:105–14.
23. Boes CJ, Capobianco DJ, Matharu MS, Goadsby PJ. Wilfred Harris' early description of cluster headache. Cephalalgia. 2002;22:320–6.
24. Kunkle EC, Pfeiffer JB Jr, Wilhoit WM, Hamrick LW Jr. Recurrent brief headache in "cluster" pattern. Trans Am Neurol Assoc. 1952;77:240–3.
25. Kudrow L. Cluster headache. Mechanisms and management. New York: Oxford University Press; 1980.
26. Ekbom K. A clinical comparison of cluster headache and migraine. Acta Neurol Scand. 1970;46(Suppl 41):1–48.
27. Sjaastad O, Saunte C, Salvesen R, Fredriksen TA, Seim A, Roe OD, Fostad K, Lobben O-P, Zhaon JM. Short-lasting unilateral neuralgiform headache attacks with conjunctival injection, tearing, sweating, and rhinorrhea. Cephalalgia. 1989;9:147–56.
28. Sjaastad O, Spiering ELH. "Hemicrania continua": another headache absolutely responsive to indomethacin. Cephalagia. 1984;4:65–70.

Chapter 2
Epidemiology of Cluster Headache

Michael Bjørn Russell

2.1 Definition of Cluster Headache

The first complete description of cluster headache was made by Gerhard von Swieten, a physician to the Empress Marie Theresa [1]. Then followed many years were cluster headache was named ciliary neuralgia, erythromelalgia of the head, erythroprosopalgia of Bing, hemicranias neuralgiformis chronica, histaminic cephalalgia, Horton's headache, Harris-Horton's disease, migrainous neuralgia (of Harris), or petrosal neuralgia (of Gardner) [2]. The periodicity of attacks was described as a main feature in 1947 and inspired to the name cluster headache [3, 4].

The distinction between cluster headache and migraine has previously caused controversies whether they were separate entities or not, since many considered cluster headache as a subtype of migraine. Different clinical features [2, 5–7], different gender distribution (see below), and the fact that the prevalence of migraine among those with cluster headache is similar to that of migraine in the general population indicate that cluster headache is a specific subtype of headache [8].

The definition of cluster headache has changed during the years. Schiller and Ekbom based their generally accepted definitions of cluster headache on explicit diagnostic criteria [9, 10]. The first edition of the International Classification of Headache Disorders was based on these diagnostic criteria [2]. Since the first International Classification of Headache Disorders from 1988 to the current third version from 2018, the definition of cluster headache has changed slightly [2, 5–7].

M. B. Russell (✉)
Head and Neck Research Group, Research Center, Akershus University Hospital, Oslo, Norway

Institute of Clinical Medicine, Campus Akershus University Hospital, University of Oslo, Oslo, Norway
e-mail: m.b.russell@medisin.uio.no

© Springer Nature Switzerland AG 2020
M. Leone, A. May (eds.), *Cluster Headache and other Trigeminal Autonomic Cephalgias*, Headache, https://doi.org/10.1007/978-3-030-12438-0_2

7

Firstly, pain-free intervals in episodic cluster headache have been expanded from at least 14 days to at least 3 months [2, 7]. Secondly, chronic cluster headache unremitting from onset and chronic cluster headache evolved from episodic cluster headache are merged to chronic cluster headache [2, 5]. Thirdly, remission periods in chronic cluster headache have been expanded from <14 days to <3 month per year [2, 7]. Fourthly, restlessness and agitations were added to the associated symptom list of cluster headache [5]. The latter is important, since some people with otherwise typical cluster headache lack autonomic symptoms [11–13].

Today the diagnosis cluster headache is universally accepted, and the clinical spectrum has been expanded with other subtypes that mimic cluster headache, i.e., paroxysmal hemicranias, short-lasting unilateral neuralgiform headache with conjunctival injection and tearing (SUNCT), and hemicranias continua [14–16].

2.2 Epidemiology

Epidemiological surveys of cluster headache are hampered by the fact that cluster headache is rare as compared to migraine and tension-type headache. Thus, many thousands of people need to be included in epidemiological surveys of cluster headache and even thought the prevalence figures have wide confidence intervals.

An epidemiological survey of 9803 18-year-old men from east central Sweden found 9 males with cluster headache, corresponding to a prevalence of 92 per 100,000 people (95% confidence interval 42–174) [17]. Thus, the "real prevalence" of cluster headache in the general population is considerably higher, since onset of cluster headache is generally after age 20 years and men have cluster headache twice as often as women.

Two epidemiological surveys were done in the Republic of San Marino 15 years apart including 21,792 and 26,628 people, respectively [18, 19]. An extensive data search was done in both San Marino surveys, i.e., the medical records of neurological, ophthalmological, and otorhinolaryngological services from the past 15 years were reviewed, family practitioners were contacted, and a letter was posted to all households of San Marino. Both surveys identified 15 people with cluster headache. The prevalence in the later survey was 64 per 100,000 people (95% confidence interval 36–106) (calculation by authors since two persons who no longer had attacks of cluster headache were not included in the papers' calculations).

An American survey of Olmsted County, Minnesota, is imprecise, because people were included with only one attack and with attacks not clearly of 15–180 min duration [20]. Thus, patients did not necessarily fulfill the International Classification of Headache Disorders criteria for cluster headache. Furthermore, the diagnosis was based on case records and was not confirmed by a clinical interview. The suspected diagnosis of cluster headache was confirmed in only 13 of 30 neurological case records in the second San Marino survey [19].

A Norwegian epidemiological survey of 1838 people in Vågå county was based on a neurologist interview and classified according to the criteria of the International

Headache Society [2, 21]. The prevalence was 326 per 100,000 people (95% confidence interval 153–783), i.e., five times higher than the prevalence in San Marino. However, three of those classified as cluster headache did not fulfill the strict criteria for cluster headache [2], since one had cluster periods of less than 1 week duration and two had only had one cluster period. Whether these persons later developed cluster headache or not is unknown. Change of cluster headache by time can be exemplified by a pair of monozygotic twins who were initially described as discordant but later became concordant for cluster headache [22, 23]. The cluster periods were very short in the beginning, and one of the twins had attacks of very short duration. Later the characteristics changed to be typical episodic cluster headache.

An Italian epidemiological survey included 10,071 people age above 14 years old [24]. The participants were all interviewed by an experienced neurologist and classified according to the International Classification of Headache Disorders [2]. The prevalence was 279 per 100,000 people (95% confidence interval 171–427).

A Swedish epidemiological survey of twins from the general population included 31,750 people [25]. Structured lay interviews identified 250 people with possible cluster headache, but only 45 of the 218 persons who were interviewed by the neurologist had cluster headache. Two screening negative twins and one index twin had their cluster headache diagnosis confirmed. The prevalence was 151 per 100,000 people (95% confidence interval 108–194).

The epidemiological survey included only people of European descent, but cluster headache has also been described in Africans, African-Americans, Japanese, and Chinese [26–29].

2.3   Conclusion

The true prevalence of cluster headache is likely to be 1 per 500–1000 people.

References

1. Isler H. Historical background. In: Olesen J, Tfelt-Hansen P, Welch KMA, editors. The headaches. New York: Raven Press; 1993. p. 1–9.
2. Headache Classification Committee of the International Headache Society. Classification and diagnostic criteria for headache disorders, cranial neuralgias and facial pain. Cephalalgia. 1988;8(suppl 7):1–96.
3. Ekbom KA. Ergotamine tartrate orally in Horton's "histaminic cephalgia" (also called Harris's "ciliary neuralgia"). Acta Psychiatr Neurol Scand. 1947;46:105–13.
4. Kunkle EC, Pfeiffer JB Jr, Wilhoit WM, Hamrick LW Jr. Recurrent brief headache in "cluster" pattern. Trans Am Neurol Assoc. 1952;77:240–3.
5. Headache Classification Committee of the International Headache Society. The international classification of headache disorders. Cephalalgia. 2004;24(suppl 1):1–160.
6. Headache Classification Committee of the International Headache Society (IHS). The international classification of headache disorders, 3rd edition (beta version). Cephalalgia. 2013;33:629–808.

7. Headache Classification Committee of the International Headache Society (IHS). The international classification of headache disorders, 3rd edition (beta version). Cephalalgia. 2018;38:1–211.

8. Russell MB. Genetic epidemiology of migraine and cluster headache. Cephalalgia. 1997;17:683–701.

9. Schiller F. Prophylactic and other treatment for "histaminic", "cluster", or "limited" variants of migraine. JAMA. 1960;173:1907–11.

10. Ekbom K. A clinical comparison of cluster headache and migraine. Acta Neurol Scand. 1970;46:1–48.

11. Ekbom K. Evaluation of clinical criteria for cluster headache with special reference to the classification of the International Headache Society. Cephalalgia. 1990;10:195–7.

12. Nappi G, Micieli G, Cavallini A, Zanferrari C, Sandrini G, Manzoni GC. Accompanying symptoms of cluster attacks: their relevance to the diagnostic criteria. Cephalalgia. 1992;12:165–8.

13. Russell MB, Andersson PG. Clinical intra- and interfamilial variation of cluster headache. Eur J Neurol. 1995;1:253–7.

14. Sjaastad O, Dale I. Evidence for a new (?) treatable headache entity. Headache. 1974;14:105–8.

15. Sjaastad O, Saunte C, Salvesen R, Fredriksen TA, Seim A, Roe OD, Fostad K, Lobben O-P, Zhaon JM. Short-lasting unilateral neuralgiform headache attacks with conjunctival injection, tearing, sweating, and rhinorrhea. Cephalalgia. 1989;9:147–56.

16. Sjaastad O, Spiering ELH. "Hemicrania continua": another headache absolutely responsive to indomethacin. Cephalalgia. 1984;4:65–70.

17. Ekbom K, Ahlborg B, Schéle R. Prevalence of migraine and cluster headache in Swedish men of 18. Headache. 1978;18:9–19.

18. D'Alessandro R, Gamberini G, Benassi G, Morganti G, Cortelli P, Lugaresi E. Cluster headache in the Republic of San Marino. Cephalalgia. 1986;6:159–62.

19. Tonon C, Guttmann S, Volpini M, Naccarato S, Cortelli P, D'Alessandro R. Prevalence and incidence of cluster headache in the Republic of San Marino. Neurology. 2002;58:1407–9.

20. Swanson JW, Yanagihara T, Stang PE, O'Fallon WM, Beard CM, Melton LJ 3rd, Guess HA. Incidence of cluster headaches: a population-based study in Olmsted County, Minnesota. Neurology. 1994;44:433–7.

21. Sjaastad O, Bekketeig LS. Cluster headache. Vågå study of headache epidemiology. Cephalalgia. 2003;23:528–33.

22. Sjaastad O, Salvesen R. Cluster headache: are we only seeing the tip of the iceberg? Cephalalgia. 1986;6:127–9.

23. Sjaastad O, Shen JM, Stovner LJ, Elsas T. Cluster headache in identical twins. Headache. 1993;33:214–7.

24. Torelli P, Beghi E, Manzoni GC. Cluster headache prevalence in the Italian general population. Neurology. 2005;64:469–74.

25. Ekbom K, Svensson DA, Pedersen NL, Waldenlind E. Lifetime prevalence and concordance risk of cluster headache in the Swedish twin population. Neurology. 2006;67:798–803.

26. Tekle Haimanot R, Seraw B, Forsgren L, Ekbom K, Ekstedt J. Migraine, chronic tension-type headache, and cluster headache in an Ethiopian rural community. Cephalalgia. 1995;15:449–50.

27. Dousset V, Henry P, Michel P. Épidemiologie des céphalées. Rev Neurol (Paris). 2000;156(suppl 4):24–9.

28. Tomita M, Suzuki N, Igarashi H, Endo M, Sakai F. Evidence against strong correlation between chest symptoms and ischemic coronary changes after subcutaneous sumatriptan injections. Intern Med. 2002;41:599–600.

29. Wheeler SD, Carrazana EJ. Delayed diagnosis of cluster headache in African-American women. J Natl Med Assoc. 2001;93:31–6.

Chapter 3
Classification and Clinical Features

Pietro Cortelli, Sabina Cevoli, Jesica Garcia, and Miguel J. A. Láinez

3.1 Classification

Cluster headache (CH) and other trigeminal autonomic cephalgias (TACs) are primary headaches, and their clinical diagnosis depends on the classification system of the International Headache Society (IHS) [1]. Goadsby and Lipton were the first to propose the term "Trigeminal Autonomic Cephalgias" in 1997 [2]. The headache field has enjoyed a systematic hierarchical classification system and associated explicit (operational) diagnostic criteria since 1988 [3]. Currently, after much field testing of the previous editions, the third edition of the *International Classification of Headache Disorders* is in force. It is named ICHD-3, and it will be coordinated with the forthcoming International Classification of Diseases edition 11 (ICD-11) of the World Health Organization [1]. According to this hierarchical classification, patients can be diagnosed in groups and subgroups with various levels of diagnostic refinement. With such a system, patients can be diagnosed according to the first or

P. Cortelli
Department of Biomedical and NeuroMotor Sciences (DiBiNeM), Alma Mater Studiorum—University of Bologna, Bologna, Italy
e-mail: pietro.cortelli@unibo.it

S. Cevoli (✉)
IRCCS Institute of Neurological Sciences of Bologna, UOC Clinica Neurologica, AUSL Bologna, Bologna, Italy
e-mail: sabina.cevoli@unibo.it

J. Garcia
Department of Neurology, Hospital Clínico Univesitario, Valencia, Spain

M. J. A. Láinez
Department of Neurology, Hospital Clínico Univesitario, Valencia, Spain

Department of Neurology, Universidad Católica de Valencia, València, Spain
e-mail: miguel.lainez@sen.es

© Springer Nature Switzerland AG 2020
M. Leone, A. May (eds.), *Cluster Headache and other Trigeminal Autonomic Cephalgias*, Headache, https://doi.org/10.1007/978-3-030-12438-0_3

second digit in general clinical practice and to third or fourth digit for specialist or research purposes.

CH and the other TACs fall into group 3 of the ICHD-3. This group includes CH, paroxysmal hemicrania (PH), short-lasting unilateral neuralgiform headache attacks (SUN) with its variants, and hemicrania continua (HC). Tables 3.1, 3.2, 3.3 and 3.4 list the ICHD-3 criteria for TACs.

TACs are a group of relatively uncommon headaches that share the clinical features of head pain, which is usually unilateral and severe, and prominent cranial autonomic features, which are generally ipsilateral to the pain. Duration of attacks and response to indomethacin are the principal characteristics useful to distinguish each form. At one end of the TAC spectrum lie the SUN syndromes, in which patients experience the most frequent and shortest attacks. At the other end is CH, in which attacks are the longest and least frequent of the TACS, while PH is at the midpoint of the spectrum. HC represents an exception because it is not characterized by individual attacks per se [4].

CH is the principal form of TAC, and, possibly because of its severe debilitating pain, it has been described in exquisite detail by authors dating as far back as 1641 [5]. CH was previously named in very different ways that have now been abandoned because confusing: ciliary neuralgia, erythromelalgia of the head, erythroprosopalgia of Bing, hemicrania angioparalytica, hemicrania neuralgiformis chronica, histaminic cephalalgia, Horton's headache, Harris-Horton's disease, migrainous neuralgia (of Harris), petrosal neuralgia (of Gardner), Sluder's neuralgia, phenopalatine neuralgia, and vidian neuralgia [1].

PH was first described by Sjaastad and Dale in 1974 in its chronic form as a separate entity from cluster CH [6].

Table 3.1 International headache classification for cluster headache

3.1 Cluster headache
3.1.1 Episodic cluster headache
3.1.2 Chronic cluster headache
A. At least five attacks fulfilling criteria B–D
B. Severe or very severe unilateral orbital, supraorbital, and/or temporal pain lasting 15–180 min (when untreated)
C. Either or both of the following
1. At least one of the following symptoms or signs, ipsilateral to the headache
(a) Conjunctival injection and/or lacrimation
(b) Nasal congestion and/or rhinorrhea
(c) Eyelid edema
(d) Forehead and facial sweating
(e) Miosis and/or ptosis
2. A sense of restlessness or agitation
D. Occurring with a frequency between one every other day and eight per day
E. Not better accounted for by another ICHD-3diagnosis

Table 3.2 International headache classification for paroxysmal hemicrania

3.2 Paroxysmal hemicranias
3.2.1 Episodic paroxysmal hemicrania
3.2.2 Chronic paroxysmal hemicrania
A. At least 20 attacks fulfilling criteria B–E
B. Severe unilateral orbital, supraorbital, and/or temporal pain lasting 2–30 min
C. Either or both of the following
1. At least one of the following symptoms or signs, ipsilateral to the headache
(a) Conjunctival injection and/or lacrimation
(b) Nasal congestion and/or rhinorrhea
(c) Eyelid edema
(d) Forehead and facial sweating
(e) Miosis and/or ptosis
2. A sense of restlessness or agitation
D. Occurring with a frequency of >5 per day
E. Prevented absolutely by therapeutic doses of indomethacin
F. Not better accounted for by another ICHD-3 diagnosis

SUN was initially described as SUNCT (short-lasting unilateral neuralgiform headache attacks with conjunctival injection and tearing) by Sjaastad in 1989, due to the prominence of conjunctival injection and tearing [7], but some patients were noted to lack either one of these, and therefore the term SUNA (short-lasting unilateral neuralgiform headache attacks with cranial autonomic symptoms) was coined. It is still debated if SUNCT is the major subset of SUNA or if the two forms are separate subtypes [8].

CH, as with PH and SUN, may be episodic or chronic according to the presence of remission periods. In the episodic forms, there are at least two bouts of attacks lasting from 7 days to 1 year (when untreated) and separated by pain-free remission periods of ≥3 months. In the chronic forms, there are attacks occurring without a remission period, or remission lasting <3 months, for at least 1 year. On the contrary, HC is characterized by continuous pain with exacerbations [1].

HC was previously classified in group 4 ("other primary headache"), but, for the presence of ipsilateral cranial autonomic symptoms and the resolution with indomethacin, it was finally considered a form of TAC [9].

PH and HC respond absolutely by therapeutic doses of indomethacin and a trial with this drug is mandatory for the diagnosis. In an adult, oral indomethacin should be used initially in a dose of at least 150 mg daily and increased if necessary up to 225 mg daily. The dose by injection is 100–200 mg. Smaller maintenance doses are often employed [1].

Headache attacks, which are believed to be a type of TAC but are missing one of the features required to fulfill all criteria for any of the subtypes coded into group 3

Table 3.3 International headache classification for SUN

3.3 Short-lasting unilateral neuralgiform headache attacks
A. At least 20 attacks fulfilling criteria B–D
B. Moderate or severe unilateral head pain, with orbital, supraorbital, temporal, and/or other trigeminal distribution, lasting for 1–600 s and occurring as single stabs, series of stabs or in a sawtooth pattern
C. At least one of the following cranial autonomic
1. Symptoms or signs, ipsilateral to the pain
2. Conjunctival injection and/or lacrimation
3. Nasal congestion and/or rhinorrhea
4. Eyelid edema
5. Forehead and facial sweating
6. Miosis and/or ptosis
D. Occurring with a frequency of at least one a day
E. Not better accounted for by another ICHD-3 diagnosis
3.3.1 Short-lasting unilateral neuralgiform headache attacks with conjunctival injection and tearing (SUNCT)
3.3.1.1 Episodic SUNCT
3.3.1.2 Chronic SUNCT
A. Attacks fulfilling criteria for 3.3 Short-lasting unilateral neuralgiform headache attacks
B. Both of the following, ipsilateral to the pain
1. Conjunctival injection
2. Lacrimation (tearing)
3.3.2 Short-lasting unilateral neuralgiform headache attacks with cranial autonomic symptoms (SUNA)
3.3.2.1 Episodic SUNA
3.3.2.2 Chronic SUNA
A. Attacks fulfilling criteria for 3.3 Short-lasting unilateral neuralgiform headache attacks and criterion B
B. Not more than one of the following, ipsilateral to the pain
1. Conjunctival injection
2. Lacrimation (tearing)

of the ICHD-3, do not fulfill all criteria for another headache disorder, therefore they should be classified as "3.5 Probable trigeminal autonomic cephalalgia" [1].

Finally in the appendix of the ICHD-3, a new entity named "A3.6 Undifferentiated trigeminal autonomic cephalalgia" was reported for a TAC-like disorder occurring in children and adolescents with characteristics of the disorder not fully developed [1].

The unilateral trigeminal distribution of the pain, the ipsilateral autonomic manifestations, and the overlaps in duration of attacks and response to treatment suggested the hypothesis that these primary headaches share a common pathophysiology [10]. Moreover, it was reported that more than one TAC may coexist in a single patient in different moment, justifying the choice of grouping TACs in Chap. 3 of the current classification. The observation of hypothalamic activation, and the

Table 3.4 International headache classification for hemicrania continua

3.4 Hemicrania continua
3.4.1 Hemicrania continua, remitting subtype
3.4.2 Hemicrania continua, unremitting subtype
A. Unilateral headache fulfilling criteria B–D
B. Present for >3 months, with exacerbations of moderate or greater intensity
C. Either or both of the following
1. At least one of the following symptoms or signs, ipsilateral to the headache
(a) Conjunctival injection and/or lacrimation
(b) Nasal congestion and/or rhinorrhea
(c) Eyelid edema
(d) Forehead and facial sweating
(e) Miosis and/or ptosis
2. A sense of restlessness or agitation or aggravation of the pain by movement
D. Responds absolutely to therapeutic doses of indomethacin
E. Not better accounted for by another ICHD-3 diagnosis
3.4.1 Hemicrania continua, remitting subtype
A. Headache fulfilling criteria for 3.4 Hemicrania continua and criterion B below
B. Headache is not daily or continuous but interrupted (without treatment) by remission periods of 24 h
3.4.2 Hemicrania continua, unremitting subtype
A. Headache fulfilling criteria for 3.4 Hemicrania continua and criterion B below
B. Headache is daily and continuous for at least 1 year, without remission periods of 24 h

fact that hypothalamic stimulation is effective in different TACs, suggests that hypothalamus might be the pathogenic link among TACs [11].

It is known that trigeminal neuralgia may coexist with a TAC: PH, 9 SUNCT, 4,6 or CH, 8 and the coexistence of multiple TAC forms and trigeminal neuralgia in a single patient has also been reported, ten prompting the suggestion that TACs and trigeminal neuralgia share a common pathophysiology.

3.2 Clinical Features

3.2.1 Cluster Headache

Cluster headache (CH) is the most common type of the TACs and is considered one of the most severe and debilitating pain syndromes in humans [12]. The pain is so severe that female patients describe each attack as worse than childbirth. The severity of the pain has earned it the nickname "suicide headache," and a suicidal risk exists in this condition [13].

With a prevalence of around 0.1% in general population, this headache is more common in men than in women at a rate of 3:1, although currently it is increasing in women. The typical age of onset of the disease is around 20–40 years; nevertheless, it can occur at almost any age.

CH attacks recur during active periods with complete remissions among the cluster bouts. Due to the high frequency of attacks, the syndrome has a substantial impact on the patient's quality of life. The clinical features of CH attacks are orbital and periorbital unilateral pain attacks, with very high intensity and deep, expansive, or burning quality. The pain is maximal in around or behind the eye and may radiate into the ipsilateral temple, jaw, upper teeth, and neck.

The excruciating headache is associated with one or more autonomic symptoms and signs ipsilateral to the pain: ptosis, miosis, conjunctival injection, tearing, facial and frontal sweating, nasal obstruction, rhinorrhea, and increased intraocular pressure. Even if pain and autonomic symptoms recur strictly unilaterally in the same patient, side exchange is reported by 15% of patients in different active periods and only by 5% in the same cluster bout.

Characteristically, CH patients have a very restless behavior with great agitation sometimes. In 80–90% of cases, patients are restless and constantly moving in a vain attempt to relieve pain. They often perform complex, stereotyped actions. During attacks, CH sufferers do not want to be touched, stroked, or comforted and frequently moan a great deal, cry, or even scream. They sometimes indulge in violent, self-hurting behavior. Restlessness is a highly sensitive and highly specific parameter for CH, and, in the absence of autonomic features, it is required for the diagnosis. Moreover, stillness during attacks can be used as a distinguishing behavior for the differential diagnosis with migraine. The possibility of a visual aura, identical to migraine aura, was rarely reported. During an active cluster cycle, acute headaches may be triggered by alcohol, nitroglycerine, pungent odors, and daytime naps. Obstructive sleep apnea syndrome is more common in CH patients than in the general population, and treatment with continuous positive airway pressure can resolve attacks in some individuals.

The attacks last from 15 to 180 min, while the frequency of paroxysms in the symptomatic phases varies between one attack every 2 days and eight times per day.

Other than the severe pain and autonomic symptoms, the most distinguishing feature is the striking rhythms with which cluster attacks occur. The chronobiological features of CH have been systematically studied since the 1980s. Recently an increased risk peak was found at 21:41, 02:02, and 06:23 h (Chronorisk) [14]. Previously, in an Italian population, Manzoni et al. found the highest peak during the afternoon, not the night [15]. The temporal profile of attacks depends on the population studied, and the same authors hinted that different factors may influence this timing, such as light exposition in different latitudes and habits. For attacks arising from sleep, a correlation with REM phase was postulated, since they appear between 60 and 90 min after falling asleep [16].

The most common presentation of cluster headache is the episodic form: in 85–90% of patients, attacks appear as a series of daily attacks lasting for weeks or months, followed by a complete remission for months or years [13, 17]. Typically, patients report one or two episodes a year, usually in the spring or autumn, although the reasons underlying this circannual rhythm remain unknown. About 25% of patients have only a single episode throughout their lifetime. If the episode does not remit within 12 months, which is the case in 10–15% of patients with cluster headache, the disease is classified as chronic cluster headache. There is some interchange between chronic and episodic forms [18], since 13% of patients with episodic CH become chronic, and 33% of patients with chronic CH have seasons of episodic cluster.

Predictive factors have been identified that are correlated with an increased risk of unfavorable evolution from the episodic form to the chronic form of cluster headache. Late onset, the presence of sporadic attacks, a high frequency of cluster periods, and short-lived duration of remission periods when the headache is still in its episodic form all correlate with a possible worsening of the clinical picture over time [19, 20]. The reasons for the evolution of episodic cluster headache to chronic are still unknown, but some factors, such as head trauma and other lifestyle factors, e.g., cigarette smoking and alcohol intake, have been suggested as having a negative influence on the course of cluster headache over time [21].

Cluster headache is frequently associated with psychiatric comorbidities, which can substantially increase the disease burden and the complexity of its treatment. Depression, anxiety, and aggressive behavior are among the most commonly observed psychiatric comorbidities. Despite the high prevalence of depression and suicidal thoughts in patients with cluster headache, suicidal attempts are rare [4].

Clinical experience and previous research suggest that CH patients have a higher prevalence than the general population of a number of comorbidities other than psychiatric ones, including coronary artery disease, peptic ulcer disease, and alcohol and tobacco use. Interestingly, CH patients had traumatic head injuries more frequently than migraineurs and were more often responsible for them, perhaps due to particular behaviors related to their lifestyles [21].

The diagnosis of cluster headache is based on clinical criteria, although a neuroimaging study is recommended, preferably magnetic resonance imaging, with sequences that accurately assess pituitary and cavernous sinuses to reject secondary forms. In fact, CH-type symptoms have been described in association with cervical, midline, intracranial lesions, and arterious-venous-malformations of the carotid territory [22]. Many cases of pituitary tumors have been described associated with CH [1, 22]. Resolution of the pain after surgical treatment suggests a pathogenetic correlation between CH attacks and previously reported lesions.

3.2.2 *Paroxysmal Hemicrania*

Paroxysmal hemicrania (PH) is a rare disorder with an estimated prevalence of 1/50,000 headache patients. PH was originally considered to be a female disease, but afterward the female to male ratio was established to be 2:1. The typical age of onset is around 30–40 years, but PH may begin at any time [4, 12]. It is characterized by unilateral, short, excruciating head pain, with accompanying ipsilateral autonomic signs. The maximal pain is most often in the ocular, temporal, maxillary, or forehead areas; less frequently neck or occipital pain is reported. The most common autonomic symptoms are lacrimation and nasal congestion, but all the CH autonomics signs can occur, even bilaterally in very few cases. Interictal discomfort or mild pain is present in up to one-third of subjects [4, 12].

Several significant differences exist between cluster headache and paroxysmal hemicrania: PH has a higher daily attack frequency (with a mean of 11 attacks per day), shorter duration of individual attacks (usually 10–30 min), and fewer nocturnal attacks; it is more often chronic versus episodic; it has less propensity to be triggered by alcohol but greater propensity to mechanical (e.g., neck movement) trigger factors; finally, it is responsive to treatment with indomethacin [4, 12].

About 10% of attacks may be induced mechanically by bending or rotating the head; external pressure against the transverse processes of C4–5, the C2 root or the greater occipital nerve can all induce the headache [13], probably due to reflex mechanisms involving connections between the trigeminovascular system and brainstem.

Episodic PH is rare in comparison to chronic PH. There is sexual equality (men = women) in the episodic form, while the chronic form has a female predominance. Generally, when a woman presents with features of cluster headache, especially the chronic subtype, paroxysmal hemicrania should be strongly considered.

The diagnosis of PH is demonstrated by its absolute responsiveness to indomethacin.

3.2.3 Short-Lasting Unilateral Neuralgiform Headache Attacks

This syndrome is a rare form of TAC. The current terminology of SUNCT (short-lasting unilateral neuralgiform headache attacks with conjunctival injection and tearing) and SUNA (short-lived unilateral neuralgiform headache, with cranial autonomic signs) has evolved from the initial description and acronym (SUNCT) to include both syndromes; however, in headache clinical practice, it is clear that many patients do not manifest both conjunctival injection and tearing [23]; therefore, SUNCT and SUNA are probably clinical phenotypes of the same syndrome.

It is the least frequent disease in the TAC group, although SUNCT is more frequent than SUNA. It has a slightly higher prevalence in men (male/female ratio: 1.5–1), and the typical age of onset is between 35 and 65 years [8]. It is characterized by attacks of moderate-severe pain, with unilateral orbital, supraorbital, or temporal location and sometimes extending to the other side. The pain is accompanied by conjunctival injection and ipsilateral tearing and sometimes by rhinorrhea and other autonomic manifestations. During the episodes, the ipsilateral eye pressure increases, and vascular congestion and palpebral edema can be observed, suggesting a false ptosis. The attacks can cause increased blood pressure, bradycardia, and hyperventilation. The SUNCT and SUNA attacks have a sudden onset and end, lasting from 1 to 600 s; they can appear in isolation or in cluster. Between attacks patients are usually asymptomatic, although someone may have residual pain in the affected area.

Usually, attacks are precipitated by mechanical stimulation in trigeminal or extratrigeminal areas, but do not present a refractory period as in trigeminal neuralgia. The crises predominate during the day, and the pattern is episodic at first, although it can become chronic. During active periods, the frequency of attacks can range from less than one attack every 2–3 days to 30 attacks per hour. Patients with SUNCT and SUNA who have a personal or family history of migraine are more likely to have photophobia, phonophobia, and persistent pain between attacks [1].

SUNCT and SUNA require a good differential diagnosis with neuralgia of the first trigeminal branch. One of the keys to differentiate them is the low response to carbamazepine, the absence of a refractory period, the longer duration of the attacks, the presence of vegetative signs, and the absence of irradiation to the other trigeminal branches. For its diagnosis, brain MRI is recommended with trigeminal nerve study, to reject secondary causes and visualize the degree of trigeminal neurovascular compression, present in the majority of cases [24, 25]. The high percentage of remission after microvascular decompression supports the pathogenetic role of neurovascular compression. The first symptomatic case of SUNCT was reported in 1991. It was due to an arteriovenous malformation in the cerebellopontine angle that was removed with clinical resolution [26].

3.2.4 Hemicrania Continua

Hemicrania continua (HC) is the second most frequent TAC. It represents 1.7% of total headache patients attending headache or neurology clinics, and it has a female preponderance [9].

It is a strictly unilateral headache, persistent, of mild-moderate intensity, with oppressive characteristics, presenting with exacerbations of pain with ipsilateral oculofacial manifestations. A continuous background pain is usually localized in V1 distribution; however, the pain may spread during the exacerbation phase to involve other areas such as occiput, neck, shoulder, maxilla, periauricular region, and oral cavity (including teeth and throat).

The intensity of pain and vegetative symptoms is lower than in the other TACs. During pain crisis the typical characteristics of migraines (photophobia, phonophobia, intolerance to movement, nausea, and vomiting) occur, and these exacerbations can last from 20 min to several days. As with cluster headache, patients are often restless or agitated during the exacerbations. Many patients with hemicrania continua also report superimposed episodes of brief stabbing pains (ice pick-like) and the sensation of a foreign body (e.g., sand, grittiness) in the eye on the side of the headache.

Approximately 51% of patients noted exacerbations after stress or relaxation after stress periods, 38% with alcohol and irregular sleep, and some patients with menstruation [9].

HC is frequently misdiagnosed; the pooled mean delay of diagnosis of HC is 8.0 ± 7.2 years. The core feature of HC is its continuous background headache. However, patients may be worried only about superimposed exacerbations. Focusing only on exacerbations and ignoring continuous background headache are the most relevant factors for the misdiagnosis of HC.

Two temporal profiles of hemicrania continua have been described: remitting and unremitting. The remitting form is characterized by headaches that are not daily or continuous but are interrupted by remission periods of 1 day or more without treatment. Most patients experience the unremitting form.

As in paroxysmal hemicrania, a complete response to indomethacin is a "sine qua non" factor for HC diagnosis [1].

References

1. Headache Classification Committee of the International Headache Society (IHS). The international classification of headache disorders, 3rd edition. Cephalalgia. 2018;38(1):1–211.
2. Goadsby PJ, Lipton RB. A review of paroxysmal hemicranias, SUNCT syndrome and other short-lasting headaches with autonomic feature, including new cases. Brain. 1997;120(Pt 1):193–209.
3. Classification and diagnostic criteria for headache disorders. Cranial neuralgias and facial pain. Headache Classification Committee of the International Headache Society. Cephalalgia. 1988;8(Suppl 7):1–96.
4. Newman LC. Trigeminal autonomic cephalalgias. Continuum (MinneapMinn). 2015;21(4):1041–57.
5. Gordon N. History of cluster headache. Curr Pain Headache Rep. 2005;9(2):132–4.
6. Sjaastad O, Dale I. Evidence for a new (?), treatable headache entity. Headache. 1974;14:105–8.
7. Sjaastad O, Saunte C, Salvesen R, Fredriksen TA, Seim A, Røe OD, Fostad K, Løbben OP, Zhao JM. Shortlasting unilateral neuralgiform headache attacks with conjunctival injection, tearing, sweating, and rhinorrhea. Cephalalgia. 1989;9:147–56.
8. Cohen AS, Matharu MS, Goadsby PJ. Short-lasting unilateral neuralgiform headache attacks with conjunctival injection and tearing (SUNCT) or cranial autonomic features (SUNA)—a prospective clinical study of SUNCT and SUNA. Brain. 2006;129:2746–60.
9. Prakash S, Patel P. Hemicrania continua: clinical review, diagnosis and management. J Pain Res. 2017;10:1493–509.
10. Leone M, Bussone G. Pathophysiology of trigeminal autonomic cephalalgias. Lancet Neurol. 2009;8:755–64.
11. Leone M, Mea E, Genco S, Bussone G. Coexistence of TACs and trigeminal neuralgia: pathophysiological conjectures. Headache. 2006;46(10):1565–70.
12. Láinez MJ, Guillamón E. Cluster headache and other TACs: pathophysiology and neurostimulation options. Headache. 2017;57(2):327–35.
13. Hoffmann J, May A. Diagnosis, pathophysiology, and management of cluster headache. Lancet Neurol. 2018;17:75–83.
14. Barloese M, Haddock B, Lund NT, Petersen A, Jensen R. Chronorisk in cluster headache: a tool for individualised therapy? Cephalalgia. 2018;38(14):2058–67.. [Epub ahead of print]

15. Manzoni GC, Terzano MG, Bono G. Cluster headache—clinical findings in 180 patients. Cephalalgia. 1983;3:21–30.
16. Barloese M, Jennum P, Knudsen S. Cluster headache and sleep, is there a connection? A review. Cephalalgia. 2012;32:481–91.
17. Manzoni GC, Micieli G, Granella F, Tassorelli C, Zanferrari C, Cavallini A. Cluster headache—course over ten years in 189 patients. Cephalalgia. 1991;11(4):169–74.
18. Burish MJ. Cluster headache: history, mechanisms, and most importantly, treatment options. Pract Neurol. 2016:34–6.
19. Torelli P, Cologno D, Cademartiri C, Manzoni GC. Application of the International Headache Society classification criteria in 652 cluster headache patients. Cephalalgia. 2001;21(2):145–50.
20. Manzoni GC, Maffezzoni M, Lambru G, Lana S, Latte L, Torelli P. Late-onset cluster headache: some considerations about 73 cases. Neurol Sci. 2012;33(Suppl 1):S157–9.
21. Lambru G, Castellini P, Manzoni GC, Torelli P. Mode of occurrence of traumatic head injuries in male patients with cluster headache or migraine: is there a connection with lifestyle? Cephalalgia. 2010;30(12):1502–8.
22. Favier I, van Vliet JA, Roon KI, Witteveen RJ, Verschuuren JJ, Ferrari MD, Haan J. Trigeminal autonomic cephalgias due to structural lesions: a review of 31 cases. Arch Neurol. 2007;64(1):25–31.
23. Weng HY, Cohen AS, Schankin C, Goadsby PJ. Phenotypic and treatment outcome data on SUNCT and SUNA, including a randomised placebo-controlled trial. Cephalalgia. 2018;38(9):1554–63.. [Epub ahead of print]
24. Pareja JA, Álvarez M, Montojo T. SUNCT and SUNA: recognition and treatment. Curr Treat Options Neurol. 2013;15:28–39.
25. Favoni V, Grimaldi D, Pierangeli G, Cortelli P, Cevoli S. SUNCT/SUNA and neurovascular compression: new cases and critical literature review. Cephalalgia. 2013;33:1337–48.
26. Bussone G, Leone M, Dalla Volta G, Strada L, Gasparotti R, Di Monda V. Short-lasting unilateral neuralgiform headache attacks with tearing and conjunctival injection: the first "symptomatic" case? Cephalalgia. 1991;11(3):123–7.

Chapter 4
Differential Diagnosis, Including Secondary Forms

Patricia Pozo-Rosich and Alessandro S. Zagami

4.1 Introduction

Cluster headache belongs to the trigeminal autonomic cephalalgias (TACs) chapter of the International Classification of Headache Disorders (ICHD-III) [1]. These are primary headaches with a trigeminal distribution of the pain which is unilateral and usually side-locked and in which the headache is accompanied by ipsilateral autonomic symptoms. The most prevalent TAC is cluster headache (CH), but the category also includes even rarer headaches such as paroxysmal hemicranias, short-lasting unilateral neuralgiform headache attacks with conjunctival injection and tearing (SUNCT), short-lasting unilateral neuralgiform headache attacks with cranial autonomic symptoms (SUNA) and hemicrania continua (see Table 4.1).

The TACs are nearly always unilateral and side-locked, with ipsilateral cranial autonomic features. The different clinical features that can help us diagnose these clinical syndromes, and differentiate between them, are shown on Table 4.2. Basically, the most prominent differences are based on three characteristics of the headache: the *duration of the attacks*, the *attack frequency* and the *response to treatment*. Practically, it is the pathochronicity of the disorders which helps us,

P. Pozo-Rosich (✉)
Headache Clinical Unit, Neurology Department, Vall d'Hebron University Hospital;
Headache Research Group, Vall d'Hebron Institute of Research, Autonomous University of Barcelona, Spain
e-mail: ppozo@vhebron.net

A. S. Zagami
Institute of Neurological Sciences, Prince of Wales Hospital, Sydney, NSW, Australia

Prince of Wales Hospital Clinical School, University of New South Wales,
Sydney, NSW, Australia
e-mail: a.zagami@unsw.edu.au

© Springer Nature Switzerland AG 2020
M. Leone, A. May (eds.), *Cluster Headache and other Trigeminal Autonomic Cephalgias*, Headache, https://doi.org/10.1007/978-3-030-12438-0_4

Table 4.1 Types of primary TACs according to the ICHD-III

3.1 Cluster headache
3.1.1 Episodic cluster headache
3.1.2 Chronic cluster headache
3.2 Paroxysmal hemicrania
3.2.1 Episodic paroxysmal hemicrania
3.2.2 Chronic paroxysmal hemicrania
3.3 Short-lasting unilateral neuralgiform headache attacks
3.3.1 Short-lasting unilateral neuralgiform headache attacks with conjunctival injection and tearing (SUNCT)
3.3.1.1 Episodic SUNCT
3.3.1.2 Chronic SUNCT
3.3.2 Short-lasting unilateral neuralgiform headache attacks with cranial autonomic symptoms (SUNA)
3.3.2.1 Episodic SUNA
3.3.2.2 Chronic SUNA
3.4 Hemicrania continua
3.4.1 Hemicrania continua, remitting subtype
3.4.2 Hemicrania continua, unremitting subtype
3.5 Probable trigeminal autonomic cephalalgia
3.5.1 Probable cluster headache
3.5.2 Probable paroxysmal hemicranias
3.5.3 Probable short-lasting unilateral neuralgiform headache attacks
3.5.4 Probable hemicrania continua

Table 4.2 Differentiating clinical features amongst the TACs

	Cluster headache	Paroxysmal hemicrania	SUNCT
Gender F:M	1:2.5–7.2	1.6–1.4:1	1:1.5
Pain type	Stabbing	Throbbing, stabbing	Severe to excruciating
Usual site	Orbit	Orbit, temple	Periorbital
Attack frequency	1/alternate day to 8/day	1–40/day (for more than half of time)	3–200/day
Duration of attack	*15–180 min*	*2–30 min*	*5–240 s*
Autonomic features	Yes	Yes	Yes
Cutaneous triggers	No	No	Yes
Migrainous features	Yes	Yes	No
Indomethacin effect	No	Yes	No
Prophylactic treatment	Verapamil Lithium	Indomethacin	Lamotrigine Gabapentin

clinicians, differentiate between the aforementioned primary TACs. Thus, the diagnosis is a clinical one and is based primarily on the patient's symptoms and the exclusion of secondary causes for the headache.

While, by definition, the TACs as primary headaches have no (as yet) identifiable cause, there are many reports of patients presenting with typical symptoms of idiopathic TACs in whom a structural lesion is found, which possibly is implicated as the cause of their symptoms. There are even more reports of "TAC-like", or probable TACs, where a structural lesion is found and is suggested as the cause of the symptoms but, in many cases, these may be a coincidental co-occurrence. Moreover, accuracy of the diagnosis is another critical issue and will obviously change over time, as the diagnostic criteria evolve. It is stated in the International Classification of Headache Disorders, third edition (beta version) [2] that "when a new headache with the characteristics of a trigeminal autonomic cephalalgia (TAC) occurs for the first time in close temporal relation to another disorder known to cause headache, or fulfils other criteria for causation by that disorder, the new headache is coded as a secondary attributed to the causative disorder".

The "truest" secondary TAC could be considered one that fulfils all the ICHD-III beta criteria for the particular TAC (including, for instance, absolute responsiveness to indomethacin in paroxysmal hemicrania and hemicrania continua), that has a demonstrable structural lesion, and that the symptoms remit once the underlying lesion is treated effectively. This has only occasionally been shown to be the case. However, it is important that secondary TACs are identified since the causative lesion will almost always need treatment in its own right, and these (relatively rare) cases may help us better understand the pathophysiology of the TACs, in general. Moreover, in some cases the patient can be rendered pain-free. In the following sections, we will briefly summarize the recent literature on secondary TACs and try to identify if there are any "red flags" that might suggest that an otherwise typical TAC might have an underlying lesion and thus which patients should have neuroimaging.

The imaging paradigm recommended by some has been brain MRI with, and without, contrast with fine cuts through the region of the hypothalamus. If a pituitary gland lesion is suspected, laboratory testing for levels of pituitary hormones has been suggested as well. The relation between cluster headache symptoms and the presence of an abnormality in the neuroimaging has been reviewed in relation with the published clinical cases in the literature particularly those cases in which it is clearly identified that a therapeutic intervention led to a significant improvement of the symptoms [3, 4].

Several reviews have highlighted the length of time between the start of the symptoms and the correct headache diagnosis, as this delay leads to suboptimal treatment and increases the patient's distress. In a study of 85 patients with CH seen in a single headache centre, the delay between onset of CH and diagnosis averaged 9 years [5], while in a recent survey of 351 patients, the average diagnostic delay was 6.2 years, with half of the patients initially receiving the wrong diagnosis [6].

In the US Cluster Headache Survey, only 25% of patients were diagnosed within 1 year and 57% within 5 years, while 22% were not diagnosed for 10 or more years. Seventy-nine percent of patients initially received an incorrect diagnosis, including migraine (34%), sinusitis (21%), allergies (6%), or tooth-related issues (5%) [7].

It is also important to take into consideration that there can also be an overlap with other headache disorders, such as migraine, and therefore, the possibility of a patient suffering from both migraine and cluster headache should not be ruled out nor that a particular patient may be suffering from cluster headache with migrainous features. Thus, the major differential for CH (other than one of the other TACs) is migraine.

4.1.1   Differentiation of Cluster Headache from Migraine

For those with an interest in, and knowledge of, headache diagnosis, it often is difficult to understand how the diagnosis of cluster headache can be missed entirely, or be delayed for so long, in so many patients, given that the phenotype of CH is so characteristic and, once learnt, should never be forgotten. However, there are several potential reasons for this. Firstly, most doctors receive very little training in headache medicine and, therefore, many may never have learnt about cluster headache, in the first place. Also, migraine is very common, especially in women, while CH is rare, but more common in men with a male/female ratio of 3.5:1 [7]. Despite the fact that the phenotype of CH is essentially the same for men and women, women with CH are more frequently misdiagnosed than men (61.1% vs. 45.5%, $p < 0.01$) [6]. As noted above, CH is most often misdiagnosed as migraine as opposed to any other headache condition, and while there are overlapping features that they share, there nevertheless remain distinct differences, even in these shared features, that clearly separate them.

Cluster headaches (and the other TACs) are unilateral, side-locked headaches in 69–92% of cases [8], whereas this only occurs in 20.8% of migraine sufferers [9]. A shift in the side of the headache within an attack occurs in only between 1 and 8% in CH [7, 10] but is more common in migraine. Cluster headache sufferers can also experience the same accompanying symptoms as in migraine, such as nausea, photophobia, and phonophobia, although less commonly. However, in CH the sensitivity to light and sound, and in particular to light, is ipsilateral to the headache much more commonly than in migraine. In one study [11], whereas only 2/54 (4%) episodic migraine patients had unilateral photophobia or phonophobia, or both, this occurred in 10/21 (48%) of chronic, and 4/5 (80%) episodic, cluster headache patients, respectively.

While the presence of ipsilateral autonomic features is one of the diagnostic criteria for the diagnosis of CH (and the other TACs) [1], autonomic features can also occur in migraine. While the frequency of autonomic features in CH ranges from 72% for rhinorrhoea to 91% for lacrimation [10], one or more autonomic features were seen in 226/841 (26.9%) in a population-based sample of migraineurs [12]. Importantly, in trying to distinguish migraine with autonomic features from

CH, it needs to be emphasized that the autonomic features are much more often lateralized, and side-locked, with the headache in CH, whereas in migraine they are more often bilateral and less prominent [13]. The presence, or not, of aura is not particularly helpful since it occurs in 14–21% of CH patients [7, 10]. Perhaps, the most telling differences in the clinical picture of a CH patient, compared to a migraine patient, are their demeanour and behaviour during an attack. In up to 97% of migraine without aura patients, movement makes the headaches worse [14] and therefore most migraine patients prefer to rest and be still. In dramatic contrast, in CH up to 93% of patients will be restless or agitated during an attack or have no worsening of the headache with movement [10] and therefore are much more likely to pace about and not be still. In another study, only 0.8% of CH patients did not have any sense of agitation during their attacks [7]. Having described the diagnostic differences between migraine and CH which help the clinician to confidently differentiate between them, the next major task when dealing with a TAC, such as CH, or a TAC-like syndrome, is whether the headache is primary or secondary. In the following sections, we will briefly summarize the recent literature on secondary TACs and try to identify if there are any "red flags" that might suggest that an otherwise typical TAC might have an underlying lesion and thus whether all, or only some, patients should have neuroimaging.

4.2   Secondary, or Symptomatic, Trigeminal Autonomic Cephalalgias

4.2.1   Summary of Previous Reviews of Symptomatic, or Secondary, Trigeminal Autonomic Cephalalgias

Since 2004 there have been five comprehensive reviews of "secondary" or "symptomatic" TACs [3, 4, 15–17]. Here we summarize the findings of these publications. Trucco et al. in 2004 [15] reviewed cases from 1980 to 2001 and identified 22 CPH, 9 HC and 7 SUNCT patients in whom coexisting pathology was identified. They did not look for symptomatic CH cases but rather referred to a review of such cases by Giraud et al. [18]. For the diagnosis of CPH, the criteria of the International Classification of Headache Disorders: second edition [19] were used, while for HC and SUNCT those suggested by Goadsby and Lipton [20] were used. Of the 22 CPH patients, 6 fulfilled all (definite CPH) and 10 fulfilled all, bar 1 (probable CPH), criteria. In the other six, there was lack of sufficient information, or else they clearly did not fulfil the required criteria. The lesions identified in the definite CPH group were a Pancoast syndrome [21]; left sella turcica gangliocytoma [22]; right cavernous sinus meningioma [23]; maxillary cyst [24], cerebral metastasis of parotid epidermoid carcinoma [25]; and Meckel's cave non-Hodgkin's lymphoma [15]. In the probable group, the lesions were right internal carotid artery aneurysm [15], vasculitis [26], intracranial hypertension [27], AV fistula [15], tuber cinereum hamartoma [28], ipsilateral occipital infarction [29], pituitary microadenoma [24], possible cerebral vasculitis [25], ipsilateral intraorbital and cavernous sinus granulomata [25], and head injury [30].

Of the nine HC cases, six cases fulfilled all, and two all but one, of the Goadsby and Lipton criteria [20]. The lesions implicated in the definite group were right mesenchymal chondrosarcoma [31] and sphenoid sinusitis [32], while in the probable group they were C7 nerve root compression [23], HIV infection [33] and head trauma in four patients [34]. Of the seven SUNCT patients, five had definite and two possible SUNCT [20]. The lesions identified in the definite group were ipsilateral AVMs in two patients [35, 36], ipsilateral para-pontine cavernous angioma [37], HIV infection [38] and craniosynostosis [39], while in the possible cases, they were ipsilateral dorsolateral brainstem infarction [40] and basilar invagination due to osteogenesis imperfecta [41].

From their review of these cases, the authors concluded that it was generally not possible to confidently establish a causal link between the pathology identified and the presenting TAC, or TAC-like, headache. They commented that posterior fossa lesions seemed somewhat common in SUNCT patients, while lesions in the region of the cavernous sinus seemed more common in CPH-like headache patients, although the numbers were small. Finally, they recommended neuroimaging in patients with "atypical" TACs, in terms of the phenotype, or with an uncharacteristic response to indomethacin in CPH or HC patients.

Favier et al. in 2007 [16] reported on 31 patients with secondary TAC, or TAC-like, headaches in whom a structural lesion was identified which, when treated successfully, resulted in a significant improvement, or even complete resolution, of the headache. They reviewed the literature from 2001 to 2005 and collated 27 cases, as well as 4 new patients from the records of their own institutions. Of the 31 patients, there were 19 patients with typical cluster, and 4 with cluster-like, headache. They also identified one PH-like, one typical CPH and one CPH-like patient and four SUNCT patients. They did not investigate patients with symptomatic, HC or HC-like, headache.

The underlying lesions in the four typical CH patients were an ipsilateral upper cervical meningioma [42], a recurrent nasopharyngeal carcinoma involving the ipsilateral internal carotid artery [43], an ipsilateral temporal lobe AVM [44] and an aspergilloma of the sphenoid sinuses [45]. The single CH-like patient had a mycotic aneurysm of the intracavernous portion of the ipsilateral internal carotid artery [46].

In the four typical ECH cases, the lesions were an infected foreign body in the ipsilateral maxillary sinus [47], a thrombosed aneurysm of the ipsilateral posterior communicating artery [48], an AVM of the ipsilateral frontal lobe [44] and a pituitary adenoma (prolactinoma) extending into the ipsilateral cavernous sinus [49], while in the three ECH-like patients, the lesions were an ipsilateral occipital lobe AVM [50] and two ipsilateral pituitary adenomas: one prolactinoma [16] and one growth hormone-secreting [51].

In the six typical chronic CH patients, the following abnormalities were identified: pituitary adenomas (prolactinomas) in three patients [16, 52, 53], a parasellar meningioma extending ipsilaterally [54], an ipsilateral meningioma of the tentorium cerebelli [55] and a benign tumour of the ipsilateral posterior fossa [56], while in the three chronic CH-like patients, there were an aneurysm of the ipsilateral vertebral artery [57], an ipsilateral subclavian steal syndrome [58], and a cavernous haemangioma of the ipsilateral orbit [16]. Both the typical cluster-tic syndrome patient [16] and the chronic cluster-tic-like patient [59] had pituitary adenomas (both prolactinomas).

There was a single patient with PH-like headaches with bilateral attacks with an AVM of the parietal lobe [60], a typical CPH patient with an aneurysm of the con-tralateral carotid artery and a dilated ipsilateral carotid artery [53], a typical CPH patient previously reported [22] and a patient with CPH-like headache with a muco-coele of the ipsilateral maxillary sinus [61]. Three of the four SUNCT patients had ipsilateral pituitary adenomas (two prolactinomas and one non-functioning) [62–64] and the other, a brainstem pilocytic astrocytoma extending to the ipsilateral cerebro-pontine cistern [65].

The authors concluded from their study that typical TACs, even those that respond to the usual pharmacologic TAC treatments, such as indomethacin, can be due to structural lesions. Moreover, only 10 of the 31 patients had atypical features. The other striking finding they noted was that 11 of the 31 patients had pituitary tumours, 10 of which were secretory and 9 of these were prolactinomas. On the basis of these observations, they recommended neuroimaging in *all* patients pre-senting with TACs or TAC-like headaches.

In 2009 Cittadini and Matharu published a review of 37 cases of symptomatic TACs [3]. These included 24 CH patients, 3 PH patients and 10 SUNCT patients. They selected cases where they believed the associated, underlying lesion was likely to be causal to the TAC, as evidenced by the fact that the lesion was ipsilateral to the TAC in all cases, although in 3 CH patients (1 cerebral vein thrombosis (CVST), 1 idiopathic granulomatous hypophysitis and 1 sphenoidal aspergilloma) and 1 SUNCT patient (metastatic carcinoid), the lesion involved the other side as well and that, in all cases, treatment of the underlying lesion resulted in significant improve-ment in the headache. In fact, in all of the CH and PH patients and in 8 of the 10 SUNCT patients, there was complete resolution of the headache, although reported follow-up times varied considerably. One SUNCT patient with a prolactinoma [63] had a marked, but not complete, response to treatment (partial resection and radio-therapy), while another SUNCT patient with bilateral intraorbital metastatic bron-chial carcinoid had only transient improvement for 1 month after radiotherapy [66].

Twenty-four of the 37 cases had already been described in 1, or other, of the 2 previous reviews [15, 16]. Thus, there were 13 new cases identified: 6 CH (4 sub-types unclear and 2 CCH), 1 PH and 6 SUNCT patients. Interestingly, three of the four unclassifiable CH (duration of headache less than a year) patients had ipsilat-eral internal carotid artery dissections [67, 68], while the fourth had CVST [69]. In the single new CPH patient [70] and in four of the six SUNCT patients [71–74], the underlying lesion was a pituitary tumour. In the CPH patient, this was a macroade-noma (prolactinoma) and in the SUNCT patients there were two microadenomas (both prolactinomas), one growth hormone-secreting adenoma and a non-functioning macroadenoma. The lesions in the two other SUNCT patients were an orbital cystic lesion [75] and a pilocytic astrocytoma [76], both ipsilateral.

The authors again highlighted the predilection for pituitary lesions in all three of the TACs studied, with 8/24 (33%) of CH patients, 2/3 (66%) PH and 7/10 (70%) of

SUNCT patients having these. They also emphasized that in more than half of CH and SUNCT patients, and in all cases of PH, an atypical headache phenotype and/or abnormal physical examination was noted. Finally, they noted that a poor response to, or the need for higher than usual doses of, appropriate medication should be a red flag for a secondary, or symptomatic, TAC. In terms of which patients should receive neuroimaging, they concluded that MR imaging should be done in all patients with "an atypical symptomatology, abnormal examination, and poor response to the appropriate treatments" [3].

The most recently published review of symptomatic TACs and TAC-like headaches is by de Coo et al. and was published in 2015 [17]. It was the first to use the ICHD-III beta criteria when evaluating reports of symptomatic TACs. They reviewed cases from 2009 to 2015 and separated them into probably secondary, possibly secondary and unknown. Probably secondary was used when there was a "dramatic improvement of the headache after treatment of the underlying lesion" and possibly secondary, when there was improvement but not complete resolution of the headache or when a causal effect was deemed possible by the authors. We will not discuss their last category, unknown.

In the 12 probably symptomatic CH patients, there were 7 patients with tumours: 2 had ipsilateral pituitary adenomas, 1 macroprolactinoma [77] and 1 non-functioning [78], 1 an intrasellar arachnoid cyst [79], 1 a hypothalamic cystic tumour related to sarcoid [80], 1 an ipsilateral glioblastoma multiforme [81], 1 an ipsilateral carotid paraganglioma [82] and an angiomyolipoma infiltrating the ipsilateral face [83]. There were two vascular lesions: one ischaemic stroke related to moyamoya [84]; and one due to neurovascular compression of the ipsilateral C3 nerve root and vertebral artery [85]; two inflammatory cases, both due to acute ipsilateral maxillary sinusitis [86, 87]; and one attributed to obstructive sleep apnoea [88]. In the seven possibly symptomatic CH patients, the underlying lesions were tumours in 2:1 ipsilateral macroprolactinoma [89] and one angiomyolipoma infiltrating the ipsilateral face [83]; two ocular causes; recurrent posterior scleritis and aseptic meningitis [90] and post intraocular lens implant [91]; two cases of multiple sclerosis [92, 93]; and one dissection of the ipsilateral distal internal carotid artery [94].

There were 14 probable cases of symptomatic SUNCT/SUNA and 12 possible cases. As is the case with other TACs, there were four cases of probable symptomatic SUNCT/SUNA due to tumours: three pituitary lesions – one ipsilateral prolactinoma [95], one ipsilateral macroprolactinoma [96] and one ipsilateral mixed gangliocytoma and pituitary adenoma [95]—and an epidermoid tumour in the ipsilateral cerebellopontine angle [97]; and likewise, two vascular lesions affecting the internal carotid artery, one aneurysm of the cavernous portion of the ipsilateral internal carotid artery [98] and an ipsilateral cavernous dural AV fistula [99]. The striking finding, however, was the high number of cases attributed to neurovascular conflict where there was compression of the ipsilateral trigeminal nerve by the superior cerebellar [7], or anterior inferior cerebellar [1], artery, eight in total [100–102]. In the possibly symptomatic group, there were five cases due to tumours: three ipsilateral pituitary adenomas, including two prolactinomas [95], one ipsilateral meningioma [103] and one lung adenocarcinoma [104]. Again, there were four cases attributed to neurovascular conflict [101, 102]. The other three underlying lesions were lesions due to multiple sclerosis [105], viral meningitis [106] and a case of mild hypothalamic/pituitary dysfunction related to ipsilateral optic nerve hypoplasia [107]. All patients in the probably symptomatic group became pain-free, bar 1 who improved considerably, whereas only five in the possibly symptomatic group became pain-free.

There were two cases of probably symptomatic, and three cases of possibly symptomatic, HC all of whom, by definition, were absolutely responsive to indomethacin. The underlying lesions in the probable group were a cerebral vein thrombosis [108] and cerebral metastases due to lung adenocarcinoma [109]. In both of these patients, after definitive treatment of the underlying condition, they were rendered pain-free and were able to cease indomethacin completely. In the three possibly symptomatic HC patients, the lesions were post-traumatic head injury, post-craniotomy for evacuation of traumatic subdural haematoma and postabdominal surgery done under spinal anaesthesia [110]. All three patients remain headache-free, but only on indomethacin.

De Coo et al. [17] concluded from their review of a total of 53 TACs that tumours, particularly of the pituitary, especially prolactinomas and other adenomas, were relatively common. They reported only a single case of cerebral artery dissection in their CH patients, in distinct contrast to other reviews. They highlighted that 8/14 patients with probable secondary SUNCT and 4/12 with possible SUNCT, that is, more than 45% of their SUNCT/SUNA cases, had evidence of ipsilateral neurovascular conflict. Moreover, they emphasized that of those patients who underwent microvascular decompression, the vast majority had excellent outcomes, often being rendered entirely pain-free. This dramatic response to microvascular decompression is similar to that seen in classical trigeminal neuralgia, with which SUNCT and SUNA share several other features as well. Thus, in some patients first division trigeminal neuralgia will enter into the differential of SUNCT/SUNA patients. While there are clear differences, such as the presence of a refractory period in TN, but not in SUNCT/SUNA, it has been suggested that these disorders may be variants of the same disorder [111].

4.3   Update of Recent Cases of Symptomatic Trigeminal Autonomic Cephalalgias

Having reviewed the previously published reviews of symptomatic TACs, and TAC-like headaches, we wished to review the more recent literature. We performed Medline and PubMed searches from 2015 to January 2018 using the keywords trigeminal autonomic cephalalgia, cluster headache, paroxysmal hemicrania, SUNCT, SUNA, hemicrania continua, secondary and symptomatic. We only selected articles in English and that were published in full. We also reviewed only those cases in which there was an identifiable pathology, which was on the appropriate side and which when treated, or spontaneously resolved, resulted in resolution of the headache or significant improvement. We identified 18 such cases which are summarized in Table 4.3.

Table 4.3 Symptomatic trigeminal autonomic cephalalgias

Authors	Year	Headache diagnosis	Age at onset	Sex	Duration of headache till diagnosis of lesion/cause	Underlying lesion	Side of lesion	Intervention	Outcome	Duration of follow-up
Andereggen et al. [112]	2017	CH	46	M	Several years	Pituitary macroprolactinoma	Ipsilateral	Dopamine agonist	Headache-free	5 years
Bellamio et al. [113]	2017	ECH/CCH	71	M	17 years	Pontine cavernous haemangioma	Ipsilateral	Surgery	Headache-free	6 years
Bellamio et al. [113]	2017	ECH	29	M	18 weeks	Cerebral vein thrombosis	Ipsilateral	Warfarin, acetazolamide	Headache-free	1 year
Chang et al. [114]	2017	ECH	49	M	7 years	Middle meningeal artery DAVF	Ipsilateral	Endovascular embolization	Headache-free	1.5 years
Dirkx and Koehler [115]	2017	CH	67	M	Several months	Post carotid endarterectomy	Ipsilateral	Verapamil	Headache-free	8 months
Dirkx and Koehler [115]	2017	CH	63	M	7 days	Post carotid endarterectomy	Ipsilateral	Verapamil	Headache-free	2 months
Rozen and Beams [116]	2015	PH and HC	44	M	21 months	Post-traumatic	Ipsilateral	Indomethacin, melatonin	Headache-free	6 months
Choi et al. [117]	2018	CPH	43	F	1 year	Orbital metastatic leiomyosarcoma	Ipsilateral	Gamma knife surgery	Headache-free	Not stated
Ljubisavljevic et al. [118]	2017	CPH-tic syndrome	40	F	2 years	Demyelinating plaque of the trigeminal principal nucleus and DREZ	Ipsilateral	Lamotrigine, indomethacin	Headache-free	6 months
Lambru et al. [119]	2017	SUNCT and TN	58	M	16 years	Haemorrhagic infarction of the dorsolateral medulla	Ipsilateral	Carbamazepine, gabapentin	Partial response	Not stated
Berk and Silberstein [122]	2016	SUNCT	33	F	1 month	Post pituitary radiotherapy	Ipsilateral	Lamotrigine	Partial response	Not stated

Cacao et al. [121]	2016	SUNCT	46	M	Not stated	Carotico-cavernous sinus fistula	Ipsilateral	Surgery, not otherwise specified	Headache-free	Not stated
Cacao et al. [121]	2016	SUNCT	51	F	Not stated	Cavernous sinus AVM	Ipsilateral	Surgery, not otherwise specified	Headache-free	Not stated
Jin et al. [120]	2016	SUNCT	64	M		Ischaemic infarction of the dorsolateral medulla	Ipsilateral	Spontaneous resolution	Headache-free	5 months
Brilla et al. [123]	2018	HC-like	50	F	14 weeks	CAD	Ipsilateral	Indomethacin	Headache-free	1 year
Brilla et al. [123]	2018	HC-like	44	M	2 days	CAD	Ipsilateral	Indomethacin	Headache-free	3 months
Brilla et al. [123]	2018	HC-like	47	F	6 months	CAD	Ipsilateral	Spontaneous resolution	Headache-free	1 month
Brilla et al. [123]	2018	HC-like	42	M	3 weeks	CAD	Ipsilateral	Spontaneous resolution	Headache-free	7 weeks
Russo et al. [124]	2017	HC	62	M	12 months	Idiopathic hypertrophic pachymeningitis	Ipsilateral	Methylprednisolone, enoxaparin	Headache much improved	Not stated

AVM arteriovenous malformation, *CAD* carotid artery dissection, *CH* cluster headache, *CPH* chronic paroxysmal hemicrania, *DAVF* dural arteriovenous fistula, *DREZ* dorsal root entry zone, *ECH* episodic cluster headache, *HC* hemicrania continua, *PH* paroxysmal hemicrania, *SUNCT* short-lasting unilateral neuralgiform headache with conjunctival injection and tearing, *Tic* tic douloreux, *TN* trigeminal neuralgia

4.3.1 Symptomatic Cluster Headache

There were six CH patients: only one patient had a pituitary tumour, a macroprolacti-noma, which had infiltrated the cavernous sinus encasing the ipsilateral internal carotid artery [112]. Biochemically, the patient had hyperprolactinaemia and central hypogo-nadism. Treatment with cabergoline led to abrupt cessation of the CH and dramatic reduction in size of the tumour. The other five patients had vascular lesions. One patient with an ipsilateral pontine cavernous hemangioma had ECH controlled with medica-tion [113]. Several years later his ECH evolved into CCH, unresponsive to medication and repeat imaging showed enlargement of the hemangioma. Successful surgery was undertaken, and the patient became, and remained, free of medication. Another patient with ECH [113] developed visual disturbance and prolonged attacks of cluster-like headache and was found to have an ipsilateral jugular vein thrombosis extending into the sigmoid sinus. Treatment with warfarin and acetazolamide led to resolution of the thrombosis and the headache. One patient with typical ECH [114] usually had bouts that lasted for several months and which were well controlled with prophylactic therapy that could be successfully weaned once the bout had terminated. However, his head-ache pattern changed such that he could not be weaned from his medication, prompting imaging with magnetic resonance angiography. This revealed a dural arteriovenous fis-tula (DAVF) in the ipsilateral posterior fossa, supplied primarily by branches of the left middle meningeal artery. Definitive treatment of the DAVF with embolization led to complete resolution of CH without relapse at 1.5 year follow-up. Two patients, with no past history of CH, developed recurrent headaches fulfilling ICHD-III beta criteria for CH, 5 days and 7 days following ipsilateral carotid endarterectomy [115]. The head-aches continued until effective treatment with verapamil was instituted.

4.3.2 Symptomatic Paroxysmal Hemicrania

We identified one case report of PH evolving into HC, both responsive to indo-methacin, and which followed head trauma [116]; and one case of CPH-like head-ache present for 1 year before identification of an ipsilateral orbital metastatic deposit of leiomyosarcoma [117]. Definitive treatment of the tumour with gamma knife surgery resulted in complete resolution of the headache and one case of CPH-tic syndrome due to demyelinating plaques, involving the ipsilateral trigeminal principal nucleus and the dorsal root entry zone of the trigeminal nerve in a patient with a clinically isolated syndrome [118]. Her pain was eventually completely con-trolled with a combination of lamotrigine and indomethacin.

4.3.3 Symptomatic SUNCT/SUNA

We identified a case report of a patient with coexistent SUNCT and trigeminal neu-ralgia (TN) both present for 16 years following haemorrhagic infarction of the ipsilateral dorsolateral medulla [119]. On imaging there was no evidence of neuro-vascular conflict to account for the TN in this patient, suggesting that both condi-tions were caused by damage to the trigeminal nucleus caudalis and adjacent autonomic structures in the medulla. Both conditions were partially controlled with a combination of carbamazepine and gabapentin. Interestingly, Jin et al. [120] reported a case of SUNCT starting 13 days after the patient developed a lateral medullary syndrome due to ipsilateral ischaemic infarction of the dorsolateral medulla. The headache eventually resolved spontaneously. There are two recent cases of SUNCT due to vascular lesions of the cavernous sinus: one a carotico-cavernous fistula and the other an AVM [121]. Both patients became headache-free after surgery. The final case of symptomatic SUNCT developed following radio-therapy to the pituitary for recurrent macroadenoma [122].

4.3.4 Symptomatic Hemicrania Continua

Brilla et al. have very recently described five cases (four of which had not been reported previously) of hemicrania continua-like headache associated with dissec-tion of the ipsilateral internal carotid artery [123]. In three of the cases, the headaches fulfilled all, bar 1, of the ICHD-III beta diagnostic criteria for HC. The three patients treated with indomethacin responded absolutely to it, while in the other two, the headaches resolved spontaneously before indomethacin could be exhibited. In the final symptomatic HC case [124], the patient presented with headache present for a year and is completely consistent with ICHD-III beta criteria, including responsive-ness to indomethacin but who, after developing diplopia due to a sixth nerve palsy, was found to have idiopathic hypertrophic pachymeningitis requiring treatment with high-dose steroids. Both the diplopia and headache resolved with this treatment.

4.3.5 Imaging in TACs and TAC-Like Headaches

Trucco et al. [15] concluded that neuroimaging should be done in patients with "atypical" TACs, in terms of the phenotype, such as older age at onset, or with an uncharacteristic response to indomethacin in CPH or HC patients. However, Favier et al. [16] noted that typical TACs, even those that responded to the usual pharma-cologic TAC treatments, such as indomethacin, could be due to structural lesions, and moreover, that in their series, only 10 of the 31 patients had such atypical fea-tures. Consequently, they recommended neuroimaging in *all* patients presenting with TACs or TAC-like headaches. However, in many countries, imaging all patients with TACs, despite them being rare, may not be practical.

In their review, Cittadini and Matharu [3] commented that it would not be until there was a large prospective study done in patients with TACs, and TAC-like head-aches, that we would know which groups of patients should have imaging to rule out potential secondary causes. In terms of which patients should receive neuroimaging given the present level of knowledge, they concluded that MR imaging should be done in all patients with "an atypical symptomatology, abnormal examination, and poor response to the appropriate treatments" but noted that the decision as to whether to recommend imaging in patients with a typical presentation and normal clinical examination was more difficult.

Wilbrink et al. [4] specifically reviewed the role of, and indications for, neuroimaging in TACs. They too noted that clinically typical TACs could be due to an underlying structural lesion and that there were no "typical warning signs or symptoms". They concluded that neuroimaging with brain MRI should be considered in all patients with TAC, or TAC-like, presentations. In certain cases, they suggested more specific additional imaging should be also be considered, such as imaging of neck vessels (looking for arterial dissections) and of the sellar, and parasellar, regions (looking for pituitary lesions and lesions involving the cavernous sinus).

Most recently, in their 2015 review [17], de Coo et al. noted that, despite the fact that secondary causes for TACs seem rare, contrast-enhanced MRI brain should be considered, at least once, in every TAC, or TAC-like, patient and, moreover, that imaging of the neck vessels should also be considered. They also emphasized the more recent finding of the high proportion of cases of SUNCT/SUNA patients with neurovascular conflict between the trigeminal nerve and the superior, or less commonly, the anterior inferior, cerebellar artery, which when treated surgically, frequently resulted in complete resolution of pain, even in previously medically refractory cases. Moreover, a very recent report [125] described two patients with medically refractory SUNCT who had already undergone invasive neuromodulation techniques (one occipital nerve stimulation and the other deep brain stimulation) with incomplete pain relief, in whom ipsilateral neurovascular conflict was demonstrated. In both patients, microvascular decompression resulted in complete resolution of their SUNCT, without the need for either ongoing medication or further neuromodulation. In the light of these observations, we would suggest that, in addition to the recommendations made by de Coo et al., additional imaging, specifically looking for neurovascular conflict, be done in all SUNCT and SUNA patients. A recent review of all SUNCT/SUNA cases to date focusing on the presence of neurovascular conflict and the response to its treatment came to the same conclusion [102]. While we acknowledge that a significant number of patients with otherwise typical TACs may well have normal imaging, it is not often that we can offer our TAC patients the possibility of a cure, such as we can if they were to have a treatable lesion, which is all the more important given how disabling, and often refractory to treatment, these rare headaches often are.

References

1. Headache Classification Committee of the International Headache Society (IHS). The international classification of headache disorders, 3rd edition. Cephalalgia. 2018;38(1):1–211.
2. Headache Classification Committee of the International Headache Society (IHS). The international classification of headache disorders, 3rd edition (beta version). Cephalalgia. 2013;33(9):629–808.

3. Cittadini E, Matharu MS. Symptomatic trigeminal autonomic cephalalgias. Neurologist. 2009;15(6):305–12.
4. Wilbrink LA, Ferrari MD, Kruit MC, Haan J. Neuroimaging in trigeminal autonomic cephalgias: when, how, and of what? Curr Opin Neurol. 2009;22(3):247–53.
5. Jensen RM, Lynberg A, Jensen RH. Burden of cluster headache. Cephalalgia. 2007;27:535–41.
6. Lund N, Barloese M, Petersen A, Haddock B, Jensen RH. Chronobiology differs between men and women with cluster headache, clinical phenotype does not. Neurology. 2017;88:1069–76.
7. Rozen TD, Fishman RS. Cluster headache in the United States of America: demographics, clinical characteristics, triggers, suicidality, and personal burden. Headache. 2012;52:99–113.
8. Newman LC. Trigeminal autonomic cephalalgias. Continuum (Minneap Minn). 2015;21(4 Headache):1041–57.
9. D'Amico D, Leone M, Bussone G. Side-locked unilaterality and pain localization in long-lasting headaches: migraine, tension-type headache, and cervicogenic headache. Headache. 1994;34:526–30.
10. Bahra A, Goadsby PJ. Cluster headache: a prospective clinical study with diagnostic implications. Neurology. 2002;58:354–61.
11. Irimia P, Cittadini E, Paemeleire K, Cohen AS, Goadsby PJ. Unilateral photophobia or phonophobia in migraine compared with trigeminal autonomic cephalalgias. Cephalalgia. 2008;28(6):626–30.
12. Obermann M, Yoon MS, Dommes P, Kuznetsova J, Maschke M, Weimar C, et al. Prevalence of trigeminal autonomic symptoms in migraine: a population-based study. Cephalalgia. 2007;27(6):504–9.
13. Lai T-H, Fuh J-L, Wang S-J. Cranial autonomic symptoms in migraine: characteristics and comparison with cluster headache. J Neurol Neurosurg Psychiatry. 2009;80(10):1116–9.
14. Russell MB, Rasmussen BK, Fenger K, Olesen J. Migraine without aura an migraine with aura are distinct clinical entities: a study of four hundred and eighty-four male and female migraineurs from the general population. Cephalalgia. 1996;16:239–45.
15. Trucco M, Mainardi F, Maggioni F, Badino R, Zanchin G. Chronic paroxysmal hemicrania, hemicrania continua and SUNCT syndrome in association with other pathologies: a review. Cephalalgia. 2004;24(3):173–84.
16. Favier I, van Vliet JA, Roon KI, Witteveen RJW, Verschuuren JJGM, Ferrari MD, et al. Trigeminal autonomic cephalgias due to structural lesions: a review of 31 cases. Arch Neurol. 2007;64(1):25–31.
17. de Coo IF, Wilbrink LA, Haan J. Symptomatic trigeminal autonomic cephalalgias. Curr Pain Headache Rep. 2015;19(8):39.
18. Giraud P, Jouanneau E, Borson-Chazot F, Lanteri-Minet M, Chazot G. Cluster-like headache: literature review. J Headache Pain. 2002;3:71–8.
19. Headache Classification Subcommittee of the International Headache Society. The international classification of headache disorders: 2nd edition. Cephalalgia. 2004;24(Suppl 1):9–160.
20. Goadsby PJ, Lipton RB. A review of paroxysmal hemicranias, SUNCT syndrome and other short-lasting headaches with autonomic features, including new cases. Brain. 1997;120:193–209.
21. Delreux V, Kevers L, Callewaert A. Hemicranie paroxystique inaugurant un syndrome de Pancoast. Rev Neurol. 1989;145:151–2.
22. Vijayan N. Symptomatic chronic paroxysmal hemicrania. Cephalalgia. 1992;12(2):111–3.
23. Sjaastad O, Stovner LJ, Stolt-Nielsen A, Antonaci F, Fredriksen TA. CPH and hemicrania continua: requirement of high indomethacin dosages-an ominous sign? Headache. 1995;35:363–7.
24. Gatzonis S, Mitsikostas DD, Ilias A, Zournas CH, Papageorgiou C. Two more secondary headaches mimicking chronic paroxysmal hemicrania. Is this the exception or the rule? Headache. 1996;36(8):511–3.
25. Foerderreuther S, von Maydell R, Straube A. A CPH-like picture in two patients with an orbitocavernous sinus syndrome. Cephalalgia. 1997;17(5):608–11.
26. Medina JL. Organic headache mimicking chronic paroxysmal hemicrania. Headache. 1992;32:73–4.

27. Hannerz J. Trigeminal neuralgia with chronic paroxysmal hemicrania: the CPH-tic syndrome. Cephalalgia. 1993;13(5):361–4.
28. Pauri F, Tilia G, Cisternino MD, Pierelli F. Tuber cinereum hamartomas mimicking chronic paroxysmal hemicrania. Ital J Neurol Sci. 1993;14(Suppl. 7):132.
29. Broeske D, Lenn NJ, Cantos E. Chronic paroxysmal hemicrania in a young child: possible relation to ipsilateral occipital infarction. J Child Neurol. 1993;8(3):235–6.
30. Matharu MS, Goadsby PJ. Post-traumatic chronic paroxysmal hemicrania (CPH) with aura. Neurology. 2001;56(2):273–5.
31. Antonaci F, Sjaastad O. Hemicrania continua: a possible symptomatic case, due to mesenchymal tumor. Funct Neurol. 1992;7(6):471–4.
32. Meckling SK, Becker WJ. Sphenoid sinusitis presenting as indomethacin-responsive "hemicrania continua": a case report. Cephalalgia. 1997;17:303.
33. Brilla R, Evers S, Soros P, Husstedt IW. Hemicrania continua in an HIV-infected outpatient. Cephalalgia. 1998;18(5):287–8.
34. Lay CL, Newman LC. Posttraumatic hemicrania continua. Headache. 1999;39(4):275–9.
35. Bussone G, Leone M, Dalla Volta G, Strada L, Gasparotti R, Di Monda V. Short-lasting unilateral neuralgiform headache attacks with tearing and conjunctival injection: the first "symptomatic" case? Cephalalgia. 1991;11(3):123–7.
36. Morales F, Mostacero E, Marta J, Sanchez S. Vascular malformation of the cerebellopontine angle associated with "SUNCT" syndrome. Cephalalgia. 1994;14(4):301–2.
37. De Benedittis G. SUNCT syndrome associated with cavernous angioma of the brain stem. Cephalalgia. 1996;16(7):503–6.
38. Barea LM, Forcelini CM. Onset of short-lasting, unilateral neuralgiform headache with conjunctival injection and tearing (SUNCT) after acquiring human immunodeficiency virus (HIV): more than a coincidence? Cephalalgia. 2001;21:518.
39. Moris G, Ribacoba R, Solar DN, Vidal JA. SUNCT syndrome and seborrheic dermatitis associated with craniosynostosis. Cephalalgia. 2001;21(2):157–9.
40. Penart A, Firth M, Bowen JR. Short-lasting unilateral neuralgiform headache with conjunctival injection and tearing (SUNCT) following presumed dorsolateral brainstem infarction. Cephalalgia. 2001;21(3):236–9.
41. ter Berg JW, Goadsby PJ. Significance of atypical presentation of symptomatic SUNCT: a case report. J Neurol Neurosurg Psychiatry. 2001;70(2):244–6.
42. Kuritzky A. Cluster headache-like pain caused by an upper cervical meningioma. Cephalalgia. 1984;4:185–6.
43. Appelbaum J, Noronha A. Pericarotid cluster headache. J Neurol. 1989;236:430–1.
44. Munoz C, Diez-Tejedor E, Frank A, Barreiro P. Cluster headache syndrome associated with middle cerebral artery arteriovenous malformation. Cephalalgia. 1996;16(3):202–5.
45. Zanchin G, Rossi P, Licandro AM, Fortunato M, Maggioni F. Clusterlike headache. A case of sphenoidal aspergilloma. Headache. 1995;35(8):494–7.
46. Todo T, Inoya H. Sudden appearance of a mycotic aneurysm of the intracavernous carotid artery after symptoms resembling cluster headache: case report. Neurosurgery. 1991;29(4):594–9.
47. Scorticati MC, Raina G, Ferderico M. Cluster-like headache associated to a foreign body in the maxillary sinus. Neurology. 2002;59:643–4.
48. McBeath JG, Nanda A. Case reports: sudden worsening of cluster headache: a signal of aneurysmal thrombosis and enlargement. Headache. 2000;40:686–8.
49. Porta-Etessam J, Ramos-Carrasco A, Berbel-Garcia A, Martinez-Salio A, Benito-Leon J. Clusterlike headache as first manifestation of a prolactinoma. Headache. 2001;41(7):723–5.
50. Mani S, Deeter J. Arteriovenous malformation of the brain presenting as a cluster headache: a case report. Headache. 1982;22:184–5.
51. Milos P, Havelius U, Hindfelt B. Cluster like headache in a patient with a pituitary adenoma: with a review of the literature. Headache. 1996;36:184–8.
52. Tfelt-Hansen P, Paulson OB, Krabbe A. Invasive adenoma of the pituitary gland and chronic migrainous neuralgia: a rare coincidence or a causal relationship? Cephalalgia. 1982;2:25–8.

53. Greve E, Mai J. Cluster headache-like headaches: a symptomatic feature? A report of three patients with intracranial pathologic findings. Cephalalgia. 1988;8(2):79–82.
54. Hannerz J. A case of parasellar meningioma mimicking cluster headache. Cephalalgia. 1989;9:265–9.
55. Taub E, Argoff CE, Winterkorn JMS, Milhorat TH. Resolution of chronic cluster headache after resection of a tentorial meningioma: case report. Neurosurgery. 1995;37:319–21.
56. Bigal ME, Rapoport AM, Camel M. Cluster headache as a manifestation of intracranial inflammatory myofibroblastic tumour: a case report with pathophysiological considerations. Cephalalgia. 2003;23(2):124–8.
57. West P, Todman D. Chronic cluster headache associated with a vertebral artery aneurysm. Headache. 1991;31:210–2.
58. Piovesan EJ, Lange MC, Werneck LC, Kowacs PA, Engelhorn AL. Cluster-like headache. A case secondary to the subclavian steal phenomenon. Cephalalgia. 2001;21(8):850–1.
59. Leone M, Curone M, Mea E, Bussone G. Cluster-tic syndrome resolved by removal of pituitary adenoma: the first case. Cephalalgia. 2004;24:1088–9.
60. Newman LC, Herskowitz S, Lipton RB, Solomon S. Chronic paroxysmal headache: two cases with cerebrovascular disease. Headache. 1992;32:75–8.
61. Kowacs PA, Piovesan EJ, Tatsui CE, Lange MC, Werneck LC, Vincent M. Symptomatic trigeminal-autonomic cephalalgia evolving to trigeminal neuralgia: report of a case associated with dual pathology. Cephalalgia. 2001;21:917–20.
62. Ferrari MD, Haan J, van Seters AP. Bromocriptine-induced trigeminal neuralgia in patient with a pituitary tumor. Neurology. 1988;38:1482–4.
63. Massiou H, Launay JM, Levy C, El Amrani M, Emperauger B, Bousser MG. SUNCT syndrome in two patients with prolactinomas and bromocriptine-induced attacks. Neurology. 2002;58:1698–9.
64. Matharu MS, Levy MJ, Merry RT, Goadsby PJ. SUNCT syndrome secondary to prolactinoma. J Neurol Neurosurg Psychiatry. 2003;74(11):1590–2.
65. Van Vliet JA, Ferrari MD, Haan J, Laan LA. Trigeminal autonomic cephalalgia-tic-like syndrome associated with a pontine tumour in a one-year-old girl. J Neurol Neurosurg Psychiatry. 2003;74:391–2.
66. Black DF, Swanson JW, Eross EJ, Cutrer FM. Secondary SUNCT due to intraorbital, metastatic bronchial carcinoid. Cephalalgia. 2005;25(8):633–5.
67. Frigerio S, Buhler R, Hess CW, Sturzenegger M. Symptomatic cluster headache in internal carotid artery dissection--consider anhidrosis. Headache. 2003;43(8):896–900.
68. Rigamonti A, Iurlaro S, Zelioli A, Agostoni E. Two symptomatic cases of cluster headache associated with internal carotid artery dissection. Neurol Sci. 2007;28(Suppl 2):S229–31.
69. Georgiadis GS, Tsitouridis I, Paspali D, Rudolf J. Cerebral sinus thrombosis presenting with cluster-like headache. Cephalalgia. 2007;27(1):79–82.
70. Sarov M, Valade D, Jublanc C, Ducros A. Chronic paroxysmal hemicrania in a patient with a macroprolactinoma. Cephalalgia. 2006;26(6):738–41.
71. Levy MJ, Matharu M, Goadsby PJ. Prolactinomas, dopamine agonists and headache: two case reports. Eur J Neurol. 2003;10:169–73.
72. Rocha Filho PAS, Galvao ACR, Teixeira MJ, Rabello GD, Fortini I, Calderaro M, et al. SUNCT syndrome associated with pituitary tumor: case report. Arq Neuropsiquiatr. 2006;64(2B):507–10.
73. Leroux E, Schwedt TJ, Black DE, et al. SUNCT cured after resection of a pituitary microadenoma. Can J Neurol Sci. 2006;33:411–3.
74. Rozen TD. Resolution of SUNCT after removal of a pituitary adenoma in mild acromegaly. Neurology. 2006;67:724.
75. Lim ECH, Teoh HL. Headache—it's more than meets the eye: orbital lesion masquerading as SUNCT. Cephalalgia. 2003;23(7):558–60.
76. Blattler T, Capone Mori A, Boltshauser E, Bassetti C. Symptomatic SUNCT in an eleven-year-old girl. Neurology. 2003;60(12):2012–3.

77. Levy MJ, Robertson I, Howlett TA. Cluster headache secondary to macroprolactinoma with ipsilateral cavernous sinus invasion. Case Rep Neurol Med. 2012;2012:830469.
78. Edvardsson B. Cluster headache associated with a clinically non-functioning pituitary adenoma: a case report. J Med Case Rep. 2014;8:451.
79. Edvardsson B, Persson S. Cluster headache and arachnoid cyst. Springerplus. 2013;2(1):4.
80. van der Vlist SHM, Hummelink BJCM, Westerga J, Boogerd W. Cluster-like headache and a cystic hypothalamic tumour as first presentation of sarcoidosis. Cephalalgia. 2013;33(6):421–4.
81. Edvardsson B, Persson S. Cluster headache and parietal glioblastoma multiforme. Neurologist. 2012;18(4):206–7.
82. Malissart P, Ducros A, Labauge P, De Champfleur NM, Carra-Dalliere C. Carotid paraganglioma mimicking a cluster headache. Cephalalgia. 2014;34(13):1111.
83. Messina G, Rizzi M, Cordella R, Caraceni A, Zecca E, Bussone G, et al. Secondary chronic cluster headache treated by posterior hypothalamic deep brain stimulation: first reported case. Cephalalgia. 2013;33(2):136–8.
84. Sewell RA, Johnson DJ, Fellows DW. Cluster headache associated with moyamoya. J Headache Pain. 2009;10(1):65–7.
85. Creac'h C, Duthel R, Barral F, Nuti C, Navez M, Demarquay G, et al. Positional cluster-like headache. A case report of a neurovascular compression between the third cervical root and the vertebral artery. Cephalalgia. 2010;30(12):1509–13.
86. Edvardsson B. Cluster headache associated with acute maxillary sinusitis. Springerplus. 2013;2:509.
87. Edvardsson B, Persson S. Cluster headache and acute maxillary sinusitis. Acta Neurol Belg. 2013;113(4):535–6.
88. Ranieri AL, Tufik S, de Siqueira JT. Refractory cluster headache in a patient with bruxism and obstructive sleep apnea. Sleep Breath. 2009;13(4):429–33.
89. Benitez-Rosario MA, McDarby G, Doyle R, Fabby C. Chronic cluster-like headache secondary to prolactinoma: uncommon cephalalgia in association with brain tumors. J Pain Symptom Manag. 2009;37(2):271–6.
90. Choi JY, Kim Y, Oh K, Yu SW, Jung KY, Kim BJ. Cluster-like headache caused by posterior scleritis. Cephalalgia. 2009;29(8):906–8.
91. Gil-Gouveia R, Fonseca A. Cluster headache after cataract surgery. Clin J Pain. 2013;29(11):e19–21.
92. Donat J. A patient with cluster headache-due to a brainstem lesion. Headache. 2012;52(6):1035–6.
93. Mijajlovic M, Aleksic VM, Covickovic Sternic NM. Cluster headache as a first manifestation of multiple sclerosis: case report and literature review. Neuropsychiatr Dis Treat. 2014;10:2269–74.
94. Candeloro E, Canavero I, Maurelli M, Cavallini A, Ghiotto N, Vitali P, et al. Carotid dissection mimicking a new attack of cluster headache. J Headache Pain. 2013;14:84.
95. Chitsantikul P, Becker WJ. SUNCT, SUNA and pituitary tumors: clinical characteristics and treatment. Cephalalgia. 2013;33(3):160–70.
96. de Lourdes Figuerola M, Bruera O, Pozzo MJ, Leston J. SUNCT syndrome responding absolutely to steroids in two cases with different etiologies. J Headache Pain. 2009;10(1):55–7.
97. Rodgers SD, Marascalchi BJ, Strom RG, Huang PP. Short-lasting unilateral neuralgiform headache attacks with conjunctival injection and tearing syndrome secondary to an epidermoid tumor in the cerebellopontine angle. Neurosurg Focus. 2013;34(3):E1.
98. Coven I, Coban G, Koyuncu G, Ilik KM. SUNCT syndrome findings accompanied by cavernous segment aneurysm. Clin Neurol Neurosurg. 2013;115(6):781–3.
99. Domingos J, Pereira PJ, Roriz MJ, Xavier AJ, Magalhaes M, Monteiro PJ. Cavernous sinus dural fistula "mimicking" SUNCT. Cephalalgia. 2012;32(3):263–4.
100. Guerreiro R, Casimiro M, Lopes D, Marques JP, Fontoura P. Video NeuroImage: symptomatic SUNCT syndrome cured after trigeminal neurovascular contact surgical decompression. Neurology. 2009;72(7):e37.

101. Williams M, Bazina R, Tan L, Rice H, Broadley SA. Microvascular decompression of the trigeminal nerve in the treatment of SUNCT and SUNA. J Neurol Neurosurg Psychiatry. 2010;81(9):992–6.
102. Favoni V, Grimaldi D, Pierangeli G, Cortelli P, Cevoli S. SUNCT/SUNA and neurovascular compression: new cases and critical literature review. Cephalalgia. 2013;33(16):1337–48.
103. Kutschenko A, Liebetanz D. Meningioma causing gabapentin-responsive secondary SUNCT syndrome. J Headache Pain. 2010;11(4):359–61.
104. Cascella C, Rosen JB, Robbins MS, Levin M. Resident and fellow section. Teaching case: symptomatic SUNCT. Headache. 2011;51(6):1022–6.
105. Bogorad I, Blum S, Green M. A case of MS presenting with SUNCT status. Headache. 2010;50(1):141–3.
106. Ito Y, Yamamoto T, Ninomiya M, Mizoi Y, Itokawa K, Tamura N, et al. Secondary SUNCT syndrome caused by viral meningitis. J Neurol. 2009;256(4):667–8.
107. Theeler BJ, Joseph KR. SUNCT and optic nerve hypoplasia. J Headache Pain. 2009;10(5):381–4.
108. Mathew T, Badachi S, Sarma GRK, Nadig R. Cerebral venous thrombosis masquerading as hemicrania continua. Neurol India. 2014;62(5):556–7.
109. Robbins MS, Grosberg BM. Hemicrania continua-like headache from metastatic lung cancer. Headache. 2010;50(6):1055–6.
110. Prakash S, Shah ND, Soni RK. Secondary hemicrania continua: case reports and a literature review. J Neurol Sci. 2009;280(1–2):29–34.
111. Lambru G, Matharu MS. SUNCT, SUNA and trigeminal neuralgia: different disorders or variants of the same disorder? Curr Opin Neurol. 2014;27(3):325–31.
112. Andereggen L, Mono M-L, Kellner-Weldon F, Christ E. Cluster headache and macroprolactinoma: case report or a rare, but potential important causality. J Clin Neurosci. 2017;40:62–4.
113. Bellamio M, Anglani M, Mainardi F, Zanchin G, Maggioni F. Cluster headache: when to worry? Two case reports. Cephalalgia. 2016;37(5):491–5.
114. Chang YH, Luo CB, Wang SJ, Chen SP. Cluster headache and middle meningeal artery dural arteriovenous fistulas: a case report. Cephalalgia. 2018;38(11):1792–96. https://doi.org/10.1177/0333102417747229. Epub 2017 Dec 3.
115. Dirkx THT, Koehler PJ. Post-operative cluster headache following carotid endarterectomy. Eur Neurol. 2017;77(3–4):175–9.
116. Rozen TD, Beams JL. A case of post-traumatic LASH syndrome responsive to indomethacin and melatonin (a man with a unique triad of indomethacin-responsive trigeminal autonomic cephalalgias). Cephalalgia. 2015;35(5):453–6.
117. Choi HA, Lee MJ, Chung C-S. Chronic paroxysmal headache secondary to an orbital metastatic leiomyosarcoma: a case report. Cephalalgia. 2017;38(2):389–92.
118. Ljubisavljevic S, Prazic A, Lazarevic M, Stojanov D, Savic D, Vojinovic S. The rare painful phenomena—chronic paroxysmal hemicrania-tic syndrome as a clinically isolated syndrome of the central nervous system. Pain Physician. 2017;20(2):E315–E22.
119. Lambru G, Trimboli M, Tan SV, Al-Kaisy A. Medullary infarction causing coexistent SUNCT and trigeminal neuralgia. Cephalalgia. 2017;37(5):486–90.
120. Jin D, Lian Y-J, Zhang H-F. Secondary SUNCT syndrome caused by dorsolateral medullary infarction. J Headache Pain. 2016;17:12.
121. Cação G, Correia FD, Pereira-Monteiro J. SUNCT syndrome: a cohort of 15 Portuguese patients. Cephalalgia. 2015;36(10):1002–6.
122. Berk T, Silberstein S. Case report: secondary SUNCT after radiation therapy—a novel presentation. Headache. 2016;56(2):397–401.
123. Brilla R, Pawlowski M, Evers S. Hemicrania continua in carotid artery dissection—symptomatic cases or linked pathophysiology? Cephalalgia. 2018;38(2):402–5.
124. Russo A, Silvestro M, Cirillo M, Tessitore A, Tedeschi G. Idiopathic hypertrophic pachymeningitis mimicking hemicrania continua: an unusual clinical case. Cephalalgia. 2018;38(4):804–7. https://doi.org/10.1177/0333102417708773. Epub 2017 May 5.
125. Hassan S, Lagrata S, Levy A, Matharu M, Zrinzo L. Microvascular decompression or neuromodulation in patients with SUNCT and trigeminal neurovascular conflict? Cephalalgia. 2018;38(2):393–8.

Chapter 5
Genetics of Cluster Headache and Other Trigeminal Autonomic Cephalalgias

Arn M. J. M. van den Maagdenberg and Anne Ducros

5.1 Why Study Genetics in Cluster Headache and Trigeminal Autonomic Cephalalgias?

Cluster headache belongs to a group of primary headache disorders, the trigeminal autonomic cephalalgias (TACs), all of which consist of disabling unilateral pain in trigeminal distribution associated with marked ipsilateral cranial autonomic features [1–4]. Cluster headache is the commonest TAC. The majority of TACs, including cluster headache, paroxysmal hemicranias, short-lasting unilateral neuralgiform headache attacks with conjunctival injection and tearing (SUNCT) and short-lasting unilateral neuralgiform headache attacks with cranial autonomic symptoms (SUNA), manifest as daily short-lived recurrent attacks and can be distinguished one from each other by the duration of the attacks [5]. Only hemicrania continua manifests as a continuous daily unilateral pain, so it is not presented in the form of attacks. Response to therapy is different among TACs. The neurobiological mechanisms underlying cluster headache and other TACs are complex and remain incompletely understood [2, 6, 7]. The leading hypothesis incriminates hypothalamic activation with secondary activation of the trigeminal-autonomic reflex, probably via a trigeminal-hypothalamic pathway [8–10]. In contrast to migraine, cluster headache has not been considered as a familial disorder until the last decades, and

A. M. J. M. van den Maagdenberg (✉)
Departments of Human Genetics and Neurology, Leiden University Medical Centre,
Leiden, The Netherlands
e-mail: a.m.j.m.van_den_Maagdenberg@lumc.nl

A. Ducros (✉)
Department of Neurology, Gui de Chauliac Hospital, CHU de Montpellier,
University of Montpellier, Montpellier, France
e-mail: a-ducros@chu-montpellier.fr

© Springer Nature Switzerland AG 2020
M. Leone, A. May (eds.), *Cluster Headache and other Trigeminal Autonomic
Cephalgias*, Headache, https://doi.org/10.1007/978-3-030-12438-0_5

43

epidemiological studies suggested that this condition could be, at least in part, of genetic origin [11]. Thereafter, the genetics of cluster headache has become an emerging research field with the major goal to identify genes that confer disease risk. The identification of causal genes will give important clues to the molecular underpinning and insight in the pathogenesis of the disorder and may guide the development of new diagnostic and therapeutic strategies. At the moment, however, such genetic factors remain unknown for any of the TACs.

5.2 Why Is It Difficult to Identify Genes Involved in Cluster Headache and Other TACs?

Genetic studies in cluster headache and TACs encounter difficulties directly related to some of the characteristic features of the disorders, i.e. their low prevalence and the fact that diagnosis is not straightforward, assuming that the disorders are genetic in the first place.

With respect to cluster headache, the prevalence is only about 0.1% in the population, and the diagnosis is often missed. In the absence of a biological or radiological marker, the diagnosis is purely based on clinical criteria proposed by the International Classification of Headache Disorders (ICHD) [4]. The patient must have had at least five attacks of severe or very severe unilateral orbital or supraorbital and/or temporal pain lasting 15–180 min when untreated. The headache is accompanied by one ipsilateral autonomic symptom of the following: conjunctival injection and/or lacrimation, nasal congestion and/or rhinorrhoea, eyelid oedema, forehead and facial sweating, miosis and/or ptosis. Since the 2004 ICHD-2, cluster headache can be diagnosed in the absence of autonomic signs if headache is associated with restlessness or agitation [12]. Primary cluster headache is characterized by the repetition of such attacks in the absence of any underlying disorder causing secondary headaches. The clinical spectrum of cluster headache may be larger, as suggested by the description of several persons with painless attacks of unilateral autonomous signs who later on developed or who had previously suffered from typical painful cluster headache attacks [13, 14]. Recurrent cluster-like attacks may be associated with several organic cerebral disorders, including mainly pituitary tumours, other brain or cervical tumours, sinusitis and carotid artery dissection [15, 16]. Many reports have described that these structural lesions might cause symptoms that are indistinguishable from those of primary cluster headache. At present, whether the mechanisms of symptomatic cluster headache attacks are different from those of primary cluster headache attacks is an unresolved issue.

Classification of individuals as definitely 'affected' or 'unaffected', which is essential for genetic studies, does not reflect the clinical heterogeneity of cluster headache. Indeed, the frequency and severity of attacks, as well as the duration of active periods show much variability from one patient to another, complicating genetic analysis. Depending on the long-term temporal course of attacks, cluster headache is divided by clinicians in episodic and chronic forms [2–4]. Most of the cluster headache patients are episodic and may present one or two active periods per year or even go in remission for years before the next bout starts. About 20% of cluster headache patients are chronic and have ongoing attacks for 1 year or more. The distinction between episodic and chronic forms is arbitrary, which further complicates genetic studies, also because it is not unknown whether the distinction reflects differences in underlying molecular pathways. The diagnostic criteria for chronic cluster headache have been modified in the latest ICHD-3 version, stipulating that attacks must have occurred without a remission period or with remissions lasting <3 months for at least 1 year [17]. In the previous versions of the classification, chronic cluster headache was diagnosed in patients having ongoing attacks for 1 year or more without more than 1 month (ICHD-2 and ICHD-3 beta) or 14 days of remission (ICHD-1) [4, 12, 18]. Some patients may evolve from one form to the other and reverse. Future genetic findings may shed light on whether episodic and chronic cluster headaches are in fact two clinical forms of the same disease or whether they represent distinct disorders. Finally, the age of onset is highly variable ranging from early childhood to more than 80 years, and the overall male to female ratio is 4.3:1, which also has to be taken into account in family and segregation studies [19].

Similar problems are related to studying the genetics of other TACs. In brief, these conditions are very rare, and their diagnosis is also purely clinical based on the ICHD criteria [4]. The prevalence of paroxysmal hemicrania is not known, but the relationship in comparison with cluster headache is reported to range from 1 to 15% [20, 21]. Paroxysmal hemicrania differs from cluster headache by a female preponderance, the shorter length and higher frequency of attacks and an absolute response to indomethacin [22], but distinguishing the two TACs may be difficult. SUNCT has an estimated prevalence around 6.6 per 100,000 [23] and manifests as very short attacks that can occur up to 300 times a day, which can be difficult to distinguish from trigeminal neuralgia [24]. The prevalence of hemicrania continua, another indomethacin-responsive TAC, is unknown, and only a few hundred cases have been published in the literature [25, 26].

5.3 Is Cluster Headache Really a Genetic Condition?

Initially, CH was not thought to be a genetic disease. However, with the official criteria for diagnosis being published, there came increasing recognition of the disease likely having a genetic basis. A logical first approach to investigate whether a trait is genetic is to perform twin studies by comparing co-occurrence of disease (concordance) in monozygotic twins versus dizygotic twins. However, because of the low prevalence of the disease, such studies are difficult to perform. Cluster headache has been reported in five concordant monozygotic twin pairs [27–31]. The first large twin survey based on the Swedish Twin Registry and the Swedish Inpatient Registry failed to identify any concordant pair; the two monozygotic and nine dizygotic twin pairs were all discordant for cluster headache and had been discordant for 10–31 years [32]. A subsequent larger Swedish study was conducted on 31,750 registered twins and showed a higher concordance rate for cluster headache in monozygotic twins (2/12 pairs) than dizygotic twins (0/25 pairs), presenting at least some indication that the trait is genetic. The fact that most monozygotic twins are discordant for CH shows that environmental factors also play a role [33].

There have been clinical reports of cluster headache in families [34, 35]. A genetic component in cluster headache pathogenesis was further confirmed by seven systematic family studies in large samples of probands with cluster headache [36–43]. Compared with the general population, the risk of cluster headache for first-degree relatives was found increased by 14- to 46-fold and for second-degree relatives by 2- to 8-fold [38–40, 42]. Differences between studies may be explained by methodological issues, for example, only the French study included a direct interview of all first-degree relatives by a headache specialist [40]. Estimating heritability in cluster headache, which is another often-used measure of the genetic component, is not feasible given the low prevalence of the disorder.

A precise transmission mode is not established for cluster headache. All types of transmission have been observed: from father to son, father to daughter, mother to son and mother to daughter. In a large Dutch study, some 1700 patients with cluster headache were asked whether they had relatives with the disease which revealed that of the 33 parent-to-child transmissions, 22 were from father to son, 6 from mother to son, 2 from mother to daughter and 3 from father to daughter [44]. The study identified 12 families with 3 affected (3 in 1 generation, 8 in 2 generations and 1 in 3 generations) and 58 families with 2 affected (33 in 1 generation, 20 in 2 generations and 5 included second-degree relatives).

A Danish complex segregation analysis [45] and two Italian family studies [37, 39] have suggested an autosomal dominant inheritance with incomplete penetrance. Such inheritance is further suggested by two studies that found a lower male/female ratio in familial cluster headache than in cluster headache in general [40, 43]. Conversely, an analysis of a single Italian pedigree suggested autosomal recessive inheritance [46]. The French family study identified 12 vertical and 8 horizontal patterns of transmissions consistent with autosomal dominant and recessive inheritance, respectively [40]. Still, a polygenic mode of inheritance should not be excluded, as in most families with cluster headache no clear segregation pattern is observed.

Altogether, these results have confirmed that cluster headache has a genetic component but that the mode of transmission may vary while the amount of heritability is unclear.

5.4   Are Other TACs Genetic Conditions?

There have been only few reports of other TACs running in families. Familial paroxysmal hemicrania was reported in a mother and a daughter [47]. In a series of 74 patients with paroxysmal hemicrania, 80% did not report a family history of any headaches, 15% had a family history of migraine and 5% had a family history of other types of headache and facial pain including cluster headache and trigeminal neuralgia, but none had paroxysmal hemicrania [48]. There has been one report of familial hemicrania continua in a single family with a mother and a daughter both affected by hemicrania continua and migraine [49]. Familial SUNCT was reported in two families each comprising of two affected first-degree relatives, namely, a brother and a sister [50] and a mother and a son [51]. One report showed, in a cohort of 117 SUNCT/SUNA and 107 hemiplegic migraine patients, co-occurrence of both disorders in 10 patients, which is not expected given the low prevalence of both disorders, suggesting that they may be brought about by a common mechanism, although this was not supported by evidence [52].

All in all, these reports suggest that the other TACs may have a genetic component, but rarity of these conditions renders epidemiological surveys difficult to conduct.

5.5 Are Other Primary Headache Types Genetic Conditions?

Of the other primary headache disorders, the genetics of migraine is the best studied. Information about the genetics of other primary headache disorders is scarce and not further discussed here. Twin and family studies in migraine have indicated a strong genetic component. The genetic component was higher in migraine with aura than migraine without aura [4], with concordance rates in monozygotic twins being 1.5- to 2-fold higher than in dizygotic twins [53–55] and an increased risk of migraine for first-degree relatives that is 1.4- to 4-fold higher, depending on the migraine type [55, 56]. The lower fold changes in migraine compared to those in cluster headache merely reflect the higher prevalence of migraine in the population (15–20%) and not that the genetic component in migraine would be lower than in cluster headache. In fact, migraine has an estimated heritability of 42%, indicating that about half of the risk for migraine is conferred through genetic factors and which is in the range of most other complex (polygenic) disorders [57].

5.6 Which Strategies Can Be Used to Identify Genes for CH?

The epidemiological evidence that cluster headache is rare, runs in families and is brought about by both genetic and environmental factors determines chances for success of the genetic approach applied to identify causal genes.

5.6.1 Gene Identification Strategy in Case of a Monogenic Inheritance

The fact that some extended Mendelian pedigrees have been identified with multiple patients with cluster headache, at least in theory, should make them suited to identify disease-causing mutations using linkage. In a linkage approach, several hundreds of genetic markers, equally spread over all chromosomes, are tested in affected and unaffected individuals of a single family or of multiple families, and markers that best segregate with the disease reveal the likely chromosomal location of the disease gene. Next, using a positional cloning approach, the pathogenetic mutation is identified in a disease locus. In recent years, next-generation sequencing (NGS) is used to speed up the process, as it allows massive parallel sequencing of all protein-coding regions ('exome sequencing'), or in fact the whole genome ('whole genome sequencing'), in a single experiment, and has been very successful in identifying disease genes for monogenic disorders [58].

Proof of causality of a mutation comes from the fact that (1) the mutation is present in most affected family members (in case of reduced penetrance, the mutation is also found in some cases who do not (yet) express the disease) and not present in non-affected family members (although phenocopies may occur, which are defined as patients that express disease because of an unlinked cause), (2) the mutation is not found in large cohorts of control individuals and (3) follow-up functional studies provide convincing support that the mutated gene affects a pathway implicated in the disease. At the moment, no pathogenic mutation for cluster headache or any of the other TACs was identified by a linkage or NGS study. For comparison, and as demonstration of how powerful such approach can be, in familial hemiplegic migraine, three genes and in them many different mutations have been identified in hundreds of families and sporadic patients, which had a profound impact on clinical care, already because the identification of a causal mutation confirms the clinical diagnosis [59].

5.6.2   Gene Identification Strategy in Case of a Polygenic Inheritance

However, as most cluster headache patients are not part of Mendelian families, but merely singletons, or at best two or three patients in a pedigree without a clear segregation pattern, alternative approaches that take into account that one genetic factor is not sufficient to bring about disease may be more appropriate to identify genetic factors. Association-based methods are particularly suited, because they can identify susceptibility genes and DNA variants with small relative risks. However, such studies only give convincing evidence for involvement of a gene when (1) a large sample size is used (preferably many hundreds to thousands); (2) when (well-phenotyped) patients and control samples have a comparable genetic architecture, so spurious association because of population stratification is prevented; and, most importantly, (3) that promising findings are replicated in other samples.

Until recently, a genetic association study was designed based on a specific hypothesis (candidate gene association study), which entails that a gene is selected based on prior knowledge that it acts in a presumed disease pathway. The frequency of alleles of polymorphic genetic markers, typically single nucleotide polymorphisms (SNPs), in such a gene is compared between patients and healthy controls. A significant difference suggests that the polymorphism (and the gene) is involved in disease pathology or that because of linkage disequilibrium, a gene in close proximity is the causal gene. Instead of testing one SNP at a time, nowadays, because of technological advances, it is feasible to cost-effectively genotype hundreds of thousands of SNPs in the entire genome (hypothesis-free approach) in thousands of patients and controls.

5.7 What Is Currently Known About the Genetics of CH?

Almost all genetic studies in cluster headache to date used the candidate gene association approach. Genes were selected because they are believed to be involved in molecular pathways that explain clinical features, in particular the characteristic periodicity and circadian rhythm of attacks, which suggests hypothalamic dysfunction, and the fact that patients are heavy smokers and drinkers [60, 61] although the latter is debated [62].

5.7.1 Candidate Gene Association Studies in Cluster Headache

A large number of candidate genes were tested, among others, *CLOCK*, *PER3*, *HCRTR1* and *HCRTR2* that affect functioning of the biological clock, which reside in the suprachiasmatic nucleus of the hypothalamus, *ADH4* that is involved in alcohol metabolization and *CACNA1A* and *NOS1-3* genes that are involved in pain processing (for comprehensive reviews, see [11] and [63]). Except for *HCRTR2*, which will be discussed separately below, none of the candidate genes showed evidence for association with cluster headache, mainly because investigated samples were much too small—most of them had below 230 cases, a number that often was subdivided into episodic and chronic cluster headaches which reduced power even more—and, without exception, no association result could be convincingly replicated. Therefore, with the present data, no conclusion can be drawn about the involvement of any of these genes in cluster headache.

The situation is slightly better for *HCRTR2*, which encodes the hypocretin receptor 2. The hypocretin (orexin) system is thought to play an important role in cluster headache as hypocretin-containing neurons almost exclusively are located in the posterolateral hypothalamus that generates rhythms [8]. Foremost, SNP rs2653349 (G1246A), which changes a valine residue to an isoleucine at position 308 of the receptor protein, was investigated, and the first study showed promising association in an Italian cohort of patients with cluster headache [64]. The association was replicated in one [65] but not in another study [66]. A recent, larger Dutch study that investigated 575 patients with cluster headache was also not able to show association, although a meta-analysis of 1167 cases and 1618 controls was again positive [67]. In light of the fact that cluster headache patients are heavy smokers, it certainly is interesting that the same SNP was linked to increased nicotine dependence because of increased rewarding effects due to changed activity of the orexin system [68].

Finally, an association of mtDNA abnormalities with cluster headache was suggested, even though transmission of disease from the father to offspring often occurs. Evidence for mitochondrial involvement came from the fact that (1) a sporadic Japanese patient with a 3243 point mutation in platelet mitochondrial tRNALeu(UUR), known to cause MELAS (mitochondrial myopathy, encephalopathy, lactacidosis and stroke-like episodes), also had cluster headache [69] and (2) cluster headache was also reported in a patient with multiple deletions in mitochondrial DNA. It remains unclear to what extent abnormal mitochondrial function actually is involved in cluster headache [70].

5.7.2 Candidate Gene Association Studies in Other Primary Headache Disorders

Candidate gene association studies have also been performed in other primary headache disorders, mainly in migraine with an equally disappointing outcome (for reviews, see [71] and [72]). Despite overwhelming evidence from clinical, pharmacological and neuroanatomical studies that, for instance, the serotonin and dopamine systems are involved in migraine, no convincing evidence for association was found for SNPs in genes of these pathways. Using a much larger large data set of 5175 patients with migraine with or without aura and 13,972 controls, a systematic re-evaluation was conducted of the most promising 21 genes, which included the *MTHFR* gene that encodes a key enzyme in folate and homocysteine metabolism that had surfaced as the best migraine candidate gene [71, 73] and also showed suggestive association in chronic cluster headache [74]. Neither the previously implicated variants nor any other variant in a region of 500 kb surrounding the respective genes provided evidence for association [73]. The most likely conclusion, therefore, is that all published associations from candidate gene association studies, in retrospect, are false positives. Proof that this scenario indeed applies comes from the consideration that in such a large sample, the associated T allele of the *MTHFR* C677T polymorphism, with reported effect sizes of ~1.5, when assuming a minor allele frequency of 31%, should have produced a p-value ~1.5×10^{-63} instead of the non-impressive observed 9.7×10^{-3} [73]. The effect size in these small studies is very much inflated, as evidenced by the small effect size (1.08), which is more in line with the larger genome-wide association studies (GWAS) discussed below. A sobering thought perhaps is the realization that a p-value cut-off of 0.05 simply is not reliable to obtain robust results when dealing with small data sets, which had already been recognized in other areas of science [75].

5.7.3 Genome-Wide Association Study in Cluster Headache

The low prevalence of cluster headache did not stop Italian researchers from performing the first, and thus far only, genome-wide association study (GWAS) in cluster headache [76]. Admittedly, their sample of 99 clinically well-defined patients with cluster headache and 360 healthy individuals is tiny compared to the thousands to tens of thousands of cases and controls that one nowadays investigates in a GWAS [77]. Also, the male-female distribution and smoking status was not appropriately matched in the cluster headache GWA study [76]. Still, by combining single-marker (testing common SNPs) and gene-based (focussing on rare protein-altering variants in 745 candidate genes with a putative role in CH) association analyses, they claim some suggestive hits, although the observed effect sizes (<0.5 or >2.0) were more extreme than those reported in other GWA studies (between ~0.8 and ~1.2). Also observed p-values, often by orders of magnitude, did not reach the commonly accepted threshold for a genome-wide significant association ($p \leq 5 \times 10^{-8}$). Therefore, the findings can, at best, be taken as hypothesis-generating. Among their hits was an association with a variant in the PACAP receptor gene *ADCYAP1R1*, which is of interest given that PACAP induces activation of specific neurons that have been implicated in the pathophysiology of cluster headache and that higher plasmatic levels of PACAP have been detected in patients with cluster headache inside a period of attacks than outside such a period [78]. In addition, their gene-based analysis provided some evidence of association for a rare potentially damaging missense variant in *MME* that encodes the membrane metallo-endopeptidase neprilysin [76]. The fact, however, that these findings could not be replicated in a much larger sample set of over 500 Swedish cluster headache patients may suggest that the initial hits were false positives [79].

5.7.4 Genome-Wide Association Studies in Other Primary Headache Disorders

Various GWAS were performed for various migraine types in increasingly large cohorts of patients and controls [80]. The most recent, and largest, migraine GWAS investigated 59,674 migraine cases and 316,078 healthy controls and identified 38 genome-wide significant loci with 45 independent SNPs that confer migraine risk [81]. Of the 29 migraine-associated SNPs that could directly be genotyped or captured by a tag SNP in the cluster headache GWAS, only SNP rs9349379 in *PHACTR1* achieved a nominally significant p-value in cluster headache [76]. The same SNP associated with several vascular diseases (coronary heart disease, coronary artery calcification and cervical artery dissection), and through various genetic and molecular approaches, it was convincingly shown that the SNP in fact regulated endothelin-1, a potent vasoconstrictor encoded by *EDN1* located 600 kb upstream of *PHACTR1* [82]. The observation that mean endothelin-1 plasma levels were increased during attacks of cluster headache suggests that vascular or immune function, two known functions of endothelin-1, may be involved in its pathology [83].

5.8   Investigating the Genetics of Cluster Headache Through RNA-Based Approaches

RNA-based approaches have also been tried to identify genes and pathways involved in cluster headache by searching for differential gene expression in tissue from patients and controls. Microarray profiling of RNA from whole blood or immortalized lymphoblastoid cell lines from a few cluster headache patients revealed differentially expressed genes: i.e. 90 in blood [84] and 1100 in cell lines [85], albeit with very limited overlap. It remains unclear to what extent the suggested pathways (noninfectious inflammation or endoplasmic reticulum protein processing) are involved in the pathology. In a recent Dutch study, RNA-sequencing (RNA-seq), a deep sequencing-based technique that is more robust and detects a wider range of transcripts than microarray technology, was used to compare whole blood gene expression profiles of a much larger sample: 39 well-characterized patients with cluster headache (19 episodic, 20 chronic) and 20 matched controls [86]. No single cluster headache-associated gene survived false discovery rate multiple testing correction. So, unlike previous reports, differences in gene expression in cluster headache, at best, seem very modest. At the level of functional gene sets, associations were observed for genes involved in several brain-related mechanisms, such as GABA receptor function and voltage-gated channels. The analysis of genes and modules of co-expressed genes suggested a role for intracellular signalling cascades, mitochondria and inflammation [86]. A role for abnormal inflammation has been proposed before [85], although the genes identified in both studies did not overlap. In the Dutch study, no evidence was obtained for the involvement of hypocretin, by analysing custom hypocretin gene sets [86]. Clearly, even larger samples should be studied with carefully taking into account (1) the matching of patients and controls and (2) the time of blood withdrawal relative to the occurrence of attacks (i.e. for cluster headache inside or outside an attack period), to identify the full range of cluster headache-associated genes and pathways. Ideally, of course, gene expression profiling should be performed in well-characterized human postmortem brain samples, but these are extremely difficult to obtain.

5.9   Conclusion

There is compelling epidemiological evidence that cluster headache has a genetic component. Evidence is less convincing for the other TACs. Despite many efforts, it has not been possible to identify causal genetic factors for cluster headache that are undisputed. Lessons can be learnt from other primary headache disorders, foremost migraine, which has shown that it is possible to identify genetic factors. Future studies in cluster headache should perhaps take into account many of the mentioned factors for success, i.e. much larger sample sizes, less heterogeneity of phenotypes (not mixing episodic and chronic patients in the analyses), more adequately matching cases and controls and—for RNA-based studies—ideally analysing diseased brain tissue or in the case of blood optimally timing the moment of drawing blood in relation to the occurrence of attacks.

References

1. Goadsby PJ, Lipton RB. A review of paroxysmal hemicranias, SUNCT syndrome and other short-lasting headaches with autonomic feature, including new cases. Brain. 1997;120:193–209.
2. May A. Cluster headache: pathogenesis, diagnosis, and management. Lancet. 2005;366:843–55.
3. Nesbitt AD, Goadsby PJ. Cluster headache. Br Med J. 2012;344:e2407.
4. Headache Classification Committee of the International Headache Society (IHS). The international classification of headache disorders, 3rd edition (beta version). Cephalalgia. 2013;33:629–808.
5. Goadsby PJ. Trigeminal autonomic cephalalgias. Pathophysiology and classification. Rev Neurol. 2005;161:692–5.
6. Leone M, Bussone G. Pathophysiology of trigeminal autonomic cephalalgias. Lancet Neurol. 2009;8:755–64.
7. Barloese MCJ. The pathophysiology of the trigeminal autonomic cephalalgias, with clinical implications. Clin Auton Res. 2018;28(3):315–24.
8. May A, Bahra A, Buchel C, Frackowiak RS, Goadsby PJ. Hypothalamic activation in cluster headache attacks. Lancet. 1998;352:275–8.
9. May A, Goadsby PJ. The trigeminovascular system in humans: pathophysiologic implications for primary headache syndromes of the neural influences on the cerebral circulation. J Cereb Blood Flow Metab. 1999;19:115–27.
10. Malick A, Strassman RM, Burstein R. Trigeminohypothalamic and reticulohypothalamic tract neurons in the upper cervical spinal cord and caudal medulla of the rat. J Neurophysiol. 2000;84:2078–112.
11. Sjostrand C. Genetic aspects of cluster headache. Expert Rev Neurother. 2009;9:359–68.
12. Headache Classification Subcommittee of the International Headache Society. The international classification of headache disorders: 2nd edition. Cephalalgia. 2004;24(Suppl 1):9–160.
13. Salvesen R. Cluster headache sine headache: case report. Neurology. 2000;55:451.
14. Leone M, Rigamonti A, Bussone G. Cluster headache sine headache: two new cases in one family. Cephalalgia. 2002;22:12–4.
15. Favier I, van Vliet JA, Roon KI, Witteveen RJ, Verschuuren JJ, Ferrari MD, et al. Trigeminal autonomic cephalgias due to structural lesions: a review of 31 cases. Arch Neurol. 2007;64:25–31.
16. Leroux E, Ducros A. Cluster headache. Orphanet J Rare Dis. 2008;3:20.
17. Headache Classification Committee of the International Headache Society. The International Classification of Headache Disorders. 3rd edition. ICHD-3. Cephalalgia. 2018;38(1):1–211.
18. Headache Classification Committee of the International Headache Society. Classification and diagnostic criteria for headache disorders, cranial neuralgias and facial pain. Cephalalgia. 1988;8:1–96.
19. Russell MB. Epidemiology and genetics of cluster headache. Lancet Neurol. 2004;3:279–83.
20. Goadsby PJ, Cittadini E, Cohen AS. Trigeminal autonomic cephalalgias: paroxysmal hemicrania, SUNCT/SUNA, and hemicrania continua. Semin Neurol. 2010;30:186–91.

21. Prakash S, Belani P, Susvirkar A, Trivedi A, Ahuja S, Patel A. Paroxysmal hemicrania: a retrospective study of a consecutive series of 22 patients and a critical analysis of the diagnostic criteria. J Headache Pain. 2013;14:26.
22. Goadsby P, Lipton R. A review of paroxysmal hemicranias, SUNCT syndrome, and other short lasting headaches with autonomic features, including new cases. Brain. 1997;120:193–209.
23. Williams MH, Broadley SA. SUNCT and SUNA: clinical features and medical treatment. J Clin Neurosci. 2008;15:526–34.
24. Cohen AS, Matharu MS, Goadsby PJ. Short-lasting unilateral neuralgiform headache attacks with conjunctival injection and tearing (SUNCT) or cranial autonomic features (SUNA)—a prospective clinical study of SUNCT and SUNA. Brain. 2006;129:2746–60.
25. Rapoport AM, Bigal ME. Hemicrania continua: clinical and nosographic update. Neurol Sci. 2003;24(Suppl 2):S118–21.
26. Silberstein SD, Peres MF. Hemicrania continua. Arch Neurol. 2002;59:1029–30.
27. Sjaastad O, Salvesen R. Cluster headache: are we only seeing the tip of the iceberg? Cephalalgia. 1986;6:127–9.
28. Sjaastad O, Shen JM, Stovner LJ, Elsas T. Cluster headache in identical twins. Headache. 1993;33:214–7.
29. Eadie MJ, Sutherland JM. Migrainous neuralgia. Med J Aust. 1966;1:1053–7.
30. Couturier EG, Hering R, Steiner TJ. The first report of cluster headache in identical twins. Neurology. 1991;41:761.
31. Roberge C, Bouchard JP, Simard D, Gagne R. Cluster headache in twins. Neurology. 1992;42:1255–6.
32. Svensson D, Ekbom K, Pedersen NL, Traff H, Waldenlind E. A note on cluster headache in a population-based twin register. Cephalalgia. 2003;23:376–80.
33. Ekbom K, Svensson DA, Pedersen NL, Waldenlind E. Lifetime prevalence and concordance risk of cluster headache in the Swedish twin population. Neurology. 2006;67:798–803.
34. D'Amico D, Leone M, Moschiano F, Bussone G. Familial cluster headache: report of three families. Headache. 1996;36:41–3.
35. Spierings EL, Vincent AJ. Familial cluster headache: occurrence in three generations. Neurology. 1992;42:1399–400.
36. Kudrow L, Kudrow DB. Inheritance of cluster headache and its possible link to migraine. Headache. 1994;34:400–7.
37. Montagna P, Mochi M, Prologo G, Sangiorgi S, Pierangeli G, Cevoli S, et al. Heritability of cluster headache. Eur J Neurol. 1998;5:343–5.
38. Russell MB, Andersson PG, Thomsen LL. Familial occurrence of cluster headache. J Neurol Neurosurg Psychiatry. 1995;58:341–3.
39. Leone M, Russell MB, Rigamonti A, Attanasio A, Grazzi L, D'Amico D, et al. Increased familial risk of cluster headache. Neurology. 2001;56:1233–6.
40. El Amrani M, Ducros A, Boulan P, Aidi S, Crassard I, Visy JM, et al. Familial cluster headache: a series of 186 index patients. Headache. 2002;42:974–7.
41. Torelli P, Manzoni GC. Clinical observations on familial cluster headache. Neurol Sci. 2003;24:61–4.
42. Cruz S, Lemos C, Monteiro JM. Familial aggregation of cluster headache. Arq Neuropsiquiatr. 2013;71:866–70.
43. Taga A, Russo M, Manzoni GC, Torelli P. Familial cluster headache in an Italian case series. Neurol Sci. 2015;36(Suppl 1):141–3.
44. Vliet JA, Ferrari MD, Haan J. Genetic factors in cluster headache. Expert Rev Neurother. 2003;3:301–6.
45. Russell MB, Andersson PG, Thomsen LL, Iselius L. Cluster headache is an autosomal dominantly inherited disorder in some families: a complex segregation analysis. J Med Genet. 1995;32:954–6.
46. De Simone R, Fiorillo C, Bonuso S, Castaldo G. A cluster headache family with possible autosomal recessive inheritance. Neurology. 2003;61:578–9.

47. Cohen AS, Matharu MS, Goadsby PJ. Paroxysmal hemicrania in a family. Cephalalgia. 2006;26:486–8.
48. Boes CJ, Dodick DW. Refining the clinical spectrum of chronic paroxysmal hemicrania: a review of 74 patients. Headache. 2002;42:699–708.
49. Weatherall MW, Bahra A. Familial hemicrania continua. Cephalalgia. 2011;31:245–9.
50. Gantenbein AR, Goadsby PJ. Familial SUNCT. Cephalalgia. 2005;25:457–9.
51. Martins IP, Viana P, Lobo PP. Familial SUNCT in mother and son. Cephalalgia. 2016;36:993–7.
52. Lambru G, Nesbitt A, Shanahan P, Matharu MS. Coexistence of hemiplegic migraine with SUNCT or SUNA: a case series. Cephalalgia. 2012;32:258–62.
53. Honkasalo ML, Kaprio J, Winter T, Heikkila K, Sillanpaa M, Koskenvuo M. Migraine and concomitant symptoms among 8167 adult twin pairs. Headache. 1995;35:70–8.
54. Ulrich V, Gervil M, Kyvik KO, Olesen J, Russell MB. Evidence of a genetic factor in migraine with aura: a population-based Danish twin study. Ann Neurol. 1999;45:242–6.
55. Russell MB, Ulrich V, Gervil M, Olesen J. Migraine without aura and migraine with aura are distinct disorders. A population-based twin survey. Headache. 2002;42:332–6.
56. Russell MB, Iselius L, Olesen J. Migraine without aura and migraine with aura are inherited disorders. Cephalalgia. 1996;16:305–9.
57. Polderman TJ, Benyamin B, de Leeuw CA, Sullivan PF, van Bochoven A, Visscher PM, et al. Meta-analysis of the heritability of human traits based on fifty years of twin studies. Nat Genet. 2015;47:702–9.
58. Kuhlenbaumer G, Hullmann J, Appenzeller S. Novel genomic techniques open new avenues in the analysis of monogenic disorders. Hum Mutat. 2011;32:144–51.
59. Ferrari MD, Klever RR, Terwindt GM, Ayata C, van den Maagdenberg AM. Migraine pathophysiology: lessons from mouse models and human genetics. Lancet Neurol. 2015;14:65–80.
60. Manzoni GC. Cluster headache and lifestyle: remarks on a population of 374 male patients. Cephalalgia. 1999;19:88–94.
61. Levi R, Edman GV, Ekbom K, Waldenlind E. Episodic cluster headache. II: high tobacco and alcohol consumption in males. Headache. 1992;32:184–7.
62. Schurks M, Diener HC. Cluster headache and lifestyle habits. Curr Pain Headache Rep. 2008;12:115–21.
63. Schurks M. Genetics of cluster headache. Curr Pain Headache Rep. 2010;14:132–9.
64. Rainero I, Gallone S, Valfre W, Ferrero M, Angilella G, Rivoiro C, et al. A polymorphism of the hypocretin receptor 2 gene is associated with cluster headache. Neurology. 2004;63:1286–8.
65. Schurks M, Kurth T, Geissler I, Tessmann G, Diener HC, Rosskopf D. Cluster headache is associated with the G1246A polymorphism in the hypocretin receptor 2 gene. Neurology. 2006;66:1917–9.
66. Baumber L, Sjostrand C, Leone M, Harty H, Bussone G, Hillert J, et al. A genome-wide scan and HCRTR2 candidate gene analysis in a European cluster headache cohort. Neurology. 2006;66:1888–93.
67. Weller CM, Wilbrink LA, Houwing-Duistermaat JJ, Koelewijn SC, Vijfhuizen LS, Haan J, et al. Cluster headache and the hypocretin receptor 2 reconsidered: a genetic association study and meta-analysis. Cephalalgia. 2015;35:741–7.
68. Nishizawa D, Kasai S, Hasegawa J, Sato N, Yamada H, Tanioka F, et al. Associations between the orexin (hypocretin) receptor 2 gene polymorphism Val308Ile and nicotine dependence in genome-wide and subsequent association studies. Mol Brain. 2015;8:50.
69. Shimomura T, Kitano A, Marukawa H, Mishima K, Isoe K, Adachi Y, et al. Point mutation in platelet mitochondrial tRNA(Leu(UUR)) in patient with cluster headache. Lancet. 1994;344:625.
70. Odawara M, Tamaoka A, Mizusawa H, Yamashita K. A case of cluster headache associated with mitochondrial DNA deletions. Muscle Nerve. 1997;20:394–5.
71. de Vries B, Frants RR, Ferrari MD, van den Maagdenberg AM. Molecular genetics of migraine. Hum Genet. 2009;126:115–32.

72. Sutherland HG, Griffiths LR. Genetics of migraine: insights into the molecular basis of migraine disorders. Headache. 2017;57:537–69.
73. de Vries B, Anttila V, Freilinger T, Wessman M, Kaunisto MA, Kallela M, et al. Systematic re-evaluation of genes from candidate gene association studies in migraine using a large genome-wide association data set. Cephalalgia. 2016;36:604–14.
74. Schurks M, Neumann FA, Kessler C, Diener HC, Kroemer HK, Kurth T, et al. MTHFR 677C>T polymorphism and cluster headache. Headache. 2011;51:201–7.
75. Button KS, Ioannidis JP, Mokrysz C, Nosek BA, Flint J, Robinson ES, et al. Power failure: why small sample size undermines the reliability of neuroscience. Nat Rev Neurosci. 2013;14:365–76.
76. Bacchelli E, Cainazzo MM, Cameli C, Guerzoni S, Martinelli A, Zoli M, et al. A genome-wide analysis in cluster headache points to neprilysin and PACAP receptor gene variants. J Headache Pain. 2016;17:114.
77. Visscher PM, Wray NR, Zhang Q, Sklar P, McCarthy MI, Brown MA, et al. 10 years of GWAS discovery: biology, function, and translation. Am J Hum Genet. 2017;101:5–22.
78. Tuka B, Szabo N, Toth E, Kincses ZT, Pardutz A, Szok D, et al. Release of PACAP-38 in episodic cluster headache patients—an exploratory study. J Headache Pain. 2016;17:69.
79. Ran C, Fourier C, Michalska JM, Steinberg A, Sjostrand C, Waldenlind E, et al. Screening of genetic variants in ADCYAP1R1, MME and 14q21 in a Swedish cluster headache cohort. J Headache Pain. 2017;18:88.
80. Gormley P, Winsvold BS, Nyholt DR, Kallela M, Chasman DI, Palotie A. Migraine genetics: from genome-wide association studies to translational insights. Genome Med. 2016;8:86.
81. Gormley P, Anttila V, Winsvold BS, Palta P, Esko T, Pers TH, et al. Meta-analysis of 375,000 individuals identifies 38 susceptibility loci for migraine. Nat Genet. 2016;48:856–66.
82. Gupta RM, Hadaya J, Trehan A, Zekavat SM, Roselli C, Klarin D, et al. A genetic variant associated with five vascular diseases is a distal regulator of endothelin-1 gene expression. Cell. 2017;170:522–33.
83. Franceschini R, Tenconi GL, Leandri M, Zoppoli F, Gonella A, Staltari S, et al. Endothelin-1 plasma levels in cluster headache. Headache. 2002;42:120–4.
84. Sjostrand C, Duvefelt K, Steinberg A, Remahl IN, Waldenlind E, Hillert J. Gene expression profiling in cluster headache: a pilot microarray study. Headache. 2006;46:1518–34.
85. Costa M, Squassina A, Piras IS, Pisanu C, Congiu D, Niola P, et al. Preliminary transcriptome analysis in lymphoblasts from cluster headache and bipolar disorder patients implicates dysregulation of circadian and serotonergic genes. J Mol Neurosci. 2015;56:688–95.
86. Eising E, Pelzer N, Vijfhuizen LS, Vries B, Ferrari MD, t Hoen PA, et al. Identifying a gene expression signature of cluster headache in blood. Sci Rep. 2017;7:40218.

Chapter 6
Pathophysiological Considerations Regarding Cluster Headache and Trigeminal Autonomic Cephalalgias

Massimo Leone and Arne May

6.1 Introduction

When we discuss pathophysiological background regarding cluster headache, scientific progress over the last 20 years has put us in the fortunate situation that we can divide this question into "what drives cluster headache" and "where is the source of the pain." For decades these (fundamentally different) questions have been mixed as so little was known about the pathophysiology of this dreadful disease. We have learned so much about modulators and generators of cluster headache attacks and— to be frank—know still relatively little of what structure actually generates the nociceptive input. We therefore focus here on central generating factors (the why) and refer to the Chaps. 8 and 9 in this book (the where) [1, 2].

Trigeminal autonomic cephalalgias (TACs) are a group of primary headaches characterized by attacks of short-lasting unilateral head pain associated with ipsilateral craniofacial autonomic manifestations [3]. The group includes cluster headache (CH), the main form, paroxysmal hemicrania (PH), short-lasting unilateral neuralgiform headache attacks, and hemicrania continua [3]; attack duration is the main feature that distinguishes TACs [3].

For decades CH has been seen as a *vascular* headache [4] according to the vascular theory of migraine and related forms, but the term of *neurovascular* headache is now used given the wealth of evidence suggesting that migraine and related disorders mainly derive from within the brain [5]. Contemporary trigeminal nerve and craniofacial parasympathetic nerve fiber activation are thought to provoke the pain

M. Leone (✉)
Department of Neurology, Neuroalgology Unit, The Foundation of the Carlo Besta Neurological Institute, IRCCS, Milano, Italy
e-mail: Massimo.Leone.m@istituto-besta.it

A. May
Department of Systems Neuroscience, University of Hamburg, Hamburg, Germany
e-mail: a.may@uke.uni-hamburg.de

© Springer Nature Switzerland AG 2020
M. Leone, A. May (eds.), *Cluster Headache and other Trigeminal Autonomic Cephalgias*, Headache, https://doi.org/10.1007/978-3-030-12438-0_6

and the autonomic craniofacial phenomena, respectively [6–8]; this activation has been named *trigeminal-parasympathetic* or *trigeminal-facial reflex* [6]. An impressive phenomenon reported by many CH patients is the clockwork regularity of attacks as well as the seasonal recurrence of cluster periods in the episodic form of the disease [9] suggesting that the biological clock located in the hypothalamus is involved in its pathophysiology [10]. Results from a number of neuroendocrinological studies lent support to the hypothalamic hypothesis [11]. The first direct demonstration of hypothalamic involvement came from the seminal neuroimaging studies showing activation of the ipsilateral posterior hypothalamus during CH attacks [12] and structural anomalies (increased neuronal density) in the same brain region [13]. These observations suggested that the *cluster generator* could be located there [12]. It was then hypothesized that high-frequency deep brain stimulation of that brain area could inhibit neuronal activation of the stimulated area just as has been used in the treatment of Parkinson disease [14]. Efficacy of hypothalamic deep brain stimulation as a treatment for intractable chronic CH [14] as well as for other intractable TACs as short-lasting unilateral neuralgiform headache attacks [15–18] and PH [19] confirmed the crucial role of the hypothalamus in CH and other TACs.

In this chapter the main focus will be pathophysiology of CH because of the scarcity of data on the other TAC forms.

6.2   Genetics

An exhaustive and detailed description of genetics in CH and related disorders is reported in this book [20]. Both twins [21] and epidemiological [22] studies suggest a familial occurrence of CH. For instance, in twins an anticipation between generations has been observed [21].

Notwithstanding some methodological limitations, epidemiological studies all suggested an increased risk for first-degree relatives of patients with CH to develop CH: 14 times (or more) higher than that of the general population [22–26]. For second-degree relatives, the risk is much lower ranging between two and eight times above that of the general population [23–26].

A number of studies have investigated involvement of various genes in CH [for a comprehensive review, see Ref. 20].

The CACNA1A gene on chromosome 19p harboring the familial hemiplegic migraine type 1 mutation was investigated in CH because of the paroxysmal nature of both diseases, but no abnormalities were observed [27]. The hypocretin system has been advocated to be involved in CH because of its involvement in pain and in the regulation of the sleep–wake cycle [26] also affected in CH. A missense single-nucleotide polymorphism in the HCRTR2 gene coding for the hypocretin-2 (orexin-B) receptor was reported in CH [28] but not confirmed in other studies [29–31]. Given the circadian occurrence of painful attacks in CH, some studies investigated genes involved in circadian rhythmicity. Among these, the PER3 gene was studied but no association was found [32]. In one study genes linked to circadian rhythms such as the RBM3 protein binding several genes, including BMAL1 (ARTNL),

PER1, and CLOCK, seemed to involved in CH [33], but a larger study did not confirm those findings [31]. It has been shown that plasma level of pituitary adenylate cyclase-activating polypeptide (PACAP) is increased during cluster attacks [34], and a genome-wide analysis study indicated that a variant of the PACAP receptor gene ADCYAP1R1 might play a role in CH [35]. Due to the conflicting results on the topic [36], future studies are needed. In summary, the genetic mutation behind the familial occurrence in CH is likely; the exact nature of this remains to be established.

6.3   From the Trigeminal System to Hypothalamus

The main actors in the generation of headache episodes in CH and TACs are the trigeminal system, the parasympathetic system, and the hypothalamus (Fig. 6.1) [5–8]. Typically CH patients report that alcohol or other vasodilating agents such as nitroglycerine can trigger attacks [9, 10]. This happens only in patients with chronic or episodic CH during active cluster periods [9, 10] suggesting that a permissive state is necessary to start CH attacks. A (anatomically still unknown) brain dysfunction could lower the threshold leading to the simultaneous activation of the trigeminal and the parasympathetic system and the inhibition of the sympathetic system. Outside the active (cluster) period, this attack like orchestrated combination of activation and inhibition is not possible to activate. A genetic susceptibility would then explain the familial occurrence in some cases.

6.3.1   Trigeminal System

Activation of the trigeminal system in CH is strongly suggested by the increased serum concentrations of CGRP during a CH attack (Fig. 6.1) [37]. CGRP is contained in neurons of the gasserian ganglion and released from these neurons [38] with at least two targets: it is a potent vasodilator and modulates the activity of nociceptive trigeminal neurons [39]. The peripheral axons of the trigeminal pseudounipolar neurons innervate the dura mater and cranial vessels, while the central projections end onto the trigeminocervical complex in the brainstem. The trigeminocervical complex plays a key role in modulating and transmitting potentially painful stimuli from the face and head to the brain. It contains the trigeminal nucleus caudalis and the C1 and C2 dorsal horns of the spinal cord [40]. Animal models have clarified the interplay between the posterior hypothalamus and the trigeminocervical complex. The two areas of the central nervous system are connected by the trigemino-hypothalamic pathway, and a number of neurotransmitters modulate pain transmission between the posterior hypothalamus and the trigeminal nucleus caudalis [41]. In humans high-frequency deep brain stimulation of the posterior hypothalamic area activates a network of brain areas including the ipsilateral trigeminal system that seems to be interconnected and plays a crucial role in attack generation

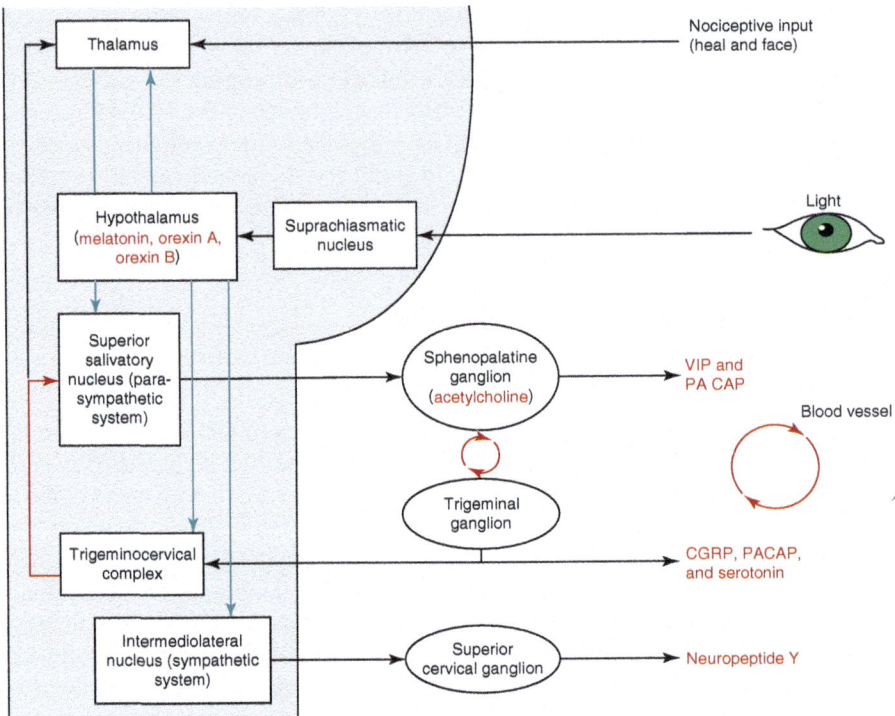

Fig. 6.1 Graphic illustrating the anatomical and neurotransmitter components of the cluster headache pathobiology. Only neurotransmitters which are known to be involved in cluster headache are shown. SSN, TCC, and ILN stand under hypothalamic control which communicates with the SCN. A strong trigeminal nociceptive input generates a signal which is transmitted to the thalamus. This signal generates in the periphery (between the trigeminal and the parasympathetic ganglion) but also centrally in a physiological reflex arch with a parasympathetic outflow. It may well be that this parasympathetic reaction (lacrimation, conjunctival injection) is facilitated due to the sympathetic deficit (miosis, ptosis) which is inherent to cluster attacks. For further explanation please see text. *ACH* acetylcholine, *CGRP* calitonin gene-related peptide, *IML* intermediolateral nucleus (sympathetic system), *SSN* superior salivatory nucleus (parasympathetic system), *TCC* trigeminocervical complex, *SCG* superior cervical ganglion, *SPG* sphenopalatine ganglion, *SCN* suprachiasmatic nucleus, *NPY* neuropeptide Y, *PACAP* pituitary adenylate cyclase-activating peptide, *VIP* vasoactive intestinal peptide, *5-HT* serotonin. *Modified after ref. [8]

[42]. Another observation questioning at least the role of the peripheral trigeminal system in CH pathophysiology is the persistence of CH after complete trigeminal nerve root section [43–45]. If these data are confirmed, the fully developed cluster picture could occur without peripheral trigeminal input, and vessels would not play any role in cluster headache generation. However, many of the clinical symptoms in CH could then not be explained. There is no question that further studies are necessary to better understand the role of the trigeminal system in pathophysiology and attack generation of CH and TACs [8].

6.3.2   Parasympathetic System

Autonomic phenomena accompanying CH attacks such as conjunctival injection, lacrimation and rhinorrhea, as well as extracranial [46] and intracranial vasodilation [47, 48] are mediated by activation of parasympathetic fibers which form the parasympathetic branch of the facial nerve, whose cell bodies originate from the superior salivatory nucleus (SSN) (Fig. 6.1). Part of the parasympathetic nerve fibers passes through the sphenopalatine ganglion (SPG) (mediating conjunctival injection, lacrimation, rhinorrhea and extracranial vasodilation) [46, 47], and part passes through the otic and carotid mini ganglia (mediating intracranial vasodilation) [47, 48].

The superior salivatory nucleus (SSN) and the trigeminal nucleus are functionally connected in the brainstem, and their contemporary activation gives rise to the trigeminal-parasympathetic reflex [6]. Nociceptive stimulation of the first division of the trigeminal nerve triggers this reflex [49]. Following this trigeminal activation, the parasympathetic neurons traveling through the SPG provoke the release of neuropeptides such as vasoactive intestinal polypeptide (VIP) [50] and pituitary adenylate cyclase-activating polypeptide (PACAP) which are raised during a CH attack (Fig. 6.1) [34]. PACAP might be a particularly interesting target for future treatments given that PACAP is a neurotransmitter of the trigeminal and the parasympathetic system [51]. The superior salivatory nucleus is, just as the trigeminal nucleus, under modulating control of the hypothalamus. Oculo-facial parasympathetic phenomena in cluster headache attacks could therefore be initiated by hypothalamic input instead of being a result of trigeminal nociceptive input, i.e., a trigeminally induced reflex phenomenon. This could explain why some CH patients report painless attacks with only autonomic phenomena [52]. Following this thought, a number of treatment interventions have been tried to stop the parasympathetic outflow and thus stop the acute attack altogether. Consequently, blockade of sphenopalatine ganglion on the pain side has been shown to be effective in CH prophylaxis in more than 50% of patients, but the recurrence rate is high [53].

In the last years, neuromodulation techniques have enlarged the armamentarium in the treatment of CH.

The efficacy produced by both sphenopalatine ganglion electrical stimulation [54, 55] and chemical inhibition of neurotransmission in the sphenopalatine ganglion by onabotulinum toxin A [56] is further evidence of the relevant role that the parasympathetic pathway has for the generation of a cluster attack [57].

In this respect the observation that CH attacks can occur without autonomic symptoms [58], and the recent finding that triggering autonomic outflow is not sufficient to provoke cluster attacks [59, 60] suggests that isolated parasympathetic activation is not the main cause of trigeminal activation.

6.3.3   Hypothalamic Activation and Stimulation

The term "cluster headache" was introduced to describe the typical seasonal recurring pattern of the disease [61]; in addition the circadian periodicity of pain attacks—more often at night and frequently starting at the same time—strongly suggests that the biological clock has a role in the pathophysiology of the disease [10]. The suprachiasmatic nucleus of the hypothalamus plays an important role in circadian synchronization of many body processes. It receives light stimuli from the retina and entrains the biological clock with the light–dark cycle (Fig. 6.1). The suprachiasmatic nucleus controls melatonin production and secretion whose plasma levels peak during the night with darkness [62]. This peak is markedly blunted in patients with CH [63–65]. This and other neuroendocrinological abnormalities lent support to the hypothesis that the hypothalamic biological clock is deranged in CH [5]. A PET study showed activation in the ipsilateral inferior hypothalamic gray matter during CH attacks [12]; and an increased neuronal density of this structure was identified in a voxel-based morphometry study [13]. Even if hypothalamic activation can occur in other painful conditions [66], the fact that application of a painful stimulus in the receptive field of the first division of the trigeminal nerve is not followed by hypothalamic activation [67] indicates that the observed hypothalamic activation is not a consequence of the pain but has a causative role in the disease. A confirmation of the prominent role of the posterior hypothalamic area in the pathophysiology of CH came from the demonstration that high-frequency deep brain stimulation of that area can improve otherwise intractable chronic CH patients [14].

In animals it has been shown that the posterior hypothalamus is a physiologic modulator of trigeminal nucleus caudalis (TNC) neuronal activity: when injected into the posterior hypothalamus, both orexins (orexin A and B) modulate neuronal activity in the TNC [41], and a disturbance in the hypothalamic orexinergic system has been hypothesized in CH [68]. Posterior hypothalamic orexins can also modulate the duration of neuronal discharge in TNC neurons [41] suggesting that these transmitters are involved in generating the various forms of TACs [68]. A significant reduction of hypocretin (orexin)-1 CSF levels has been found in both episodic and chronic CHs [69] and attributed to a reduced activity of hypothalamic descending antinociceptive pathway, but an alternative theory is that it simply represents a pain-induced phenomenon. The conflicting results of genetic studies do not allow confirming involvement of hypothalamic orexinergic system in CH [28–30]. GABA-A receptors in the posterior hypothalamus are also involved in the modulation of neuronal discharge in the TNC [41]. Involvement of hypothalamic GABA-A receptors in CH is also suggested by the efficacy of both verapamil and topiramate in CH prophylaxis [70] since both drugs inhibit GABA-A receptors in the CNS [71].

Hypothalamic deep brain stimulation takes weeks to months to exert its preventive effect [72, 73] suggesting that a mere inhibition of hypothalamic neurons is a too simplistic hypothesis to explain its mechanism of action. It has been shown that prolonged hypothalamic stimulation increases ipsilateral cold pain threshold in V1 territories [74] indicating that the continuous stimulation could restore the antinociceptive system. The periventricular posterior hypothalamic region [75], very close to that of electrode placement in hypothalamic deep brain stimulation [76], includes the A11 nucleus that contains dopamine cells, dopamine cells colocalized with CGRP, as well as CGRP-only cells [75]. Sensory and pain responses in the trigeminocervical complex (TCC) are strongly inhibited by projection from the A11 nucleus [75]. Hypothalamic stimulation could increase V1 cold pain threshold [74] by activating A11 hypothalamic neurons.

Hypothalamic stimulation could also exert its action by interfering with mechanisms leading to pain chronification. Hypothalamic stimulation induces blood flow changes in some brain areas as anterior cingulate, insula, and frontal lobe [42] involved in pain chronification [77] and long-term potentiation could be the basic mechanism of the changes [78]. An interference of hypothalamic stimulation with pain chronification is indicated by the observations that in some CH patients, long-term hypothalamic stimulation reverted chronic to episodic CH [79]. We note that in patients undergoing hypothalamic continuous stimulation, the parasympathetic system activity is normal [80], and this suggests that the stimulation could improve CH by restoring parasympathetic activity in the superior salivatory nucleus and thus preventing further activation of the trigemino-parasympathetic reflex (Fig. 6.1). It needs to be pointed out that although we start unraveling the enigma of cluster headache attacks and although the scientific consensus now is that CH is a brain disorder and not a vascular or vessel disease, many questions remain. We must understand the pathophysiology completely if we ever want to change the course of the disease and by doing so change the life of our patients to the better.

References

1. Jurgens T, Nielsen T. Leone M, May A, editors. Some observations about the origin of the pain in cluster headache. New York: Springer; 2019.
2. Sprenger T, Schulte L. Leone M, May A, editors. What role for the hypothalamus and diencephalic area. New York: Springer; 2019.
3. Headache Classification Committee of the International Headache Society (HIS). The international classification of headache disorders, 3rd edn (beta version). Cephalalgia. 2013;33:629–808.
4. Ad Hoc Committee on Classification of Headache of the National Institute of Health. Classification of headache. JAMA. 1962;179:717–8.
5. Goadsby PJ. Pathophysiology of cluster headache: a trigeminal autonomic cephalalgia. Lancet Neurol. 2002;1:251–7.
6. Goadsby PJ, Lipton RB. A review of paroxysmal hemicranias, SUNCT syndrome and other shortlasting headaches with autonomic feature, including new cases. Brain. 1997;120:193–209.
7. Leone M, Bussone G. Pathophysiology of trigeminal autonomic cephalalgias. Lancet Neurol. 2009;8:755–64.
8. Hoffmann J, May A. Diagnosis, pathophysiology, and management of cluster headache. Lancet Neurol. 2018;17:75–83.
9. Sjaastad O. Cluster headache syndrome. In: Sjaastad O, editor. Major problems in neurology, volume 23. London, UK: WB Saunders Company Ltd, 1992. Kudrow L. Cluster headache, mechanism and management. 1st ed. New York: Oxford University Press; 1980.
10. Kudrow L. Cluster headache, mechanism and management. 1st ed. New York, NY: Oxford University Press; 1980.
11. Leone M, Bussone G. A review of hormonal findings in cluster headache. Evidence for hypothalamic involvement. Cephalalgia. 1993;13:309–17.
12. May A, Bahra A, Büchel C, Frackowiak RS, Goadsby PJ. Hypothalamic activation in cluster headache attacks. Lancet. 1998;352:275–8.

13. May A, Ashburner J, Büchel C, et al. Correlation between structural and functional changes in brain in an idiopathic headache syndrome. Nat Med. 1999;5:836–8.
14. Leone M, Franzini A, Bussone G. Stereotactic stimulation of posterior hypothalamic gray matter for intractable cluster headache. N Engl J Med. 2001;345(19):1428–9.
15. Leone M, Franzini A, D'Andrea G, Broggi G, Casucci G, Bussone G. Deep brain stimulation to relieve severe drug-resistant SUNCT. Ann Neurol. 2005;57:924–7.
16. Lyons MK, Dodick DW, Evidente VG. Responsiveness of short-lasting unilateral neuralgiform headache with conjunctival injection and tearing to hypothalamic deep brain stimulation. J Neurosurg. 2008;26:1–3.
17. Bartsch T, Falk D, Knudsen K, Reese R, Raethjen J, Mehdorn HM, et al. Deep brain stimulation of the posterior hypothalamic area in intractable short-lasting unilateral neuralgiform headache with conjunctival injection and tearing (SUNCT). Cephalalgia. 2011;31:1405–8.
18. Miller S, Akram H, Lagrata S, Hariz M, Zrinzo L, Matharu M. Ventral tegmental area deep brain stimulation in refractory short-lasting unilateral neuralgiform headache attacks. Brain. 2016;139:2631–40.
19. Walcott BP, Bamber NI, Anderson DE. Successful treatment of chronic paroxysmal hemicranias with posterior hypothalamic stimulation: technical case report. Neurosurgery. 2009;65:E997.
20. van den Maagdenberg AMJM, Ducros A. Genetics of cluster headache and other trigeminal autonomic cephalalgias. In: Leone M, May A, editors. Cluster headache and other trigeminal autonomic cephalalgias. New York: Springer; 2019.
21. Sjaastad O, Shen JM, Stovner LJ, Elsås T. Cluster headache in identical twins. Headache. 1993;33:214–7.
22. Russell MB, Andersson PG. Clinical intra- and interfamilial variability of cluster headache. Eur J Neurol. 1995;1:253–7.
23. Kudrow L, Kudrow DB. Inheritance of cluster headache and its possible link to migraine. Headache. 1994;34:400–7.
24. Leone M, Russell MB, Rigamonti A, et al. Increased familial risk of cluster headache. Neurology. 2001;56:1233–6.
25. Russell MB, Andersson PG, Thomsen LL. Familial occurrence of cluster headache. J Neurol Neurosurg Psychiatry. 1995;58:341–3.
26. El Amrani M, Ducros A, Boulan P, et al. Familial cluster headache: a series of 186 index patients. Headache. 2002;42:974–7.
27. Haan J, van Vliet JA, Kors EE, et al. No involvement of the calcium channel gene (CACNA1A) in a family with cluster headache. Cephalalgia. 2001;21:959–62.
28. Rainero I, Gallone S, Valfrè W, et al. A polymorphism of the hypocretin receptor 2 gene is associated with cluster headache. Neurology. 2004;63:1286–8.
29. Baumber L, Sjöstrand C, Leone M, Harty H, Bussone G, Hillert J, Trembath R, Russell MB. A genome-wide scan and hcrtr2 candidate gene analysis in a European cluster headache cohort. Neurology. 2006;66:1888–93.
30. Weller CM, Wilbrink LA, Houwing-Duistermaat JJ, et al. Cluster headache and the hypocretin receptor 2 reconsidered: a genetic association study and meta-analysis. Cephalalgia. 2015;35:741–7.
31. Eising E, Pelzer N, Vijfhuizen LS, et al. Identifying a gene expression signature of cluster headache in blood. Sci Rep. 2017;7:40218.
32. Ofte HK, Tronvik E, Alstadhaug KB. Lack of association between cluster headache and PER3 clock gene polymorphism. J Headache Pain. 2016;17:18.
33. Costa M, Squassina A, Piras IS, et al. Preliminary transcriptome analysis in lymphoblasts from cluster headache and bipolar disorder patients implicates dysregulation of circadian and serotonergic genes. J Mol Neurosci. 2015;56:688–95.
34. Tuka B, Szabó N, Tóth E, et al. Release of PACAP-38 in episodic cluster headache patients—an exploratory study. J Headache Pain. 2016;17:69.
35. Bacchelli E, Cainazzo MM, Cameli C, et al. A genome-wide analysis in cluster headache points to neprilysin and PACAP receptor gene variant. J Headache Pain. 2016;17:114.

36. Ran C, Fourier C, Michalska JM, et al. Screening of genetic variants in ADCYAP1R1, MME and 14q21 in a Swedish cluster headache cohort. J Headache Pain. 2017;18:88.
37. Goadsby PJ, Edvinsson L. Human in vivo evidence for trigeminovascular activation in cluster headache. Neuropeptide changes and effects of acute attacks therapies. Brain. 1994;117:427–34.
38. Goldberg S, Silberstein SD. Targeting CGRP: a new era for migraine treatment. CNS Drugs. 2015;29(6):443–52.
39. Storer RJ, Akerman S, Goadsby PJ. Calcitonin gene-related peptide (CGRP) modulates nociceptive trigeminovascular transmission in the cat. Br J Pharmacol. 2004;142:1171–81.
40. May A, Goadsby PJ. The trigeminovascular system in humans: pathophysiologic implications for primary headache syndromes of the neural influences on the cerebral circulation. J Cereb Blood Flow Metab. 1999;19:115–27.
41. Bartsch T, Levy MJ, Knight YE, Goadsby PJ. Differential modulation of nociceptive dural input to [hypocretin] orexin A and B receptor activation in the posterior hypothalamic area. Pain. 2004;109:367–78.
42. May A, Leone M, Boecker H, et al. Hypothalamic deep brain stimulation in positron emission tomography. J Neurosci. 2006;26(13):3589–93.
43. Jarrar RG, Black DF, Dodick DW, Davis DH. Outcome of trigeminal nerve section in the treatment of chronic cluster headache. Neurology. 2003;60:1360–2.
44. Matharu MS, Goadsby PJ. Persistence of attacks of cluster headache after trigeminal nerve root section. Brain. 2002;125:976–84.
45. Leone M, Franzini A, Broggi G, May A, Bussone G. Long-term follow up of bilateral hypothalamic stimulation for intractable cluster headache. Brain. 2004;127:2259–64.
46. Spencer SE, Sawyer WB, Wada H, Platt KB, Loewy AD. CNS projections to the pterygopalatine parasympathetic preganglionic neurons in the rat: a retrograde transneuronal viral cell body labeling study. Brain Res. 1990;534:149–69.
47. Goadsby PJ. Autonomic nervous system control of the cerebral circulation. In: Buijis RM, Swaab DF, editors. Handbook of clinical neurology. Amsterdam: Elsevier; 2013. p. 193–201.
48. Goadsby PJ, Lambert GA, Lance JW. The peripheral pathway for extracranial vasodilation in the cat. J Auton Nerv Syst. 1984;10:145–55.
49. May A, Büchel C, Turner R, Goadsby PJ. Magnetic resonance angiography in facial and other pain: neurovascular mechanisms of trigeminal sensation. J Cereb Blood Flow Metab. 2001;21:1171–6.
50. Goadsby PJ, Macdonald GJ. Extracranial vasodilation mediated by vasoactive intestinal polypeptide (VIP). Brain Res. 1985;329:285–8.
51. Hoffmann J, Martins-Oliveira M, Akerman S, Supronsinchai W, Xu C, Goadsby PJ. PAC-1 receptor antibody modulates nociceptive trigeminal activity in rat. Cephalalgia. 2016;36(Suppl 1):141.
52. Leone M, Rigamonti A, Bussone G. Cluster headache sine headache: two new cases in one family. Cephalalgia. 2002;22:12–4.
53. Pipolo C, Bussone G, Leone M, Lozza P, Felisati G. Sphenopalatine endoscopic ganglion block in cluster headache: a reevaluation of the procedure after 5 years. Neurol Sci. 2010;31(Suppl 1):S197–9.
54. Schoenen J, Jensen RH, Lantéri-Minet M, et al. Stimulation of the sphenopalatine ganglion (SPG) for cluster headache treatment. Pathway CH-1: a randomized, sham-controlled study. Cephalalgia. 2013;33:816–30.
55. Barloese MCJ, Jürgens TP, May A, et al. Cluster headache attack remission with sphenopalatine ganglion stimulation: experiences in chronic cluster headache patients through 24 months. J Headache Pain. 2016;17:67.
56. Bratbak DF, Nordgård S, Stovner LJ, et al. Pilot study of sphenopalatine injection of onabotulinumtoxin A for the treatment of intractable chronic cluster headache. Cephalalgia. 2016;36:503–9.
57. Schytz HW, Barløse N, Guo S, et al. Experimental activation of the sphenopalatine ganglion provokes cluster-like attacks in humans. Cephalalgia. 2013;33:831–41.

58. Martins IP, Gouveia RG, Antunes JL. Double dissociation between autonomic symptoms and pain in cluster headache. Cephalalgia. 2005;25:398–400.
59. Möller M, Haji AA, Hoffmann J, May A. Peripheral provocation of cranial autonomic symptoms is not sufficient to trigger cluster headache attacks. Cephalalgia. 2018;38(8):1498–502. https://doi.org/10.1177/0333102417738248.
60. Guo S, Petersen AS, Schytz HW, Barløse M, Caparso A, Fahrenkrug J, Jensen RH, Ashina M. Cranial parasympathetic activation induces autonomic symptoms but no cluster headache attacks. Cephalalgia. 2018;38(8):1418–28. https://doi.org/10.1177/0333102417738250.
61. Kunkle EC, Pfeifer JB Jr, Wilhoit WM, Hamrick LW Jr. Recurrent brief headache in cluster pattern. N C Med J. 1954;15(10):510–2.
62. Pévet P. Melatonin receptors as therapeutic targets in the suprachiasmatic nucleus. Expert Opin Ther Targets. 2016;20(10):1209–18.
63. Chazot G, Claustrat B, Brun J, Jordan D, Sassolas G, Schott B. A chronobiological study of melatonin, cortisol growth hormone and prolactin secretion in cluster headache. Cephalalgia. 1984;4:213–20.
64. Waldenlind E, Waldenlind GE, Gustafsson SA, Ekbom K, Wetterberg L. Circadian secretion of cortisol and melatonin in cluster headache during active cluster periods and remission. J Neurol Neurosurg Psychiatry. 1987;50:207–13.
65. Leone M, Lucini V, D'Amico D, Grazzi L, Moschiano F, Fraschini F, Bussone G. Abnormal 24-hour urinary excretory pattern of 6-sulphatoxymelatonin in both phases of cluster headache. Cephalalgia. 1998;18:664–7.
66. Schulte LH, May A. The migraine generator revisited: continuous scanning of the migraine cycle over 30 days and three spontaneous attacks. Brain J Neurol. 2016;139:1987–93.
67. May A, Kaube H, Büchel C, et al. Experimental cranial pain elicited by capsaicin: a PET study. Pain. 1998;74:61–6.
68. Holland P, Goadsby PJ. The hypothalamic orexinergic system: pain and primary headaches. Headache. 2007;47(6):951–62.
69. Barloese M, Jennum P, Lund N, Knudsen S, Gammeltoft S, Jensen R. Reduced CSF hypocretin-1 levels are associated with cluster headache. Cephalalgia. 2015;35(10):869–76.
70. May A, Leone M, Áfra J, et al. EFNS guideline on the treatment of cluster headache and other trigemino-autonomic cephalalgias. Eur J Neurol. 2006;13:1066–77.
71. Das P, Bell-Horner CL, Huang RQ, et al. Inhibition of type A GABA receptors by l-type calcium channel blockers. Neuroscience. 2004;124:195–206.
72. Leone M, Proietti Cecchini A. Deep brain stimulation in headache. Cephalalgia. 2016;36(12):1143–8.
73. Akram H, Miller S, Lagrata S, Hyam J, Jahanshahi M, Hariz M, Matharu M, Zrinzo L. Ventral tegmental area deep brain stimulation for refractory chronic cluster headache. Neurology. 2016;86(18):1676–82.
74. Jürgens T, Leone M, Proietti-Cecchini A, et al. Hypothalamic deep-brain stimulation modulates thermal sensitivity and pain thresholds in cluster headache. Pain. 2009;146(1–2):84–90.
75. Charbit AR, Akerman S, Holland PR, Goadsby PJ. Neurons of the dopaminergic/calcitonin gene-related peptide A11 cell group modulate neuronal firing in the trigeminocervical complex: an electrophysiological and immunohistochemical study. J Neurosci. 2009;29(40):12532–41.
76. Fontaine D, Lanteri-Minet M, Ouchchane L, et al. Anatomical location of effective deep brain stimulation electrodes in chronic cluster headache. Brain. 2010;133(Pt 4):1214–23.
77. Zhuo M. Cortical excitation and chronic pain. Trends Neurosci. 2008;31:199–207.
78. May A. Chronic pain may change the structure of the brain. Pain. 2008;137:7–15.
79. Leone M, Franzini A, Proietti Cecchini A, Bussone G. Success, failure and putative mechanisms in hypothalamic stimulation for drug resistant chronic cluster headache. Pain. 2013;154(1):89–94.
80. Cortelli P, Guaraldi P, Leone M, et al. Effect of deep brain stimulation of the posterior hypothalamic area on the cardiovascular system in chronic cluster headache patients. Eur J Neurol. 2007;14:1008–15.

Chapter 7
Neuroimaging in Cluster Headache and Trigeminal Autonomic Cephalalgias

Laura H. Schulte and Stefania Ferraro

7.1 Introduction

Within the last 20 years, the tremendous progress of neuroimaging techniques has provided an unprecedented impact on the comprehension of pathological processes at the basis of several neurological conditions.

Cluster headache has greatly benefitted from these technical and theoretical advancements: neuroimaging indeed shifted the core understanding of this neuro-pathological condition from neurovascular mechanisms to dysfunctions of the central nervous system. Here, we present a comprehensive review of the neuroimaging studies that have revolutionized the comprehension of this neuropathology.

7.2 Structural Imaging

7.2.1 Voxel-Based Morphometry

Voxel-based morphometry (VBM) is a widely used method based on high-resolution MRI images, which aims at identifying focal morphometric changes in grey and white matter volume. Simply speaking, VBM is a comparison of grey and white

L. H. Schulte
Department of Systems Neuroscience and Clinic of Psychiatry, University Medical Center Eppendorf, Hamburg, Germany
e-mail: la.schulte@uke.de

S. Ferraro (✉)
Fondazione IRCCS Istituto Neurologico Carlo Besta, Milan, Italy
e-mail: stefania.ferraro@istituto-besta.it

© Springer Nature Switzerland AG 2020
M. Leone, A. May (eds.), *Cluster Headache and other Trigeminal Autonomic Cephalgias*, Headache, https://doi.org/10.1007/978-3-030-12438-0_7

matter concentrations between two groups of subjects [1]. To function well, high-resolution images of the single subjects have to be realigned and warped to ensure congruity of brain regions between subjects. VBM is further based on voxel-based image segmentation into grey and white matter images taking into account intrinsic intensity information of the single volumes as well as a priori information and is thus strongly depending on grey and white matter contrast of the respective images. Consequently, VBM is an apt method for cerebral structures, while performance on the level of the cerebellum and brainstem is poor. Furthermore, VBM is susceptible to a lot of confounders, such as poor image realignment or misclassification of tissue types [2]. Although grey matter changes found using VBM are usually interpreted as a local increase or decrease in grey matter volume and thus as a marker of neuronal density and plasticity, it is in fact not clear what is really the structural correlate to the so-called VBM grey matter changes. Nonetheless, VBM is until today widely used in pain and headache research.

VBM has a long history in cluster headache: it was in fact the first method ever to be used to depict changes in brain structure in cluster headache patients [3] and has since been used in multiple consecutive studies. Back in 1999, May and colleagues were able to correlate functional changes observed within the posterior hypothalamic area in acute cluster headache attacks with bilateral grey matter changes in the same area [3] in cluster headache patients both within and outside the bout. This very important early study in the field of VBM had—taken together with the functional imaging results—high therapeutic impact: in the following years, over 50 otherwise intractable cluster headache patients were treated successfully with deep brain stimulation of the posterior hypothalamic area [4–7]. This study was over the next nearly 20 years followed by various other studies: Matharu et al. conducted a VBM study of 66 episodic cluster headache patients and 96 healthy controls but did not find any structural alterations between cluster headache patients and control participants despite the fact that they used a predefined hypothalamic region of interest for statistical small volume correction. Findings of the more recent studies present a multifaceted image of structural changes in cluster headache: the most common finding is grey matter volume changes in areas unspecifically involved in pain processing and modulation of aversive stimuli, among these the thalamus, insular and cingulate cortex, cerebellum, temporal lobe, hippocampus, and frontal cortex [8–10]. Naegel et al. showed these changes to be dynamic and depending on the disease and pain state regarding their direction, location, and extent [8].

None of the studies were able to replicate the posterior hypothalamic volume changes. One possible reason could be the differences in the software used for analysis: SPM (http://www.fil.ion.ucl.ac.uk/spm) as well as the VBM toolbox for SPM have been gradually updated with huge impact on the normalization and segmentation procedures which crucially influence results in a relatively small area as the hypothalamus. However, very recently, Arkink et al. found increased grey matter values in the anterior part of the hypothalamus in chronic cluster headache patients as compared to healthy controls [11]. This VBM analysis was amended by a volume comparison of the manually segmented anterior hypothalamus leading to the finding of increased anterior hypothalamic volume in chronic as well as episodic cluster headache. Taken together, very early and very recent VBM analyses suggest some structural alterations within the hypothalamus in cluster headache patients, whereas other VBM studies in cluster headache found more unspecific changes in general pain processing areas.

7.2.2 Diffusion Tensor Imaging

The evolution of the magnetic resonance imaging (MRI) techniques has provided an extraordinary tool to characterize the microstructural organization of biological tissue in vivo: diffusion tensor imaging (DTI) [12]. DTI maps the magnitude and directionality of the water molecules diffusion by means of the diffusion tensor model. There are four major parameters that can be computed from the diffusion tensor in each voxel: mean diffusivity (MD), fractional anisotropy (FA), radial diffusivity (RD), and axial diffusivity (AD). Based on these parameters, it is possible to detect microstructural alterations of the white matter and to understand whether the investigated structures present de-myelination or dys-myelination, although some doubts still persist about the exact interpretation of these measures [13, 14]. Remarkably, the principal direction of the diffusion tensor can be used to perform tractography, a technique that allows revealing the anatomical connectivity of the brain [15].

Despite the putative importance of the study of white matter microstructural alterations in the cluster headache pathophysiology, these investigations are few and, due to the puzzling results, not conclusive. In particular, in one of the first DTI studies, Absinta et al. [9], using a 3T MRI scanner, published a convincing evidence of the absence of white matter alterations in a convenient sample of episodic cluster headache patients during the "out-of-bout" condition. However, subsequent investigations, all conducted with a 1.5T MRI scanner and mainly in small samples of patients, showed the widespread presence of microstructural alterations of the white matter in episodic cluster headache. The first study [16] of these series showed significant FA changes in frontal and subcortical areas (amygdala, hippocampus, thalamus, and basal ganglia) and in the brainstem in a small sample of episodic cluster headache individuals, mainly in "out-of-bout" condition. The authors speculated that these white matter microstructural alterations indicated pain processing abnormalities, suggesting a possible key role in the cluster headache pathophysiology of the alterations of the descending pain inhibitory pathways. Remarkably, they interpreted the alterations observed in the brainstem as abnormalities of the medial lemniscus and of the nucleus tractus trigemini, involved in the modulations of the trigemino-sensory pathways. Interestingly, the alterations observed in the upper brainstem were linked to lesions of the sympathetic pathway. Altogether these results support the well-recognized involvement of the sympathetic and trigeminal systems in the cluster headache pathophysiology, but also a role of the pain processing pathways, suggested in several neuroimaging studies [17–19].

Along the same lines, the work of Szabó et al. [20] reported widespread alterations of the white matter across all the brain areas (i.e., in the frontal, parietal, temporal and occipital lobes) in patients with episodic cluster headache. More recently, Király et al. [21] investigated white matter microstructural alterations of the subcortical structures in two different groups of patients with left or right episodic cluster headache. Interestingly, the data from these patients were not merged in a unique sample, due to the observed differences in diffusivity parameters between the left and right hemisphere. In line with the hypothesis of the involvement of the subcortical structures in pain processing, they found evidence of microstructural alterations in the right amygdala, caudate, and pallidum. Chou et al. [22] showed white matter alterations in a group of episodic cluster headache patients during "in-bout" and "out-of-bout" periods. Using tract-based spatial statistic (TBSS), they found microstructural alterations in frontal (medial prefrontal gyrus, in subgyral area of the frontal lobe), limbic (hippocampus/amygdala, insula), and cerebellar areas. These areas play an important role in the processing of the cognitive and affective dimensions of the painful experience; clearly, this result provides further support for the mass of neuroimaging data showing structural and functional alterations in the regions involved in pain processing [3, 16, 23, 24]. Notably, the observed alterations were present in both "in-bout" and "out-of-bout" conditions, suggesting possible stable white matter abnormalities. Very remarkably, the authors observed direct anatomical connections between these altered white matter areas and the ipsilateral hypothalamus. This important result shows, again, a key role of the hypothalamus in the cluster headache pathophysiology. In the light of the negative findings of the work of Absinta et al. [9] conducted with a 3T MRI scanner in a relatively large sample of patients and the different results obtained by other studies conducted with a 1.5T MRI scanner [20–22, 25], future investigations are needed to identify global microstructural white matter alterations in the cluster headache pathophysiology.

Remarkably, some studies were dedicated to the investigations of the anatomical circuits at the basis of successful hypothalamic deep brain stimulation (DBS). Although DBS of the hypothalamic region is successful in the treatment of more than 60% of patients implanted for drug-refractory cluster headache [26], the stimulated anatomical and functional networks at the basis of this efficacy are not well understood. To identify the cerebral networks associated with the DBS targets in chronic cluster headache, Clelland et al. [27] used DTI. Two important results were observed: (1) the tips of the electrodes for DBS were located in the midbrain tegmentum, near the third ventricle, and posterior to the hypothalamus, as previously suggested [28, 29]; (2) the DBS targets project to three main regions: the ipsilateral hypothalamus, reticular formation, and cerebellum. The observed anatomical projections from the DBS target to the ipsilateral hypothalamus are an important proof of concept that links the neuroimaging data, showing the activity in midbrain [30] and hypothalamic regions [24] during the attacks, with clinical, neuroendocrinological, and animal findings providing converging evidence of the hypothalamic involvement in cluster headache pathophysiology [26, 31]. Importantly, a direct pathway between the hypothalamus and cerebellum was evidenced in a previous DTI study [32]; this fits well with the observed abnormal functional connectivity between the hypothalamus and cerebellum [33, 34], and with the observation that the cerebellum and the hypothalamus/midbrain tegmentum are activated during the attacks [24, 30]. The cerebellum was suggested to be part of the pain processing network playing an important role in the nociceptive modulation [35]. Remarkably, the observed data are very consistent with studies evidencing projections from the DBS electrode target to the cerebellum and the reticular nucleus [36, 37].

7.3 Functional Imaging

7.3.1 Single-Photon Emission Tomography and Positron Emission Tomography

In functional neuroimaging, fluorodeoxyglucose-positron emission tomography (FDG-PET) is often used to measure brain metabolism. By using methods of statistical parametric mapping, groups of subjects can be compared regarding the distribution of areas with heightened glucose metabolism. Areas with such a heightened metabolism are usually interpreted as being activated in the respective group or under a respective condition. It is thus possible to identify and localize brain activations typical for a certain group of patients or for a certain condition within one group of patients (e.g., cluster headache patients inside of an attack). While FDG-PET is a widely used method in neuroimaging as an unspecific marker of brain activity, there are a lot of specific ligand-PET variants, in which radioactively marked ligands are used to measure, e.g., receptor density within certain parts of the brain [38]. Single-photon emission tomography (SPECT) on the other hand is a method that in scientific neuroimaging in the headache field has become gradually less influential. Reasons might include the poor spatial resolution and the fact that it has never really been used in voxel-based analyses in the headache field [39].

There are currently only a few SPECT studies in cluster headache available, all of which have been conducted prior to the broad establishment of voxel-based analyses. Results are mostly contradictory: whereas some studies did not find any differences in mean cerebral blood flow (CBF) when comparing the acute attack state with the state outside of attacks [40–42], other studies have found a heterogeneous pattern (increases in some patients and decreases or no changes in others during acute cluster headache attacks) [43, 44] or an increased CBF during acute attacks [45]. There is only one SPECT study to date that has not focused on overall CBF changes during attacks but has used a case-control design to compare "out-of-bout" cluster headache patients with healthy controls [46]. CBF was lower in the contralateral primary somatosensory cortex and motor cortex as well as in the thalamus. All in all, while providing some early attempts on capturing brain activity changes in cluster headache, SPECT studies have as yet not provided much insight into cluster headache pathophysiology.

Regarding other trigeminal autonomic cephalalgias, evidence from SPECT imaging is limited to two case reports: In paroxysmal hemicrania, hypoperfusion was detected bilaterally in the frontoparietal region between attacks with complete normalization of rCBF within attacks [47], whereas in two SUNCT patients, perfusion was normal during attacks [48].

Positron emission tomography (PET) on the other hand is a still widely used functional imaging method that had its main significance in the early functional studies in cluster headache. The possibility of performing voxel-based analyses in combination with PET allowed for a distinct attribution of changes in cerebral blood flow to certain areas of the brain and brainstem. Back in 1996, Hsieh et al. investigated a group of four episodic cluster headache patients during induced attacks and found increased regional cerebral blood flow in various pain processing areas such as the anterior cingulate cortex, insular region, and operculum, indicating the expected but unspecific involvement of those areas in cluster headache pain processing [49]. These brain regions however are widely involved in pain processing and not specific for cluster headache. Judging from the clinical appearance with a clear circadian and circannual rhythmicity of attacks and bouts as well as a clear autonomic involvement, the hypothalamus has long been hypothesized to be crucially involved in the pathophysiology of cluster headache. Activation within this region was thus the first finding to be seen as specific for cluster headache attacks in a PET study of nine episodic cluster headache patients during nitroglycerin-triggered attacks: a small area close to the posterior hypothalamic grey matter was strongly activated during these attacks than outside of attacks [30]. This activation was present neither in mild headaches following nitroglycerin administration nor in experimentally induced pain. This led to the conclusion of this activation being indeed not solely an epiphenomenon of severe pain during cluster attacks but really cluster attack specific—a finding of tremendous importance as it was the first with a specific link to cluster headache pathophysiology. Other PET studies have been able to replicate this finding in a spontaneous acute cluster attack in one chronic cluster patient [50] and also provided evidence for reduced availability of opioidergic receptors within the hypothalamic area depending on the disease duration: the longer the disease duration, the less receptor binding was observed [38]. Additionally, hypermetabolism in many cortical and subcortical pain processing areas could be observed in cluster headache patients during "in-bout" periods but between attacks when compared to "out-of-bout" periods [51]. Interestingly, when comparing all cluster headache patients regardless of the bout status with all healthy controls, many of these areas showed hypometabolism. This undermines the hypothesis that chronic pain conditions may functionally affect pain processing areas with the cluster-specific alterations of functional increases during "in-bout" periods. PET in combination with voxel-based analyses has thus contributed essentially to our current understanding of cluster headaches and has even paved the way for specific new treatment options: stimulation of the posterior hypothalamic grey area is a treatment option in otherwise intractable cluster headache, which makes this a great example of translational medicine.

Another advantage of PET as an imaging method as compared to functional MRI is that it operates without a strong magnetic field while providing a reasonable spatial resolution, which makes it an apt tool to investigate effects and treatment mechanisms of neurostimulation therapies: this has to date been done for occipital nerve stimulation in drug-resistant chronic cluster headache [52]. After 6–30 months of stimulation, hypermetabolism within several areas of the pain matrix including the anterior cingulate cortex, the midbrain, and pons normalized, while there was still heightened activity within the hypothalamus. This might suggest a symptomatic rather than a curing effect of occipital nerve stimulation in cluster headache. To date, there are no further PET studies on neurostimulation devices in cluster headache, although this method might be ideal to study the effects of the relatively new and effective sphenopalatine ganglion stimulation.

Regarding other trigeminal autonomic cephalalgias, similar activations of the posterior hypothalamus could be demonstrated. During the acute untreated stage of paroxysmal hemicrania, there was stronger activation of the posterior hypothalamus and midbrain contralaterally to the pain site. A similar pattern could be observed for hemicrania continua with significant activation of the posterior hypothalamic grey area and the dorsal rostral pons [53]. Noteworthy, while posterior hypothalamic activation in cluster headache usually occurred ipsilaterally to the pain site, in paroxysmal hemicrania and hemicrania continua it was detected on the contralateral site.

7.3.2 Resting State Functional Magnetic Resonance Imaging

During the resting state (RS) condition, a poorly defined state in which an individual is not actively engaged in cognitive or sensory-motor tasks, the brain shows an extraordinary highly structured intrinsic dynamic activity. fMRI during RS is able to capture the low-frequency (<0.1 Hz) large-scale spatial patterns of this ongoing activity, mapping the spontaneous blood oxygen level-dependent signal covariations in the temporal domain between distant brain regions [54, 55]. The first report that RS-fMRI signal fluctuations are highly structured dates back to 1995 with the seminal work of Biswal and colleagues [54]. In this study, the authors showed that low-frequency RS-fMRI signal fluctuations in the sensory-motor regions present a high degree of correlation in the time domain. The authors argued that this temporal coherence observed between distant areas was an epiphenomenon of the functional connectivity between brain areas. Subsequent studies confirmed that several different cortical and subcortical networks present high temporal coherence of RS-fMRI signal fluctuations. This pattern of correlated activity, defined as "functional connectivity" [54, 56], seems to have its underpinning in the anatomical connectivity of the brain [57–60]: strong evidence came from studies on corpus callosum agenesis [61], and callosotomy [62, 63], neuropathological conditions that abolish, particularly in the acute state, the interhemispheric functional connectivity. However, a seminal study investigating both the functional connectivity (using RS-fMRI) and the anatomical connectivity (using diffusion tensor imaging) showed that the functional connectivity is not completely explained by the structural connectivity; indeed functional connectivity also exists between distant brain regions with no direct anatomical pathways [56]. Based on the observation that every single functional network comprises regions that are typically co-activated during the execution of a cognitive task, it was hypothesized that the task-related activity is mirrored in this intrinsic and dynamic spontaneous process [64]. At the moment, we have no clear explanations for this pervasive phenomenon [64]; however, it was speculated that this low-frequency ongoing activity might organize and coordinate neuronal activity [65] or, in a Bayesian perspective, that it may represent a dynamic prediction of the brain regions that will be involved together in the execution of tasks [66].

7.3.2.1 The Main Resting State Functional Magnetic Resonance Imaging Networks

The analyses of the spatiotemporal coherence of low-frequency fluctuations during RS-fMRI acquisitions reveal several functional networks characterized by distinct temporal coherence features [67]. These functional networks are supposed to underlie cognitive, motor, and sensory processing [68–70] and are detected mainly by means of independent component analyses (ICA) [71, 72], the seed-based approach, and the hierarchical clustering [73]. The most investigated functional circuit is the default mode network: the seminal fMRI work of Greicius et al. [74] showed that the medial prefrontal cortex, the posterior cingulate/precuneus, and the lateral parietal cortex form a very robust functional network, which increases its activity during rest and decreases its activity during the execution of tasks. This particular pattern of activity led to hypothesize that the brain presents a baseline functional state [75] whose activity is suppressed or reduced when the subject is engaged in the goal-directed behavior, although there are still some debates [76]. Beyond the default mode network, other very consistent neural functional networks, each one characterized by specific BOLD signal time-courses [71, 77], were identified. These networks comprise primary sensory networks, such as the visual [71, 78]; auditory [55] and the sensorimotor network [67]; and networks mediating several other cognitive functions, such as the temporoparietal network, the executive control network, and the salience network, particularly important in the cluster headache pathophysiology. In addition, hippocampus [79], thalamus [80], cerebellum [81], basal ganglia [81], and hypothalamic [82] networks were also identified.

7.3.3   The Main RS-fMRI Networks in Cluster Headache

A summary of the studies investigating functional connectivity with RS-fMRI in cluster headache pathophysiology is presented in Table 7.1.

In the past, the investigations of neurological disorders have greatly benefited from localization-based approaches; however, the relatively recent advances in acquisition techniques, in data analyses, and in the theoretical frameworks opened new venues for the investigation of the brain activity more focused on the complexity and interactions between cerebral regions. Along these lines, RS-fMRI, investigating large-scale brain networks in the low-frequency domain, offered new and successful perspectives in various neurological and psychiatric diseases, such as

Table 7.1 Summary of the studies investigating cerebral functional connectivity in cluster headache pathophysiology using resting state functional magnetic resonance imaging (RS-fMRI) with independent component analyses (ICA)

Resting state—independent component analyses

Authors	Participants	Identified networks	Between-groups differences	Other analyses
Rocca et al. [17]	13 episodic CH "out-of-bout" patients (8 with right-sided, 5 with left-sided attacks)	1. Visual networks 2. Auditory network 3. Sensorimotor network 4. Frontoparietal-temporal areas 5. Frontoparietal areas L & R 6. Default mode network	*CH vs. CTRL:* 1. Sensorimotor network: decreased RS-FC in primary sensorimotor cortex, supplementary motor area, and anterior cingulate cortex 2. Primary visual network: decreased RS-FC in V1	Inverse correlations between RS-FC and disease duration in: 1. Sensorimotor network (in left primary sensory-motor cortex) 2. Primary visual network (in left V1)
Faragò et al. [33]	17 episodic CH "out-of-bout" patients (with right-sided attacks after flipping MRI images)	1. Visual networks 2. Auditory network 3. Sensorimotor network 4. Salience network 5. Ipsilateral and contralateral attentional network 6. Default mode network 7. Cerebellar networks	*CH vs. CTRL:* 1. Ipsilateral attentional network: increased RS-FC in superior frontal gyrus and middle frontal gyrus 2. Increased RS-FC in ipsilateral/ contralateral cerebellar network	Inverse correlations between RS-FC and cumulative headache days in controlateral attentional network (in frontal pole)
Chou et al. [27]	17 episodic CH "in-bout" and "out-of-bout" (with right-sided attacks after flipping MRI images)	1. Visual networks 2. Sensorimotor network 3. Default mode network 4. Salience network 5. Frontal attentional network 6. Dorsal attentional network 7. Parietal, cerebellar, temporal, and subcortical networks	*CH vs. CTRL:* RS-FC differences in several networks, in particular in DMN (in left precuneus) and in the salience network (L and R and L insula); *CH "in-bout" vs. CH "out-of-bout":* RS-FC differences in frontal network (R inferior frontal gyrus) and L attentional network (L postcentral gyrus)	Inverse correlations between RS-FC and disease duration in the frontal attentional network (R cingulate gyrus) during "in-bout" condition

CH cluster headache patients, *CTRL* control group, *RS-FC* resting state functional connectivity, *L* left, *R* right

Alzheimer's disease, depression, and schizophrenia [83–88]. More importantly, alterations in the low-frequency coherence of specific networks were showed to have diagnostic and prognostic value for specific neurological diseases [89, 90]. This suggests that the more consistent RS-fMRI networks, such as the default mode network, might be sensitive biomarkers of the pathological dynamic organization of the brain.

What is the role of the investigations of the functional connectivity of the RS-fMRI networks in revealing the neuropathological bases of the cluster headache?

Cluster headache is characterized by extremely severe unilateral head pain and ipsilateral cranial-facial autonomic symptoms [91]. Clinical, neuroendocrinological, and animal findings [26, 31] together with the already mentioned neuroimaging studies of May et al. [30, 92] strongly suggest the ipsilateral (to the head side of attack) posterior hypothalamus as the generator of cluster headache attacks. These findings led to the pioneering successful treatment of refractory chronic cluster headache with hypothalamic deep brain stimulation (DBS) [93]. As the electrode tip is in fact usually located posterior to the hypothalamus in the diencephalon–mesencephalic junction, where it possibly stimulates several fasciculi and regions [94] and DBS is also successful when stimulating the ventral tegmental area [95] and the posterior wall of the third ventricle [96], the hypothalamus could have a modulatory role on some functional networks, possibly comprising the hypothalamo-trigeminal pathway [26, 97], pointing clearly to the possible presence of a dysfunctional network, normalized or modulated by DBS [26].

In line with this very important hypothesis, the study of RS-fMRI functional connectivity is very promising in the investigation of the neuropathological bases of the cluster headache condition. In this framework, since 2010, neuroimaging studies have begun to shed lights on the presence of several abnormal functional networks in the cluster headache condition: in particular, the hypothalamic network, the salience network, and the default mode network might play a key role in the cluster headache pathophysiology.

7.3.3.1 The Salience Network

The salience network is one of the most interesting functional RS-fMRI circuits in regard to cluster headache pathophysiology. The seminal work of Seeley et al. [98] showed that the areas typically involved during the execution of a variety of demanding fMRI tasks and comprising the dorsal anterior cingulate cortex, the frontoinsular cortex, the dorsolateral prefrontal cortex, and the lateral parietal cortex are dissociable into two functional circuits when appreciated with RS-fMRI: the salience network and the executive control network. The key nodes of the salience network comprise the dorsal anterior cingulate cortex and the orbital frontoinsular cortex, with projections to subcortical structures such as the thalamus, hypothalamus, and ventral tegmental area/substantia nigra. Previous works have shown that the dorsal anterior cingulate cortex and the frontoinsular cortex represent salient stimuli, such as hunger [99] and pain [100], and respond to emotional pain, such as during social rejection; it was therefore hypothesized that these areas are the neural substrate of the interoceptive feedbacks [101]. In agreement, Seeley et al. [98] proposed that the salience network identifies relevant homeostatic stimuli, by integrating sensory information with visceral and autonomic functions, supporting a capital role of this network in pain processing. Notably, the identified salience network comprises brain regions involved in the central processing of the autonomic functions [102]. Indeed, the anterior cingulate cortex, the insular cortex, the amygdala, and the hypothalamus were shown to be key components of the autonomic function network. It is important to note that the parasympathetic and the sympathetic system present divergent central processing pathways: the parasympathetic system maps onto areas of the default mode network, while the sympathetic system maps onto areas of the salience and the executive network [102]. The possible involvement of the salience network in the cluster headache pathophysiology is well suggested by its clinical features and neuroimaging investigations. The typical clinical features of this condition (severe head pain and cranial-facial autonomic symptoms) directly call in cause areas involved in pain and in central autonomic processing; neuroimaging investigations provided convincing evidence of the involvement of the hypothalamus, the anterior cingulate cortex, and the insular cortex, areas belonging to the salience network, during spontaneous and induced cluster headache attacks [18, 23, 24, 50, 103]. Similarly, RS-fMRI studies also reported abnormal functional connectivity between these same cortical regions (i.e., anterior cingulate cortex and insular cortex) and the hypothalamus in "out-of-bout" conditions [17] and during CH attacks [104]. Based on these pieces of evidence, Qiu et al. [105] directly investigated the functional connectivity of the salience network in a relatively large sample of episodic cluster headache patients during the "in-bout" condition but outside the attacks. The results of this study suggest that episodic cluster headache patients present, in comparison to healthy individuals, a decreased functional connectivity between regions of the salience network and the bilateral hypothalamus, independent from the site of recurrent attacks. The authors suggested that the presence of a defective functional connectivity within the salience network might indicate an abnormal pain control, with possible dysregulation of the antinociceptive pathways, leading to the generation of the cluster headache attacks. Functional alterations of the salience network were replicated in a more recent study [19] showing a decreased functional connectivity in the insular cortex within this network in cluster headache patients during "in-bout" and "out-of bout" conditions. This last observation seems to indicate that the functional alterations in the salience network are relatively stable and not related to the shift from "in-bout" to "out-of bout" condition and vice versa.

7.3.3.2 The Default Mode Network

The default mode network comprises the ventral medial prefrontal cortex, the dorsomedial prefrontal cortex, the posterior cingulate cortex, the precuneus, and the lateral parietal cortex [76]. The entorhinal cortex is frequently described as a structure belonging to this functional network. According to Raichle [76], the default mode network integrates the sensory-visceromotor processing (occurring in the ventral medial prefrontal cortex), with the self-referential activity (occurring in the medial prefrontal cortex) and the recalling of the previous experience (occurring in the precuneus/parietal cortex and in the hippocampus). Importantly in the context of the cluster headache, as we have noted above, the central processing of the parasympathetic activity occurs in the default mode network [102]. Given the above characteristics, it is not unexpected that default mode network presents abnormal functional connectivity in chronic pain conditions [106–108] and in several neuropsychiatric [77] and neurodegenerative [74] diseases. Notably, the dysfunctional connectivity of default mode network in the context of chronic pain processing seems to mediate pain rumination [109]. Based on these observations, it is plausible that the cluster headache, as recurrent (chronic) and severe pain, may induce alterations of the default mode network functional connectivity. Rocca et al. [17], investigating the intrinsic functional connectivity in episodic cluster headache patients during the out-of-bout condition, reported no alterations in the default mode network. This lack of evidence was possibly related to the relatively small sample size investigated. Indeed, in a larger dataset of cluster headache patients, Chou et al. [19] observed functional alterations of the default mode network (in left precuneus) in both the "in-bout" and "out-of-bout" conditions with no differences between the two. As for the salience network, this work suggests that the default mode network is dysfunctional in episodic cluster headache patients; however, this dysfunction is not affected differently by the "in-bout" and "out-of-bout" conditions, indicating relatively stable functional alterations in this network.

7.3.3.3 Hypothalamic RS-fMRI Functional Connectivity

A summary of the studies investigating hypothalamic functional connectivity with RS-fMRI is presented in Table 7.2.

Hypothalamic functional connectivity was recently investigated [82] in a large sample of healthy and overweight participants. Using a seed-based approach, lateral and medial hypothalamus were shown to present an overlapping functional connectivity with the striatum, the thalamus, the brainstem, and with some cortical regions, such as the orbitofrontal cortex, the cingulum, and the temporal areas. However, the two hypothalamic subnuclei also revealed distinct patterns of functional connectivity: in particular, the lateral hypothalamus was shown to be part of the functional network comprising the dorsal striatum, the thalamus, the midbrain, the operculum, the anterior cingulate, and the prefrontal cortex. It is interesting to note that some cortical areas (the operculum and the anterior cingulate cortex) of the lateral hypothalamic network map onto regions belonging to the salience network (frontoinsular cortex and anterior cingulate cortex), while the prefrontal cortex maps onto the executive control network, as observed in the work of Seeley et al. [98]. The authors speculated that the lateral hypothalamus works in concert with regions involved in goal-directed behaviors (dorsal striatum and cingulo-opercular network) and with regions responding to stimulus salience (opercular and

Table 7.2 Summary of the studies investigating hypothalamic functional connectivity in cluster headache pathophysiology using resting state functional magnetic resonance imaging (RS-fMRI) with seed-based analyses (seed in left or right hypothalamus, or * in hypothalamus ipsilateral to the pain or controlateral to the pain)

Hypothalamic functional connectivity—seed-based analyses				
	Patients	Seed characteristic	RS-FC of R (or ipsilateral*) hypothalamus	RS-FC of L (or contralateral*) hypothalamus
Rocca et al. [17]	13 episodic CH patients: "out-of-bout" patients (8 with right-sided, 5 left-sided attacks)	5 mm spherical volume, centered at [2/−2, −18, −8] in SPM space	*CH vs. CTRL:* Increased RS-FC with anterior cingulate cortex, bilateral secondary sensorimotor cortex, left V1, right middle occipital gyrus, right thalamus and right insula	*CH vs. CTRLs:* Increased RS-FC with anterior cingulate cortex, bilateral secondary sensorimotor cortex, left V1, right middle occipital gyrus, right thalamus and right insula
Qiu et al. [104]	12 episodic CH patients: "in-attack" and "out-of-attack" (all right-sided)	6 mm spherical volume, centered at [2, −18, −8] in Talairach space	*In-attack CH vs. out-of-attack CH:* increased RS-FC with anterior cingulate cortex, posterior cingulate cortex, superior frontal gyrus, middle frontal gyrus, inferior frontal gyrus, superior temporal gyrus, inferior parietal lobule, gyrus, amygdala. *Out-of attack vs. CTRL:* increased RS-FC with inferior frontal gyrus, superior temporal gyrus, middle temporal gyrus, temporal pole, insula cortex, parahippocampal gyrus and uncus; decreased RS-FC with precuneus, inferior parietal lobule, occipital lobe	
Yang et al. [34]	18 episodic CH patients: "in-bout" and "out-of-bout" (with right-sided attacks after flipping images)	4 mm spherical volume, centered at [4/−4, −18, −8] in MNI space	*CH (in-bout and out-of-bout) vs. CTRL:* RS-FC* alterations with L middle frontal gyrus and bilateral inferior temporal gyri	*CH (in-bout and out-of-bout) vs. CTRL:* RS-FC* alterations with R fusiform gyrus, L middle frontal gyrus, L inferior semi-lunar lobule, and L inferior temporal gyrus
		Visual identification of hypothalamus in MNI space	*CH (in-bout and out-of-bout) vs. CTRL:* RS-FC* alterations with L medial frontal gyrus, R cuneus *CH in-bout vs. CH out-of-bout:* RS-FC* alterations with bilateral cerebellar areas, L precuneus	*CH (in-bout and out-of-bout) vs. CTRL:* RS-FC* alterations with right cuneus. *CH in-bout vs. CH out-of-bout:* RS-FC* alterations with L cerebellar tonsil, R medial frontal areas

(continued)

Table 7.2 (continued)

Hypothalamic functional connectivity—seed-based analyses

	Patients	Seed characteristic	RS-FC of R (or ipsilateral*) hypothalamus	RS-FC of L (or contralateral*) hypothalamus
Qiu et al. [105]	21 episodic CH patients: "in-bout" outside attacks (13 with right-sided, 8 left-sided attacks)	10-mm cubic volume, centered at [5/−5, −18, −8] in MNI space	*CH vs. CTRL*: decreased RS-FC with salience network (dorsal anterior cingulate cortex and anterior insula-frontal operculum) in both right- and left-sided CH	*CH vs. CTRL*: decreased RS-FC with salience network (dorsal anterior cingulate cortex and anterior insula-frontal operculum) in both right- and left-sided CH
Ferraro et al. [111]	17 chronic CH patients outside attacks (with right-sided attacks after flipping images)	Visual identification of hypothalamus in native space	*CH vs. CTRL*: RS-FC* alterations with diencephalic-mesencephalic junction regions	

CH cluster headache patients, *CTRL* control group, *RS-FC* resting state functional connectivity, *L* left, *R* right

anterior cingulate cortex) [98]. As we have discussed above, the hypothalamus seems to play an important role in the modulation of a possible dysfunctional network in the cluster headache pathophysiology [31]. Based on this rationale, some studies have investigated the hypothalamic functional connectivity by means of RS-fMRI. However, there is an important consideration that needs to be done when interpreting these studies: the most part of the previous literature using RS-fMRI [17, 104, 105], with the exception of a few [34], used regions of interest defined by the standard coordinates of posterior hypothalamic activation as reported in the study of May et al. [30]; reconsideration of these coordinates led to hypothesize that they really relate to midbrain areas [29, 110]. Therefore it is possible that some of these results truly investigated functional connectivity of midbrain areas and not of the hypothalamus.

Rocca et al. [17] complemented the ICA analyses using a seed-based approach to investigate the hypothalamic functional connectivity. The authors showed that episodic CH patients in out-of-bout conditions present an increased functional connectivity between the hypothalamus and the anterior cingulate cortex, but also with the secondary somatosensory cortex and the occipital regions, confirming the results obtained with ICA, which showed functional connectivity alterations beyond the pain processing regions [17] and involving the visual regions.

Qiu et al. [104], directly testing the functional connectivity of the hypothalamus network, showed that episodic cluster headache patients during "attack" condition in comparison to "out-of-attack" condition present increased functional connectivity between the ipsilateral-to-the-pain hypothalamus and several cortical and subcortical areas such as the anterior cingulate cortex, the posterior cingulate cortex, the superior, middle, and inferior frontal gyrus and ventral medial prefrontal cortex, the superior temporal gyrus, the inferior parietal lobule, the parahippocampal gyrus, and the amygdala. It is interesting to note that some of the identified areas belong to the default mode network (posterior cingulate cortex, inferior parietal lobule, ventral medial prefrontal cortex and parahippocampal gyrus). Two observations are important in this regard: (1) the central processing of the parasympathetic activity occurs in regions of the default mode network [102], as we have discussed above; therefore the typical autonomic symptoms of the cluster headache during the attack well explain the dysfunctional connectivity in the default mode network; (2) the observed abnormal functional connectivity in the default mode network occurs in areas involved in the recalling of the past experience, namely the posterior cingulate cortex/precuneus, the parietal cortex, and the hippocampus [76]. The different dysfunctional connectivity observed in the "attack" condition in comparison to the "out-of-attack" condition suggests that during the attack the central processing of the parasympathetic activity and pain processing might have a direct effect on the functional connectivity of the default mode network. However, as we have discussed in the previous sections, cluster headache patients seem to present a relatively stabilized dysfunctional connectivity within the default mode network, with no difference between the "in-bout" and out-of-bout conditions [19]. Altogether these results indicate that the acute modulations in the default mode network during the cluster headache attacks might be the cause of the permanent dysfunction of this circuit; however, this dysfunctional activity is not at the basis of the shift from the "in-bout" to the "out-of-bout" condition or vice versa. Notably, Yang et al. [34] showed that the hypothalamic dysfunctional connectivity is different between the "in-bout" and "out-of-bout" conditions: interestingly, "in-bout" condition revealed decreased hypothalamic functional connectivity with regions of the default mode network (i.e., the precuneus) but also with the middle frontal gyrus, and the cerebellar areas. Interestingly, the episodic cluster headache patients differed from healthy participants in hypothalamic functional connectivity in visual region (i.e., the cuneus) and in the middle frontal gyrus, further confirming that the functional connectivity abnormalities are well beyond the pain matrix. Additionally, the annual bout frequency correlated significantly with the hypothalamic functional connectivity in the cerebellar areas, suggesting that this might be an effect of the pathophysiological condition. It is important to note that in this study, the authors used as seed the anatomical hypothalamus.

A more recent study [111] investigated the functional connectivity in chronic cluster headache patients (out of the attacks) using as seed the anatomical hypothalamus. The authors showed an increased functional connectivity between the ipsilateral posterior hypothalamus and a number of diencephalic–mesencephalic structures, comprising the ventral tegmental area, the dorsal nuclei of raphe, and the bilateral substantia nigra, the subthalamic nucleus, and the red nucleus. They concluded that in chronic cluster headache patients, there is a deranged functional connectivity between the posterior ipsilateral hypothalamus and diencephalic–mesencephalic regions that mainly involves structures that are part of (i.e., ventral tegmental area, substantia nigra) or modulate (dorsal nuclei of raphe, subthalamic nucleus) the midbrain dopaminergic systems [111]. These results suggest that the midbrain dopaminergic systems could play a role in cluster headache pathophysiology and in particular in the chronicization process.

7.3.3.4 Other RS-fMRI Networks

Beyond the involvement of the salience network and the default mode network, several studies presented evidence that episodic cluster headache patients present important alterations in other functional networks. The study by Rocca et al. [17] showed that episodic cluster headache individuals in out-of-bout condition present abnormalities in the visual and the sensorimotor networks. In particular, episodic CH patients showed reduced functional connectivity bilaterally in V1 (visual network), and in the primary sensory-motor cortex, the supplementary motor area, and the anterior cingulate cortex (sensorimotor network). These results indicate that episodic cluster headache patients present dysfunctional connectivity in networks comprising regions involved in the sensory discrimination processing (primary and secondary somatosensory area, posterior insula and thalamus) and in the affective-cognitive processing (anterior cingulum) of the painful experience. Notably, the anterior cingulate cortex is part of the salience network [98, 112]: alteration of functional connectivity in this region, again, reinforces the hypothesis of a strong involvement of this circuit in the cluster headache pathophysiology.

These results clearly showed that the alteration of the functional connectivity in the cluster headache brain is well beyond the regions involved in pain processing: this is evidenced by the dysfunctional connectivity observed in the visual networks. Possibly, photophobia and retro-orbital pain, frequently observed in cluster headache [113], might lead to functional connectivity alterations of the visual system.

Remarkably, the disease duration was negatively correlated with the strength of the functional connectivity in V1 and in the primary sensory-motor cortex: it is possible that these abnormalities might be the consequence of prolonged and severe painful condition, known to induce alterations of the central nervous system [114]. Chou et al. [19] confirmed functional alterations in the visual and the somatosensory networks in episodic cluster headache patients investigated during "in-bout" and "out-of-bout" conditions. Notably, this study found evidence of functional alterations also in several other networks such as the temporal, frontal, and dorsal attention network, and, as we have discussed so far, also in default mode network (in left precuneus) and in the salience network (in left insula). Importantly, differences in functional connectivity between the "in-bout" and "out-of-bout" conditions were not observed in the classical regions of the pain matrix, but in the frontal network (in the right inferior frontal gyrus) and the dorsal attention network (in the left postcentral gyrus). Further supporting widespread functional connectivity alterations, Faragò et al. [33] showed that episodic cluster headache patients during out-of-bout condition present dysfunctional connectivity within the attention network (in the ipsilateral superior frontal gyrus and medial frontal cortex) and the cerebellar network. Interestingly the cumulative headache days showed negative correlation within the controlateral attention network and the frontal pole, suggesting that these abnormalities are possible effects of the cluster headache pathophysiology.

7.3.3.5 Concluding Remarks

Since 2010, relatively few studies were conducted to determine the putative dysfunctional neural networks involved in cluster headache pathophysiology. Moreover, the different conditions investigated ("in-bout," "out-of-bout," "in-attacks") and the different coordinates used to investigate the hypothalamic functional connectivity (in midbrain tegmentum or in the hypothalamus) make difficult to have a coherent picture of the resting state functional connectivity in the cluster headache.

However, several, although not conclusive, considerations can be done.

First of all, the episodic cluster headache patients present widespread functional connectivity alterations in several networks. This suggests that the cluster headache brain is functionally reorganized, in a maladaptive or adaptive way, across multiple networks and multiple areas (i.e., visual networks, salience network, and default mode network), not only confined in regions involved in pain processing.

Second, the salience network seems to play a capital role in the cluster headache pathophysiology: the reported studies suggest that this network presents a relatively stable functional alteration during the "in-bout" and "out-of-bout" conditions. It is tempting to speculate that the dysfunctional connectivity of the salient network might be a neural "tract" of these patients and it might constitute the basis of the chronification of the disease. However, this circuit does not play a role in the shift between the "in-bout" and "out-of-bout" conditions. Notably, alteration of this network suggests that cluster headache patients present a dysfunctional ability in the elaboration of salient stimuli. In this regard, it is important to note that alterations of the salient network are present in several pain conditions, such as headache [115] and irritable bowel syndrome [117], headache [116, 117], and irritable bowel syndrome [118]. Moreover, disruption of the integrity of the salience network was observed in several neuropsychiatric conditions, such as autism [119], schizophrenia [120], and addiction [121]. Therefore, the observed alterations are clearly not cluster headache-specific. This clearly opens an important question: is there a specific role of the salience network in cluster headache pathophysiology? Is it a specific effect of the disease or is it an epiphenomenon?

Third, the default mode network seems to be involved in cluster headache pathophysiology, as the salience network, with functional alterations not related to the conditions of the cluster headache patients ("in-bout" or "out-of-bout" condition), but stabilized as neural "tract." The dysfunctional activity of this circuit during the attacks might be at the basis of these stabilized alterations across the different conditions. Due to the role of the default mode network in the integration of the sensory-visceromotor processing, self-referential activity, and recalling of previous experience [76], these results suggest that cluster headache presents disturbances in the social-emotional spheres.

Future studies should confirm these results and should clarify if the observed dysfunctional networks are specific neurophysiological patterns of the cluster headache or are an unspecific response to or a cause of pain processing.

7.3.4 Event-Related Functional Magnetic Resonance Imaging

Currently no functional imaging studies exist that used a stimulation paradigm during a functional MRI (fMRI) session in trigeminal autonomic cephalalgias to detect distinct neuronal mechanisms of stimulus processing. However, a few studies used fMRI in a quasi-event-related setting by repeatedly recording echo-planar images during attacks and outside attacks and modeling the attacks as events that could then be compared to the scans outside attacks as some kind of baseline condition. Thus it might be possible to detect attack-specific activation patterns using fMRI—an imaging technique that is due to its nonquantitative characteristic usually not apt to detect simple activations at rest. In cluster headache, studying the attack, the attack-free state, and the state shortly after pain relieved by sumatriptan using such a semi-event-related setting could replicate the activation of the posterior hypothalamus previously identified in PET studies [24, 122]. Furthermore, different brainstem centers could be identified as being active during the acute pain stage of cluster headache attacks, including the red nucleus and the ventral pons [122]. A similar experimental approach was used in a patient with an atypical trigeminal autonomic cephalalgia (paroxysmal hemicrania might possibly be the closest fit), demonstrating a similar activation within the posterior hypothalamic grey as demonstrated in cluster headache [123]. In one case of SUNCT, activations corresponding to various brain and brainstem pain processing areas could be detected [124], whereas two other cases detected hypothalamic activation during attacks of SUNCT [92, 125].

Semi-event-related functional magnetic resonance imaging has thus proven to be useful in the detection of pathophysiologic mechanisms underlying trigeminal autonomic cephalalgias, although most studies are limited to very few patients or even single case reports.

7.4 Conclusion

Within the past 30 years, neuroimaging studies have broadened our understanding of cluster headache and TAC pathophysiology. Especially early PET studies are here of vast importance as they were the first to identify the hypothalamus as the region specifically involved in cluster headache pathophysiology and differentiating the acute pain stage of cluster headache from experimentally inflicted pain. Our current understanding of cluster headache is fundamentally based upon these findings and most of the following studies emanated from the knowledge obtained here. Technical advances both regarding image acquisition and analyzing methods have led to more refined approaches and will in the future further advance our comprehension of these debilitating diseases.

References

1. Ashburner J, Friston KJ. Voxel-based morphometry—the methods. NeuroImage. 2000;11:805–21.
2. Ashburner J. Computational anatomy with the SPM software. Magn Reson Imaging. 2009;27:1163–74.
3. May A, et al. Correlation between structural and functional changes in brain in an idiopathic headache syndrome. Nat Med. 1999;5:836–8.
4. Leone M, Franzini A, Broggi G, May A, Bussone G. Therapeutic stimulation of the hypothalamus: pathophysiological insights and prerequisites for management. Brain. 2005;128:E35.
5. Leone M, Franzini A, Broggi G, Bussone G. Hypothalamic deep brain stimulation for intractable chronic cluster headache: a 3-year follow-up. Neurol Sci. 2003;24(Suppl 2):S143–5.
6. Leone M, et al. Lessons from 8 years' experience of hypothalamic stimulation in cluster headache. Cephalalgia. 2008;28:787–97; discussion 798
7. Leone M, Franzini A, Proietti Cecchini A, Bussone G. Success, failure, and putative mechanisms in hypothalamic stimulation for drug-resistant chronic cluster headache. Pain. 2013;154:89–94.
8. Naegel S, et al. Cortical plasticity in episodic and chronic cluster headache. Neuroimage Clin. 2014;6:415–23.
9. Absinta M, et al. Selective decreased grey matter volume of the pain-matrix network in cluster headache. Cephalalgia. 2012;32:109–15.
10. Yang F-CC, et al. Altered gray matter volume in the frontal pain modulation network in patients with cluster headache. Pain. 2013;154:801–7.
11. Arkink EB, et al. The anterior hypothalamus in cluster headache. Cephalalgia. 2017;37:1039–50.
12. Pierpaoli C, Jezzard P, Basser PJ, Barnett A, Di Chiro G. Diffusion tensor MR imaging of the human brain. Radiology. 1996;201:637–48.
13. Feldman HM, Yeatman JD, Lee ES, Barde LHF, Gaman-Bean S. Diffusion tensor imaging: a review for pediatric researchers and clinicians. J Dev Behav Pediatr. 2010;31:346–56.
14. Alexander AL, et al. Characterization of cerebral white matter properties using quantitative magnetic resonance imaging stains. Brain Connect. 2011;1:423–46.
15. Taoka T, et al. Diffusion anisotropy and diffusivity of white matter tracts within the temporal stem in Alzheimer disease: evaluation of the "tract of interest" by diffusion tensor tractography. AJNR Am J Neuroradiol. 2006;27:1040–5.
16. Teepker M, et al. Diffusion tensor imaging in episodic cluster headache. Headache. 2012;52:274–82.
17. Rocca MA, et al. Central nervous system dysregulation extends beyond the pain-matrix network in cluster headache. Cephalalgia. 2010;30(11):1383–91. https://doi.org/10.1177/0333102410365164.
18. Qiu E-C, et al. Altered regional homogeneity in spontaneous cluster headache attacks: a resting-state functional magnetic resonance imaging study. Chin Med J. 2012;125:705–9.
19. Chou K-H, et al. Bout-associated intrinsic functional network changes in cluster headache: a longitudinal resting-state functional MRI study. Cephalalgia. 2017;37:1152–63.
20. Szabó N, et al. White matter disintegration in cluster headache. J Headache Pain. 2013;14:64.

21. Király A, et al. Macro- and microstructural alterations of the subcortical structures in episodic cluster headache. Cephalalgia. 2018;38(4):662–73.
22. Chou KH, et al. Altered white matter microstructural connectivity in cluster headaches: a longitudinal diffusion tensor imaging study. Cephalalgia. 2014;34:1040–52.
23. May A, et al. Hypothalamic activation in cluster headache attacks. Lancet. 1998;352:275–8.
24. Morelli N, et al. Functional magnetic resonance imaging in episodic cluster headache. J Headache Pain. 2009;10:11–4.
25. Teepker M, et al. Diffusion tensor imaging in episodic cluster headache. Headache. 2011;52:274–82.
26. Leone M, Bussone G. Pathophysiology of trigeminal autonomic cephalalgias. Lancet Neurol. 2009;8:755–64.
27. Clelland CD, Zheng Z, Kim W, Bari A, Pouratian N. Common cerebral networks associated with distinct deep brain stimulation targets for cluster headache. Cephalalgia. 2014;34:224–30.
28. Del Rio MS, Alvarez LJ. Functional neuroimaging of headaches. Lancet Neurol. 2004;3:645–51.
29. Matharu MS, Zrinzo L. Deep brain stimulation in cluster headache: hypothalamus or midbrain tegmentum? Curr Pain Headache Rep. 2010;14:151–9.
30. May A, Bahra A, Büchel C, Frackowiak RS, Goadsby PJ. Hypothalamic activation in cluster headache attacks. Lancet. 1998;352:275–8.
31. Leone M, Proietti Cecchini A. Advances in the understanding of cluster headache. Expert Rev Neurother. 2017;17:165–72.
32. Lemaire J-J, et al. White matter connectivity of human hypothalamus. Brain Res. 2011;1371:43–64.
33. Faragó P, et al. Ipsilateral alteration of resting state activity suggests that cortical dysfunction contributes to the pathogenesis of cluster headache. Brain Topogr. 2017;30:281–9.
34. Yang F, Chou KH, Fuh JL, Lee PL, Lirng JF, Lin YY, Lin CP, Wang SJ. Altered hypothalamic functional connectivity in cluster headache: a longitudinal resting-state functional MRI study. J Neurol Neurosurg Psychiatry. 2015;86(4):437–45.
35. Helmchen C, Mohr C, Erdmann C, Binkofski F. Cerebellar neural responses related to actively and passively applied noxious thermal stimulation in human subjects: a parametric fMRI study. Neurosci Lett. 2004;361:237–40.
36. Owen SLF, et al. Connectivity of an effective hypothalamic surgical target for cluster headache. J Clin Neurosci. 2007;14:955–60.
37. Seijo F, et al. Neuromodulation of the posterolateral hypothalamus for the treatment of chronic refractory cluster headache: experience in five patients with a modified anatomical target. Cephalalgia. 2011;31:1634–41.
38. Sprenger T, et al. Opioidergic changes in the pineal gland and hypothalamus in cluster headache: a ligand PET study. Neurology. 2006;66:1108–10.
39. Massimo F. Oxford textbook of neuroimaging. Oxford: Oxford University Press; 2015.
40. Norris JW, Hachinski VC, Cooper PW. Cerebral blood flow changes in cluster headache. Acta Neurol Scand. 1976;54:371–4.
41. Henry PY, Vernhiet J, Orgogozo JM, Caille JM. Cerebral blood flow in migraine and cluster headache. Compartmental analysis and reactivity to anaesthetic depression. Res Clin Stud Headache. 1978;6:81–8.
42. Krabbe AA, Henriksen L, Olesen J. Tomographic determination of cerebral blood flow during attacks of cluster headache. Cephalalgia. 1984;4:17–23.
43. Nelson RF, et al. Cerebral blood flow studies in patients with cluster headache. Headache. 1980;20:184–9.
44. Afra J, Ertsey C, Jelencsik H, Dabasi G, Pánczél G. SPECT and TCD studies in cluster headache patients. Funct Neurol. 1995;10:259–64.
45. Sakai F, Meyer JS, Ishihara N, Naritomi H, Deshmukh VD. Noninvasive 133XE inhalation measurements of regional cerebral blood flow in migraine and related headaches. Acta Neurol Scand Suppl. 1977;64:196–7.

46. Di Piero V, Fiacco F, Tombari D, Pantano P. Tonic pain: a SPET study in normal subjects and cluster headache patients. Pain. 1997;70:185–91.
47. Schlake HP, Böttger IG, Grotemeyer KH, Husstedt IW, Schober O. Single photon emission computed tomography (SPECT) with 99mTc-HMPAO (hexamethyl propylenamino oxime) in chronic paroxysmal hemicrania—a case report. Cephalalgia. 1990;10:311–5.
48. Poughias L, Aasly J. SUNCT syndrome: cerebral SPECT images during attacks. Headache. 1995;35:143–5.
49. Hsieh JC, Hannerz J, Ingvar M. Right-lateralised central processing for pain of nitroglycerin-induced cluster headache. Pain. 1996;67:59–68.
50. Sprenger T, et al. Specific hypothalamic activation during a spontaneous cluster headache attack. Neurology. 2004;62:516–7.
51. Sprenger T, et al. Altered metabolism in frontal brain circuits in cluster headache. Cephalalgia. 2007;27:1033–42.
52. Magis D, et al. Central modulation in cluster headache patients treated with occipital nerve stimulation: an FDG-PET study. BMC Neurol. 2011;11:25.
53. Matharu MS, et al. Posterior hypothalamic and brainstem activation in hemicrania continua. Headache. 2004;44:747–61.
54. Biswal B, Yetkin FZ, Haughton VM, Hyde JS. Functional connectivity in the motor cortex of resting human brain using echo-planar MRI. Magn Reson Med. 1995;34:537–41.
55. Cordes D, et al. Frequencies contributing to functional connectivity in the cerebral cortex in "resting-state"; data. AJNR Am J Neuroradiol. 2001;22:1326–33.
56. Honey CJ, et al. Predicting human resting-state functional connectivity from structural connectivity. Proc Natl Acad Sci U S A. 2009;106:2035–40.
57. Vincent JL, et al. Intrinsic functional architecture in the anaesthetized monkey brain. Nature. 2007;447:83–6.
58. Passingham RE, Stephan KE, Kötter R. The anatomical basis of functional localization in the cortex. Nat Rev Neurosci. 2002;3:606–16.
59. Cohen AL, et al. Defining functional areas in individual human brains using resting functional connectivity MRI. NeuroImage. 2008;41:45–57.
60. Skudlarski P, et al. Measuring brain connectivity: diffusion tensor imaging validates resting state temporal correlations. NeuroImage. 2008;43:554–61.
61. Quigley M, et al. Role of the corpus callosum in functional connectivity. AJNR Am J Neuroradiol. 2003;24:208–12.
62. Johnston JM, et al. Loss of resting interhemispheric functional connectivity after complete section of the corpus callosum. J Neurosci. 2008;28:6453–8.
63. Uddin LQ. Brain connectivity and the self: the case of cerebral disconnection. Conscious Cogn. 2011;20:94–8.
64. Fox MD, Raichle ME. Spontaneous fluctuations in brain activity observed with functional magnetic resonance imaging. Nat Rev Neurosci. 2007;8(9):700–11. https://doi.org/10.1038/nrn2201.
65. Salinas E, Sejnowski TJ. Correlated neuronal activity and the flow of neural information. Nat Rev Neurosci. 2001;2:539–50.
66. Pouget A, Dayan P, Zemel RS. Inference and computation with population code. Annu Rev Neurosci. 2003;26:381–410.
67. Xiong J, Parsons LM, Gao JH, Fox PT. Interregional connectivity to primary motor cortex revealed using MRI resting state images. Hum Brain Mapp. 1999;8:151–6.
68. Beckmann CF, DeLuca M, Devlin JT, Smith SM. Investigations into resting-state connectivity using independent component analysis. Philos Trans R Soc Lond Ser B Biol Sci. 2005;360:1001–13.
69. Cordes D, et al. Mapping functionally related regions of brain with functional connectivity MR imaging. AJNR Am J Neuroradiol. 2000;21:1636–44.
70. Lowe MJ, Mock BJ, Sorenson JA. Functional connectivity in single and multislice echoplanar imaging using resting-state fluctuations. NeuroImage. 1998;7:119–32.

71. De Luca M, Beckmann CF, De Stefano N, Matthews PM, Smith SM. fMRI resting state networks define distinct modes of long-distance interactions in the human brain. NeuroImage. 2006;29:1359–67.
72. Bartels A, Zeki S. Brain dynamics during natural viewing conditions—a new guide for mapping connectivity in vivo. NeuroImage. 2005;24:339–49.
73. Cordes D, Haughton V, Carew JD, Arfanakis K, Maravilla K. Hierarchical clustering to measure connectivity in fMRI resting-state data. Magn Reson Imaging. 2002;20:305–17.
74. Greicius MD, Krasnow B, Reiss AL, Menon V. Functional connectivity in the resting brain: a network analysis of the default mode hypothesis. Proc Natl Acad Sci U S A. 2003;100(1):253–8.
75. Raichle ME, et al. A default mode of brain function. Proc Natl Acad Sci U S A. 2001;98(2):676–82.
76. Raichle ME. The brain's default mode network. Annu Rev Neurosci. 2015;38:433–47.
77. Greicius M. Resting-state functional connectivity in neuropsychiatric disorders. Curr Opin Neurol. 2008;21:424–30.
78. Power JD, et al. Functional network organization of the human brain. Neuron. 2011;72:665–78.
79. Rombouts SA, Stam CJ, Kuijer J, et al. Identifying confounds to increase specificity during a 'no task condition': evidence for hippocampal connectivity using fMRI. NeuroImage. 2003;20(2):1236–45.
80. Zhang D, Snyder AZ, Fox MD, Sansbury MW, Shimony JS, Raichle ME. Intrinsic functional relations between human cerebral cortex and thalamus. J Neurophysiol. 2008;100(4):1740–8.
81. O'Reilly JX, Beckmann CF, Tomassini V, Ramnani N, Johansen-Berg H. Distinct and overlapping functional zones in the cerebellum defined by resting state functional connectivity. Cereb Cortex. 2010;20(4):953–65.
82. Kullmann S, et al. Resting-state functional connectivity of the human hypothalamus. Hum Brain Mapp. 2014;35:6088–96.
83. Greicius MD, Flores BH, Menon V, Glover GH, Solvason HB, Kenna H, Reiss AL, Schatzberg AF. Resting-state functional connectivity in major depression: abnormally increased contributions from subgenual cingulate cortex and thalamus. Biol Psychiatry. 2007;62:429–37.
84. Wang L, et al. Changes in hippocampal connectivity in the early stages of Alzheimer's disease: evidence from resting state fMRI. NeuroImage. 2006;31:496–504.
85. Zang YF, He Y, Zhu CZ, Cao QJ, Sui MQ, Liang M, Tian LX, Jiang TZ, Wang YF. Altered baseline brain activity in children with ADHD revealed by resting-state functional MRI. Brain and Development. 2007;29(2):83–91.
86. Zhou Y, et al. Functional dysconnectivity of the dorsolateral prefrontal cortex in first-episode schizophrenia using resting-state fMRI. Neurosci Lett. 2007;417:297–302.
87. Wu Q-Z, et al. Abnormal regional spontaneous neural activity in treatment-refractory depression revealed by resting-state fMRI. Hum Brain Mapp. 2011;32:1290–9.
88. Rosazza C, et al. Multimodal study of default-mode network integrity in disorders of consciousness. Ann Neurol. 2016;79:841–53.
89. Greicius MD, Menon V. Default-mode activity during a passive sensory task: uncoupled from deactivation but impacting activation. J Cogn Neurosci. 2004;16:1484–92.
90. Filippini N, et al. Distinct patterns of brain activity in young carriers of the APOE-epsilon4 allele. Proc Natl Acad Sci U S A. 2009;106:7209–14.
91. Headache Classification Committee of the International Headache Society (IHS). The international classification of headache disorders, 3rd edition (beta version). Cephalalgia. 2013;33:629–808.
92. May A, Bahra A, Büchel C, Turner R, Goadsby PJ. Functional magnetic resonance imaging in spontaneous attacks of SUNCT: short-lasting neuralgiform headache with conjunctival injection and tearing. Ann Neurol. 1999;46:791–4.
93. Franzini A, et al. Stimulation of the posterior hypothalamus for treatment of chronic intractable cluster headaches: first reported series. Neurosurgery. 2003;52:1095–101.
94. Fontaine D, et al. Anatomical location of effective deep brain stimulation electrodes in chronic cluster headache. Brain. 2010;133:1214–23.

95. Akram H, et al. Ventral tegmental area deep brain stimulation for refractory chronic cluster headache. Neurology. 2016;86:1676–82.
96. Chabardès S, et al. Endoventricular deep brain stimulation of the third ventricle. Neurosurgery. 2016;0:1.
97. May A, et al. Hypothalamic deep brain stimulation in positron emission tomography. J Neurosci. 2006;26:3589–93.
98. Seeley WW, et al. Behavioral/systems/cognitive dissociable intrinsic connectivity networks for salience processing and executive control. J Neurosci. 2007;27:2349–56.
99. Craig AD. How do you feel? Interoception: the sense of the physiological condition of the body. Nat Rev Neurosci. 2002;3:655–66.
100. Peyron R, Laurent B, García-Larrea L. Functional imaging of brain responses to pain. A review and meta-analysis (2000). Neurophysiol Clin. 2000;30(5):263–88.
101. Critchley HD, Wiens S, Rotshtein P, Ohman A, Dolan RJ. Neural systems supporting interoceptive awareness. Nat Neurosci. 2004;7(2):189–95.
102. Beissner F, Meissner K, Bär K-J, Napadow V. The autonomic brain: an activation likelihood estimation meta-analysis for central processing of autonomic function. J Neurosci. 2013;33:10503–11.
103. May A, Bahra A, Büchel C, Frackowiak RS, Goadsby PJ. PET and MRA findings in cluster headache and MRA in experimental pain. Neurology. 2000;55:1328–35.
104. Qiu E, et al. Abnormal brain functional connectivity of the hypothalamus in cluster headaches. PLoS One. 2013;8:e57896.
105. Qiu E, Tian L, Wang Y, Ma L, Yu S. Abnormal coactivation of the hypothalamus and salience network in patients with cluster headache. Neurology. 2015;84:1402–8.
106. Baliki MN, Geha PY, Apkarian AV, Chialvo DR. Beyond feeling: chronic pain hurts the brain, disrupting the default-mode network dynamics. J Neurosci. 2008;28:1398–403.
107. Napadow V, La Count L, Park K, As-Sanie S, Clauw DJ, Harris RE. Intrinsic brain connectivity in fibromyalgia is associated with chronic pain intensity. Arthritis Rheum. 2010;62(8):2545–55.
108. Loggia M, et al. Default mode network connectivity encodes clinical pain: an arterial spin labeling study. Pain. 2013;154(1):24–33.
109. Kucyi A, et al. Enhanced medial prefrontal-default mode network functional connectivity in chronic pain and its association with pain rumination. J Neurosci. 2014;34:3969–75.
110. Del Rio MS, et al. Reviews functional neuroimaging of headaches. Lancet Neurol. 2004;3:645–51.
111. Ferraro S, et al. Defective functional connectivity between posterior hypothalamus and regions of the diencephalic-mesencephalic junction in chronic cluster headache. Cephalalgia. 2018;38(13):1910–8. https://doi.org/10.1177/0333102418761048.
112. Borsook D, Edwards R, Elman I, Becerra L, Levine J. Pain and analgesia the value of the salience circuit. Prog Neurobiol. 2013;104:93–105.
113. Bahra A, May A, Goadsby PJ. Cluster headache: a prospective clinical study with diagnostic implications. Neurology. 2002;58:354–61.
114. Tracey I. Imaging pain. Br J Anaesth. 2008;101:32–9.
115. Adamson MM, et al. Higher landing accuracy in expert pilots is associated with lower activity in the caudate nucleus. PLoS One. 2014;9:e112607.
116. Uddin LQ. The self in autism: an emerging view from neuroimaging. Neurocase. 2011;17:201–8.
117. Elsenbruch S, et al. Patients with irritable bowel syndrome have altered emotional modulation of neural responses to visceral stimuli. Gastroenterology. 2010;139:1310–9.
118. Eck J, Richter M, Straube T, Miltner WHR, Weiss T. Affective brain regions are activated during the processing of pain-related words in migraine patients. Pain. 2011;152:1104–13.
119. Maleki N, Becerra L, Borsook D. Migraine: maladaptive brain responses to stress. Headache. 2012;52:102–6.

120. Palaniyappan L, Simmonite M, White TP, Liddle EB, Liddle PF. Neural primacy of the salience processing system in schizophrenia. Neuron. 2013;79:814–28.
121. Geng X, et al. Salience and default mode network dysregulation in chronic cocaine users predict treatment outcome. Brain. 2017;140:1513–24.
122. Morelli N, et al. Brainstem activation in cluster headache: an adaptive behavioural response? Cephalalgia. 2013;33:416–20.
123. Sprenger T, et al. Hypothalamic activation in trigeminal autonomic cephalgia: functional imaging of an atypical case. Cephalalgia. 2004;24:753–7.
124. Auer T, et al. Attack-related brainstem activation in a patient with SUNCT syndrome: an Ictal fMRI study. Headache. 2009;49:909–12.
125. Sprenger T, et al. SUNCT: bilateral hypothalamic activation during headache attacks and resolving of symptoms after trigeminal decompression. Pain. 2005;113:422–6.

Chapter 8
Some Observations About the Origin of the Pain in Cluster Headache

Trine Nielsen, Arne May, and Tim P. Jürgens

8.1   Introduction

Given the clinical presentation and neuroscientific evidence, it is undisputed that the hypothalamus plays a central role in cluster headache (CH) pathogenesis [1, 2]. But does an activation of the hypothalamus suffice in generating the perception of pain or are peripheral structures required? This chapter revolves around the question of nociceptive input: where does the pain in CH originate from? This is a question which, as of yet, has no conclusive answer [2–5]. However, looking at previous research and clinical observations, we might be able to make some assumptions and pose some qualified guesses.

In order for an anatomical structure to come into consideration as the origin of the pain, it must have an effect on the trigeminocervical complex (TCC) [6]: an extension of the spinal nucleus of the trigeminal nerve into the adjacent column of grey matter from the brainstem into the upper cervical cord receiving nociceptive intra- and extracranial afferents from the trigeminal nerve and the upper cervical spinal nerves (C1 and C2) converging onto second-order neurons. These neurons project cranially and form a most complex network throughout the brainstem, diencephalic and cortical areas [7, 8]. Signals are relayed to medullary pontine nuclei [9], to hypothalamic nuclei via the trigeminohypothalamic tract [10] and along the quintothalamic tract to areas in the thalamus such as the ventral posterior medial nucleus (VPM) [11]. Higher central structures, such as the somatosensory cortex and insular cortex, take part in the integration and processing of nociception [8, 12].

T. Nielsen (✉) · A. May
Department of Systems Neuroscience, University Medical Centre Hamburg-Eppendorf, Hamburg, Germany
e-mail: trine.nielsen.11@regionh.dk

T. P. Jürgens
Department of Neurology, University Medical Center Rostock, Rostock, Germany
e-mail: Tim.Juergens@med.uni-rostock.de

© Springer Nature Switzerland AG 2020   91
M. Leone, A. May (eds.), *Cluster Headache and other Trigeminal Autonomic Cephalgias*, Headache, https://doi.org/10.1007/978-3-030-12438-0_8

However, they also convey descending, direct and indirect modulatory signals via several anatomical structures [13], including the hypothalamus [14, 15] and, in turn, through other medullary pontine nuclei.

Also contributing to the rich brainstem network is the connection between the TCC and the superior salivatory nucleus (SSN) as the main parasympathetic nucleus. Efferent parasympathetic fibres project through the greater petrosal branch of the facial nerve and the sphenopalatine ganglion (SPG), where they synapse to secondary neurons, to the lacrimal gland, nasal mucosa and the cranial vasculature [16]. This connection allows for a reflex response to trigeminal stimuli on the cranial vasculature, dura mater and the lacrimal gland (the trigeminal-autonomic reflex) [3]. Other efferent fibres project to the parotid and buccal secretory glands via the otic ganglion [16].

This anatomical construct leads to the question of whether the pain originates from a peripheral structure, in which case it would have to be within the receptive fields of the aforementioned nociceptive afferents, or whether it originates centrally.

Any structure considered must, in addition, fit into a pathophysiological model which provides a satisfactory explanation to some of the main features of the disease, namely the severe pain intensity, the strict unilaterality and mainly retro-orbital location of the pain, the symptoms of parasympathetic activation and sympathetic deficit and the striking circadian and circannual rhythmicity [17]. Furthermore, one would expect excitatory and inhibitory stimulation of the structure to lead to initiation and termination of a CH attack, respectively.

Taken together, this leaves the following structures to be considered:

- The eye and retro-orbital tissue
- Intra- and extracranial vessels including the cavernous sinus and the internal carotid artery
- Peripheral nervous tissue such as the trigeminal nerve and trigeminal ganglion, the parasympathetic branch of the facial nerve and the sphenopalatine ganglion and the vagal nerve
- Central nervous structures such as brainstem networks and the hypothalamus.

In the following, the above-mentioned structures will be discussed as possible origins of pain. Clinical and pathophysiological aspects regarding the attack generation and oscillating systems are described in other chapters; hence their mention will be kept to a minimum in this chapter.

8.2   The Possible Sites of Pain Origin

8.2.1   The Eye and Retro-Orbital Tissue

The most pronounced symptom in CH is the severe pain located mainly supra- or retro-orbitally. Some patients describe a feeling of having their eye pushed out of its socket [5], which entails the question whether CH could be an ocular disease.

Intraictal intraocular pressure measurements in CH patients show increased pressure bilaterally but predominantly ipsilateral to the symptomatic side [18]. The change in intraocular pressure happens swiftly, which points more towards a changed intraorbital blood volume than a change in aqueous humour, as this is a slower process [18]. However, neither pain nor autonomic symptoms experienced during a CH attack could be elicited by an experimentally induced increase in intraocular pressure (Valsalva manoeuvre) interictally in CH patients within a cluster bout. However, the intraocular pressure increases significantly more on the symptomatic side when the patient is within a bout [19]. As CH still occurs after removal of the orbital bulb [20, 21], it is safe to assume that cluster headache is not an ocular disease. The increased intraorbital pressure could, however, point towards a dysfunction of the orbital vascular bed, either as a vascular disturbance or as an epiphenomenon occurring due to a nervous malfunction [19].

8.2.2   Vascular Structures

Cluster headache, as first described by Horton et al., has long been referred to as a vascular headache [22]. Vasodilation within the trigeminovascular system has been observed during attacks [23, 24], and experimentally induced attacks with vasodilating agents such as nitroglycerin and histamine have been reported [25, 26]. However, as vasodilatation is not necessary for an attack to occur [27] and as vasodilating agents cannot elicit an attack in patients outside of a bout [25], CH is now recognised as a *neuro*-vascular disease [3].

A multitude of vascular structures have been placed under scrutiny in the search of a peripheral origin of pain in CH. Of the intra- and extracranial vessels investigated, especially the cavernous sinus and the internal carotid artery have been given much attention.

8.2.2.1   Cavernous Sinus

The cavernous sinus is, with its parasellar location and close relation with a myriad of vascular and nervous structures, an intriguing anatomical location when considering the origin of pain in CH. In fact, given its distinct anatomical features the cavernous sinus has been mentioned early in the literature as the possible source of the pain in CH [28–30]. The sinus is a dural cavity receiving venous output from the superior and inferior ophthalmic veins. Various structures traverse the sinus, such as the internal carotid artery densely innervated with sympathetic autonomic fibres, the oculomotor nerve, the trochlear nerve, the ophthalmic and maxillary branch of the trigeminal nerve and the abducens nerve. A malady in this area could affect the ophthalmic division of the trigeminal nerve and thereby explain the location of the headache pain. Moreover, it could explain the sympathetic deficit as an undermining of the sympathetic fibres located along the wall of the internal carotid artery.

In the late 1980s it was postulated that the pain in CH originates as an intracavernous inflammatory process [30]. It had been shown that irritative stimuli on the cavernous sinus amongst other vascular structures could produce pain in or behind the eye. Moreover, studies using orbital phlebography had pointed towards an inflammatory process in the cavernous sinus during CH attacks [29].

It was thought that an inflammation in this area would obliterate venous outflow from the sinus and, in cases with insufficient drainage, thereby causing venous congestion, which was argued to be painful [28]. Furthermore, the inflammation was thought to cause damage to poorly myelinated sympathetic fibres, causing symptoms of sympathetic deficit, which in turn afflicted the duration of the attack. The explanation being that a regeneration of the myelin would cause an attack to cease, whereas a prolonged inflammation could cause a chronification of the disease. Moreover, the tendency of a CH attack to initiate during sleep in a circadian pattern was explained with the increase in venous load due to horizontal positioning [28].

The theory was dismissed [16, 31] after several studies had shown either no signs of inflammation in magnetic resonance imaging (MRI) [32], similar findings with orbital phlebography in patients with other diseases [33, 34] or no differences in frequency of pathology between CH patients and patients with tension-type headache (TTH) or migraine [35].

If the cavernous sinus is the pain origin in CH, it is not because of inflammation [31]. But could it be due to another dysfunction in the area? The characteristic ipsilateral location would still remain enigmatic, considering the anastomoses connecting the bilateral cavernous sinuses. Moreover, how it is possible that none of the other cranial nerves crossing the sinus are affected and causing symptoms?

8.2.2.2 Internal Carotid Artery

Along with the cavernous sinus the internal carotid artery (ICA) has been argued to be a peripheral drive in the CH pain [36]. The ICA arises from the common carotid artery bilaterally as it bifurcates into an external and internal part. A sympathetic nervous plexus, the carotid plexus, surrounds the artery which protrudes cranially.

A case study reported two cases of CH following carotid endarterectomy. It was argued that, in patients with existing hypothalamic dysfunction, damage to the trigeminal nerve roots, along with damage to the sympathetic plexus on the ICA, could present a peripheral trigger mechanism for CH, causing pain, vasodilatation and in turn reflex parasympathetic activation of the trigeminal-autonomic reflex [3, 36].

Secondary cluster-like headache following carotid endarterectomy is rarely reported, however, often enough for it to be listed in the IHS classifications system [17]. Moreover, carotid dissection has been reported to elicit symptoms mimicking CH attacks [37].

It is worth noticing that changes in blood flow through the ICA are an epiphenomenon to nociceptive input on the first trigeminal branch [3].

If one considers the carotid artery as the source of the pain, one implies that damage of the trigeminal C-fibres travelling along the vessel wall into the cranium is responsible. There is no definite answer why this cannot be the case and this theory therefore must stand at the moment. However, the strict side-locked and retro-orbital spatial distribution pain would be difficult to explain.

8.2.3   The Trigeminal Nerve and Ganglion

The pain in CH is mainly distributed within an area innervated by the trigeminal nerve. The pseudounipolar trigeminal nerve provides the sensory innervation of structures such as the frontal dura mater, the meningeal vessels and the most components of the eye. Providing afferent somatosensory information from these structures via the trigeminal ganglion to the TCC in the brainstem, this nerve plays a central role in the speculations about the origin of the CH pain.

Activation of the trigeminovascular system in CH has been demonstrated by means of increased jugular blood levels of calcitonin gene-related peptide (CGRP) within CH attacks [24]. Moreover, triptans, one of the key therapeutics in the acute treatment of CH, exert their effects on the 5-hydroxytryptamine (5-HT) 1B/1D receptors mainly on trigeminal nerve endings and blood vessels, respectively, causing diminished release of neurotransmitter and vasoconstriction. This indicates that the trigeminal nerve could be an important nociceptive component of CH. However, CH has been shown to persist despite complete trigeminal nerve root section in two case reports [27, 38] where continued effects of triptans were reported in one patient. This data must be regarded with caution, as there are no more than these two reports. In addition, though, it has been shown that some newer triptans able to cross the blood-brain barrier might also have an inhibitory effect on neurons within the TCC [7, 39]. Taken together, it seems unlikely that activation of the trigeminal system alone can explain the pain in CH [4].

8.2.4   The Parasympathetic Fibres of the Facial Nerve
and the Sphenopalatine Ganglion

Parasympathetic activation and resulting symptoms closely accompany the pain in CH [24]. The parasympathetic fibres of the facial nerve form the efferent component of the trigeminal-autonomic reflex [3], innervating the lacrimal gland, mucosa of the nasopharynx and the meningeal vessels [40]. Activation of the SSN near the TCC results in signals relayed via preganglionic fibres projecting to the sphenopalatine ganglion (SPG) where most fibres synapse onto postganglionic fibres. Sympathetic fibres from the carotid plexus follow the same path but only bypass the SPG without synapsing [41]. Whether trigeminal nociception causes parasympathetic activation in CH or vice versa is still unknown. However, the close relation between the structures is evident through the trigeminal-autonomic reflex and furthermore through an anatomic link between the SPG and the trigeminal ganglion [42]. A hypothesis is that, as a consequence of SPG stimulation, subsequent activation of trigeminal nociceptors relays signals to the TCC which in turn activates the SSN via the trigeminal-autonomic reflex, thus forming a self-reinforcing mechanism [41] which generates and maintains the CH pain.

High frequency stimulation of the SPG with an implanted neurostimulator has shown a significant effect in aborting acute attacks as well as in reducing attack frequency [43, 44]. Moreover, low frequency stimulation of the SPG induced cluster-like attacks in three of six chronic CH patients within 30 min after stimulation, which in turn could be treated with high frequency stimulation [45]. This indicates that neurotransmitters released from parasympathetic fibres may activate or modulate trigeminal nociception. This is supported by the fact that SPG blockade [46] or ablation reduces attack frequency [47] and alleviates pain in CH patients [44].

The role of the SPG in CH is intriguing. Most of the initially listed criteria for a peripheral structure to act as a drive for the pain in CH are fulfilled. However, although rare, CH without autonomic symptoms is well known [48] and does indicate that the parasympathetic activation is more likely an epiphenomenon to trigeminal activation than vice versa.

8.2.5   The Vagal Nerve

The vagal nerve is a mixed nerve with both afferent and efferent components. The majority of the cervical vagus nerve fibres carry sensory afferents which relay their input to the nucleus tractus solitarius (NTS) in the brainstem [49, 50]. From here afferents project to different nuclei related to primary headaches such as the locus coeruleus (LC), the dorsal raphe nucleus (DRN) [51], the paraventricular hypothalamus (PVN) [52] and the trigeminal nucleus [53]. Non-invasive vagus nerve stimulation (nVNS) has been proved effective in CH treatment of acute attacks in episodic CH but not in chronic CH patients [54]. The exact mechanism for the pain-relieving as well as frequency-reducing effects is not known. However, animal studies and human fMRI studies have shown that VNS has an inhibitory effect on areas including the spinal trigeminal nucleus [55, 56]. It has moreover been speculated that VNS has an indirect modulatory mechanism on the trigeminovascular system [53]. For example, through activation of areas such as the PVN and LC which lead to an anti-nociceptive modulation on the trigeminal-autonomic system [57].

8.2.6   Brainstem Networks

Several brainstem nuclei are involved in pain transmission in general and trigeminal nociception [8] and headache [58] in particular. However, whereas the brainstem has been repeatedly been discussed as being pivotal in migraine pathophysiology

[58, 59], it has never been shown in neuroimaging to be involved in generating cluster headache attacks [60].

8.2.7   Hypothalamus

Involvement of the hypothalamus in CH has become evident through findings in CH patients such as abnormal structural changes in the inferior posterior hypothalamus with neuronal dysfunction [61, 62] and, more importantly, hypothalamic activation of the ipsilateral inferior hypothalamic grey matter during CH attacks [63]. It has therefore been suggested that the hypothalamus serves as a central generator of CH attacks with a focus in the inferior posterior hypothalamus. The theory has led to trials with deep brain stimulation in CH patients with intractable CH [64–66]. Clinical improvement was found in 60% of the cases; however, the effect of hypothalamic high frequency stimulation is only preventive and occurs after prolonged stimulations of weeks to months [67]. As there is no effect of deep brain stimulation on acute CH attacks [66] and as hypothalamic stimulation have never been reported to have triggered attacks, another mechanism of the hypothalamus than a mere inhibitory or excitatory mechanism [68] is sought. It has been suggested that the hypothalamus provides a permissive state for the trigeminal-autonomic reflex and is to a higher degree implicated in terminating rather than triggering CH attacks [67].

8.3   Conclusion

The exact anatomical structure generating the nociceptive input in cluster headache cannot, as of yet, be unequivocally identified. However, there are several reasons why it should be located in the periphery rather than just in the brain:

- Stimulation of the hypothalamus does not evoke cluster attacks [64, 68].
- Sumatriptan penetrates the blood-brain barrier poorly but has excellent therapeutic efficacy in acute attacks of CH. Likewise, monoclonal CGRP antibodies probably have a site of action outside of the CNS as they do not cross the BBB to a relevant extent under normal conditions [1].
- SPG stimulation disrupts the trigeminal-autonomic reflex and offers acute pain relief in CH patients [69].
- Peripheral mechanisms alone cannot satisfactorily explain the complete symptomatology of CH [2].

If one accepts the notion that the central brain signals, involving the hypothalamus, are attack-generating rather than pain-producing, one also has to conclude that the pain must come from the periphery. This excludes (as pointed out above) the parasympathetic system, the sinus cavernosus and, most likely, the carotid arteries and also the eye itself. From all the above data and considerations we propose that the nociception, i.e. activation of nociceptors generating the pain signal, is probably generated from structures behind the eye and has an arterial and/or venous origin. However, what exactly excites trigeminal input in the retro-orbital space, be it vessel calibre or aseptic inflammation or both, remains uncertain. It is intriguing that all known cluster headache triggers (nitroglycerin, alcohol, histamine, warmth) involve vessel calibre change [1, 70]. However, it needs to be pointed out that, whatever the source, it can only lead to pain signals when the hypothalamic area drifts into a permissive state in episodic as well as in chronic cluster headache.

References

1. Hoffmann J, May A. Diagnosis, pathophysiology, and management of cluster headache. Lancet Neurol. 2018;17(1):75–83.
2. Barloese MCJ. The pathophysiology of the trigeminal autonomic cephalalgias, with clinical implications. Clin Auton Res. 2018;28(3):315–24.
3. Goadsby PJ. Pathophysiology of cluster headache: a trigeminal autonomic cephalgia. Lancet Neurol. 2002;1(4):251–7.
4. Leone M, Proietti CA. Advances in the understanding of cluster headache. Expert Rev Neurother. 2017;17(2):165–72.
5. May A. Cluster headache: pathogenesis, diagnosis, and management. Lancet. 2005;366(9488):843–55.
6. Bogduk N. Anatomy and physiology of headache. Biomed Pharmacother. 1995;49(10):435–45.
7. Goadsby PJ, Holland PR, Martins-Oliveira M, Hoffmann J, Schankin C, Akerman S. Pathophysiology of migraine: a disorder of sensory processing. Physiol Rev. 2017;97(2):553–622.
8. Schulte LH, Sprenger C, May A. Physiological brainstem mechanisms of trigeminal nociception: an fMRI study at 3T. NeuroImage. 2016;124(Pt A):518–25.
9. Liu Y, Broman J, Zhang M, Edvinsson L. Brainstem and thalamic projections from a craniovascular sensory nervous centre in the rostral cervical spinal dorsal horn of rats. Cephalalgia. 2009;29(9):935–48.
10. Malick A, Burstein R. Cells of origin of the trigeminohypothalamic tract in the rat. J Comp Neurol. 1998;400(1):125–44.
11. Williams MN, Zahm DS, Jacquin MF. Differential foci and synaptic organization of the principal and spinal trigeminal projections to the thalamus in the rat. Eur J Neurosci. 1994;6(3):429–53.
12. DaSilva AFM, Becerra L, Makris N, Strassman AM, Gonzalez RG, Geatrakis N, Borsook D. Somatotopic activation in the human trigeminal pain pathway. J Neurosci. 2002;22(18):8183–92.
13. Tracey I, Mantyh PW. The cerebral signature for pain perception and its modulation. Neuron. 2007;55(3):377–91.
14. Malick A, Strassman RM, Burstein R. Trigeminohypothalamic and reticulohypothalamic tract neurons in the upper cervical spinal cord and caudal medulla of the rat. J Neurophysiol. 2000;84(4):2078–112.
15. Bartsch T, Levy MJ, Knight YE, Goadsby PJ. Differential modulation of nociceptive dural input to [hypocretin] orexin A and B receptor activation in the posterior hypothalamic area. Pain. 2004;109(3):367–78.
16. May A, Goadsby PJ. The trigeminovascular system in humans: pathophysiologic implications for primary headache syndromes of the neural influences on the cerebral circulation. J Cereb Blood Flow Metab. 1999;19(2):115–27.

17. Headache Classification Committee of the International Headache Society (IHS). The international classification of headache disorders, 3rd edition (beta version). Cephalalgia. 2013;33(9):629–808.
18. Horven I, Sjaastad O. Cluster headache syndrome and migraine. Ophthalmological support for a two-entity theory. Acta Ophthalmol. 1977;55(1):35–51.
19. Barriga FJ, Sánchez-del-Río M, Barón M, Dobato J, Gili P, Yangüela J, Bueno A, Pareja JA. Cluster headache: interictal asymmetric increment in intraocular pressure elicited by Valsalva manoeuvre. Cephalalgia. 2004;24(3):185–7.
20. Evers S, Sörös P, Brilla R, Gerding H, Husstedt IW. Cluster headache after orbital exenteration. Cephalalgia. 1997;17(6):680–2.
21. Rogado AZ, Graham JR, Graham P. Headache rounds—through a glass darkly. Headache. 1979;19(2):058–62.
22. Fanciullacci M. When cluster headache was called histaminic cephalalgia (Horton's headache). J Headache Pain. 2006;7(4):231–4.
23. May A, Bahra A, Büchel C, Frackowiak RS, Goadsby PJ. PET and MRA findings in cluster headache and MRA in experimental pain. Neurology. 2000;55(9):1328–35.
24. Goadsby PJ, Edvinsson L. Human in vivo evidence for trigeminovascular activation in cluster headache. Neuropeptide changes and effects of acute attacks therapies. Brain J Neurol. 1994;117(Pt 3):427–34.
25. Ekbom K. Nitroglycerin as a provocative agent in cluster headache. Arch Neurol. 1968;19(5):487–93.
26. Horton BT. Histaminic cephalgia. J Lancet. 1952;72(2):92–8.
27. Matharu MS, Goadsby PJ. Persistence of attacks of cluster headache after trigeminal nerve root section. Brain. 2002;125(5):976–84.
28. Hardebo JE. How cluster headache is explained as an intracavernous inflammatory process lesioning sympathetic fibers. Headache. 1994;34(3):125–31.
29. Hannerz J. Orbital phlebography and signs of inflammation in episodic and chronic cluster headache. Headache. 1991;31(8):540–2.
30. Moskowitz MA. Cluster headache: evidence for a pathophysiologic focus in the superior pericarotid cavernous sinus plexus. Headache. 1988;28(9):584–6.
31. Remahl IN, Waldenlind E, Bratt J, Ekbom K. Cluster headache is not associated with signs of a systemic inflammation. Headache. 2000;40(4):276–82.
32. Sjaastad O, Rinck P. Cluster headache: MRI studies of the cavernous sinus and the base of the brain. Headache. 1990;30(6):350–1.
33. Hannerz J, Greitz D, Hansson P, Ericson K. SUNCT may be another manifestation of orbital venous vasculitis. Headache. 1992;32(8):384–9.
34. Hannerz J. Pathoanatomic studies in a case of Tolosa-Hunt syndrome. Cephalalgia. 1988;8(1):25–30.
35. Bovim G, Jenssen G, Ericson K. Orbital phlebography: a comparison between cluster headache and other headaches. Headache. 1992;32(8):408–12.
36. Dirkx THT, Koehler PJ. Post-operative cluster headache following carotid endarterectomy. Eur Neurol. 2017;77(3–4):175–9.
37. Candeloro E, Canavero I, Maurelli M, Cavallini A, Ghiotto N, Vitali P, Micieli G. Carotid dissection mimicking a new attack of cluster headache. J Headache Pain. 2013;14:84.
38. Jarrar RG, Black DF, Dodick DW, Davis DH. Outcome of trigeminal nerve section in the treatment of chronic cluster headache. Neurology. 2003;60(8):1360–2.
39. Classey JD, Bartsch T, Goadsby PJ. Distribution of 5-HT1B, 5-HT1D and 5-HT1F receptor expression in rat trigeminal and dorsal root ganglia neurons: relevance to the selective antimigraine effect of triptans. Brain Res. 2010;1361:76–85.
40. Uddman R, Hara H, Edvinsson L. Neuronal pathways to the rat middle meningeal artery revealed by retrograde tracing and immunocytochemistry. J Auton Nerv Syst. 1989;26(1):69–75.
41. Jürgens TP, May A. Role of sphenopalatine ganglion stimulation in cluster headache. Curr Pain Headache Rep. 2014;18(7):433.

42. Csati A, Tajti J, Tuka B, Edvinsson L, Warfvinge K. Calcitonin gene-related peptide and its receptor components in the human sphenopalatine ganglion—interaction with the sensory system. Brain Res. 2012;1435:29–39.
43. Schoenen J, Jensen RH, Lantéri-Minet M, Láinez MJA, Gaul C, Goodman AM, et al. Stimulation of the sphenopalatine ganglion (SPG) for cluster headache treatment. Pathway CH-1: a randomized, sham-controlled study. Cephalalgia. 2013;33(10):816–30.
44. Jürgens TP, Barloese M, May A, Láinez JM, Schoenen J, Gaul C, Goodman AM, Caparso A, Jensen RH. Long-term effectiveness of sphenopalatine ganglion stimulation for cluster headache. Cephalalgia. 2017;37(5):423–34.
45. Schytz HW, Barløse M, Guo S, Selb J, Caparso A, Jensen R, Ashina M. Experimental activation of the sphenopalatine ganglion provokes cluster-like attacks in humans. Cephalalgia. 2013;33(10):831–41.
46. Sanders M, Zuurmond WW. Efficacy of sphenopalatine ganglion blockade in 66 patients suffering from cluster headache: a 12- to 70-month follow-up evaluation. J Neurosurg. 1997;87(6):876–80.
47. Narouze S, Kapural L, Casanova J, Mekhail N. Sphenopalatine ganglion radiofrequency ablation for the management of chronic cluster headache. Headache. 2009;49(4):571–7.
48. Martins IP, Gouveia RG, Antunes JL. Double dissociation between autonomic symptoms and pain in cluster headache. Cephalalgia. 2005;25(5):398–400.
49. Nemeroff CB, Mayberg HS, Krahl SE, McNamara J, Frazer A, Henry TR, George MS, Charney DS, Brannan SK. VNS therapy in treatment-resistant depression: clinical evidence and putative neurobiological mechanisms. Neuropsychopharmacology. 2006;31(7):1345–55.
50. Foley JO, DuBois FS. Quantitative studies of the vagus nerve in the cat. I. The ratio of sensory to motor fibers. J Comp Neurol. 1937;67(1):49–67.
51. Dorr AE, Debonnel G. Effect of vagus nerve stimulation on serotonergic and noradrenergic transmission. J Pharmacol Exp Ther. 2006;318(2):890–8.
52. Cunningham JT, Mifflin SW, Gould GG, Frazer A. Induction of c-Fos and DeltaFosB immunoreactivity in rat brain by Vagal nerve stimulation. Neuropsychopharmacology. 2008;33(8):1884–95.
53. Gwyn DG, Leslie RA, Hopkins DA. Observations on the afferent and efferent organization of the vagus nerve and the innervation of the stomach in the squirrel monkey. J Comp Neurol. 1985;239(2):163–75.
54. Goadsby PJ, de Coo IF, Silver N, Tyagi A, Ahmed F, Gaul C, et al. Non-invasive vagus nerve stimulation for the acute treatment of episodic and chronic cluster headache: a randomized, double-blind, sham-controlled ACT2 study. Cephalalgia. 2018;38(5):959–69.
55. Akerman S, Simon B, Romero-Reyes M. Vagus nerve stimulation suppresses acute noxious activation of trigeminocervical neurons in animal models of primary headache. Neurobiol Dis. 2017;102:96–104.
56. Frangos E, Komisaruk BR. Access to vagal projections via cutaneous electrical stimulation of the neck: fMRI evidence in healthy humans. Brain Stimul. 2017;10(1):19–27.
57. Robert C, Bourgeais L, Arreto C-D, Condes-Lara M, Noseda R, Jay T, Villanueva L. Paraventricular hypothalamic regulation of trigeminovascular mechanisms involved in headaches. J Neurosci. 2013;33(20):8827–40.
58. Schulte LH, May A. The migraine generator revisited: continuous scanning of the migraine cycle over 30 days and three spontaneous attacks. Brain J Neurol. 2016;139(Pt 7):1987–93.
59. Schulte LH. Hypothalamus as a mediator of chronic migraine: evidence from high-resolution fMRI. Neurology. 2017;88(21):2011–6.
60. May A. New insights into headache: an update on functional and structural imaging findings. Nat Rev Neurol. 2009;5(4):199–209.
61. May A, Ashburner J, Büchel C, McGonigle DJ, Friston KJ, Frackowiak RS, Goadsby PJ. Correlation between structural and functional changes in brain in an idiopathic headache syndrome. Nat Med. 1999;5(7):836–8.
62. Lodi R, Pierangeli G, Tonon C, Cevoli S, Testa C, Bivona G. Study of hypothalamic metabolism in cluster headache by proton MR spectroscopy. Neurology. 2006;66(8):1264–6.

63. May A, Bahra A, Büchel C, Frackowiak RS, Goadsby PJ. Hypothalamic activation in cluster headache attacks. Lancet. 1998;352(9124):275–8.
64. Leone M, Franzini A, Bussone G. Stereotactic stimulation of posterior hypothalamic gray matter in a patient with intractable cluster headache. N Engl J Med. 2001;345(19):1428–9.
65. Bartsch T, Pinsker MO, Rasche D, Kinfe T, Hertel F, Diener HC, et al. Hypothalamic deep brain stimulation for cluster headache: experience from a new multicase series. Cephalalgia. 2008;28(3):285–95.
66. Leone M, Franzini A, Broggi G, Mea E, Cecchini AP, Bussone G. Acute hypothalamic stimulation and ongoing cluster headache attacks. Neurology. 2006;67(10):1844–5.
67. Leone M, Bussone G. Pathophysiology of trigeminal autonomic cephalalgias. Lancet Neurol. 2009;8(8):755–64.
68. Leone M, Franzini A, Broggi G, May A, Bussone G. Long-term follow-up of bilateral hypothalamic stimulation for intractable cluster headache. Brain J Neurol. 2004;127(Pt 10):2259–64.
69. Schoenen J. Sphenopalatine ganglion stimulation in neurovascular headaches. Prog Neurol Surg. 2015;29:106–16.
70. May A, Schwedt TJ, Magis D, Pozo-Rosich P, Evers S, Wang S-J. Cluster headache. Nat Rev Dis Primers. 2018;4:18006.

Chapter 9
Animals Models for Trigeminal Autonomic Cephalalgias

Simon Akerman and Cristina Tassorelli

9.1 Introduction

Trigeminal autonomic cephalalgias (TACs) are highly disabling primary headache disorders. Their pathophysiology is characterised by three major clinical features as classified by the International Classification of Headache Disorders 3rd edition [1]:

1. Severe or very severe, unilateral, trigeminal distribution of pain, sometimes described as the worst pain experienced by humans [2]
2. Lateralised-associated symptoms, including cranial autonomic features [3], such as lacrimation, conjunctival injection, and nasal congestion, and a local third-order sympathetic lesion due to carotid swelling [4]
3. Recurrent pattern of attacks [2, 5]

They are rare compared to other primary headaches, such as migraine and tension-type headache. Cluster headache is the most common, with a prevalence in the general population of about 0.1% [6, 7], similar to other debilitating neurological disorders, such as multiple sclerosis. Whereas paroxysmal hemicranias is approximately 1:50,000, while short-lasting unilateral neuralgiform headache attacks with conjunctival injection and tearing (SUNCT) and short-lasting unilateral neuralgiform headache (SUNA) have a prevalence of approximately 1:15,000. The TACs are differentiated from each other by their highly individual characteristic attack patterns, and also to some extent by their response to treatments, as sum-

S. Akerman (✉)
Department of Neural and Pain Sciences, University of Maryland Baltimore, Baltimore, MD, USA
e-mail: sakerman@umaryland.edu

C. Tassorelli
Headache Science Centre, IRCCS. C. Mondino Foundation, Pavia, Italy

Department of Brain and Behavioural Sciences, University of Pavia, Pavia, Italy
e-mail: cristina.tassorelli@unipv.it

© Springer Nature Switzerland AG 2020
M. Leone, A. May (eds.), *Cluster Headache and other Trigeminal Autonomic Cephalgias*, Headache, https://doi.org/10.1007/978-3-030-12438-0_9

Table 9.1 Clinical features and treatments of trigeminal autonomic cephalalgias [5, 8, 9]

	Cluster headache	Paroxysmal hemicrania/CPH	SUNCT/SUNA
Sex F:M	1:3	1:1/7:1	1:1.2
Prevalence	0.1%	1/50,000	1/15,000
Pain type Severity Site	Stabbing, boring Excruciating Orbit, temple	Throbbing, boring, stabbing Excruciating Orbit, temple	Burning, stabbing, sharp Severe to excruciating Periorbital
Attack frequency	1/alternate days to 8/ day	1–40/day (>5/day most of the time)	3–200/day
Duration of attack	15–180 min	2–30 min	5–240 s
Autonomic features	Yes	Yes	Yes (mainly conjunctival injection and lacrimation –SUNCT)
Abortive treatments	Sumatriptan, oxygen	None	None
Preventive treatments	Verapamil, methysergide, lithium	Indomethacin (absolute response)	Lamotrigine, topiramate, gabapentin

CPH chronic paroxysmal hemicranias, *SUNCT* short-lasting unilateral neuralgiform headache attacks with conjunctival injection and tearing, *SUNA* short-lasting unilateral neuralgiform headache

marised in Table 9.1 [5, 8, 9]. Cluster headache attacks tend to have the longest duration with lower attack frequency per day and seem to respond specifically to oxygen and sumatriptan treatment [10]. Paroxysmal hemicrania has an intermediate duration and attack frequency per day and is specifically defined by its response to indomethacin [11]. SUNCT and SUNA have the shortest duration with many attacks per day [12], while hemicrania continua has unremitting pain [13].

9.2   Animal Models: Putative Mechanisms

Generally, the development of animal models for a particular disorder has two major aims: to help understand its pathophysiology and to aid in the identification, development and screening of novel and effective therapeutic targets. It is therefore important that these models clearly translate the clinical features of a disorder, using what is currently known about its pathophysiology. These include the anatomy, physiology, pharmacology, molecular biology and genetics, as well as response to treatments. Translating all of these components into a single preclinical approach is often complex, so that only one or two may be captured in a single model. However, the likelihood is that the more features that are translated, the more accurate and reliable the animal approach. In the case of TACs, the very clear classification of symptoms for diagnosis [1] and the well-defined clinical features represent a huge advantage when trying to develop a translational preclinical approach. However, with that being said, historically, there has been a dearth of animal models for TACs. The majority of our understanding comes from clinical research and studies in patients experiencing headache attacks, as well as preclinical studies into generalised primary headache mechanisms, where the anatomy and physiology of the trigeminovascular and cranial autonomic systems are likely shared across many headache disorders.

9.2.1 Evidence from Clinical Studies

A defining feature of TACs compared to other primary headaches is a very clear and reproducible activation in the posterior hypothalamic grey matter, demonstrated in cluster headache [14], paroxysmal hemicrania [15], SUNCT [16] and hemicrania continua [17]. Furthermore, deep brain stimulation of this region has been shown to relieve symptoms in cluster headache [18], chronic paroxysmal hemicrania [19] and SUNCT [20, 21]. In an experimental clinical approach for TACs, capsaicin injection into the forehead produces pain, and many of the vascular changes present during TACs, but no hypothalamic (or even brainstem) activation [22]. The implication is that the trigeminally mediated pain and vascular changes are not the cause of the hypothalamic activation; rather hypothalamic activation causes the subsequent activation of trigeminovascular and cranial autonomic pathways, resulting in TAC symptoms. There is also evidence of release of calcitonin gene-related peptide (CGRP) and vasoactive intestinal peptide (VIP) into the extracranial vasculature during attacks of cluster headache [23] and of chronic paroxysmal hemicrania [24], and release of pituitary adenylate cyclase-activating peptide (PACAP) during cluster headache attacks [25]. The different TACs also have very specific response to treatments (Table 9.1), which can be used as a tool in developing an animal model of TACs. Indeed, CGRP release during cluster headache attacks is normalised by treatment with oxygen or sumatriptan, but not by opioids [23], indicative of the important role of this peptide in cluster headache pathophysiology.

9.2.2 Evidence from Preclinical Studies

The anatomy and physiology of the trigeminovascular and cranial autonomic systems is now well described and is likely shared across many primary headache disorders, including TACs. The pain associated with TACs is mainly located in and around the orbit, peri-orbitally or temporally. This localised pain is thought to be mediated by trigeminal inputs that originate at the dural superior sagittal sinus and middle meningeal artery [26, 27]. Stimulation of these sites in preclinical studies results in neuronal activation in trigeminocervical neurons [28, 29]. Therefore, the excruciating trigeminal distribution of pain is likely a consequence of activation of the trigeminovascular system innervation of the dura mater. Dural-nociceptive stimulation also leads to ascending neuronal activation in higher brainstem and diencephalic nuclei [30–32] involved in pain processing, including the superior salivatory nucleus (SuS) within the pons [33], via a reflex connection from the trigeminal nucleus caudalis (TNC). Lateralised cranial autonomic features are believed to result from activation of this trigeminal autonomic reflex arc to the SuS and its projection to the cranial vessels and lacrimal glands. As a defining feature in TACs, it is therefore thought that this projection plays a far more significant role in their pathophysiology. The last defining characteristic of TACs is the episodic and circadian nature of attacks, believed to be related to the internal control of biological rhythms. This is likely via hypothalamic activation, previously alluded to in the clinical section of this chapter. Anatomically, reciprocal functional connections between the TNC and various hypothalamic nuclei that receive dural nociceptive information and provide descending control of trigeminovascular nociceptive traffic have been described. The SuS also receives descending projections from various hypothalamic nuclei, including the paraventricular hypothalamic nuclei (PVN) [34], as well as limbic and cortical areas [35–37]. It therefore seems the SuS is ideally placed to integrate and relay nociceptive and autonomic information to and from the trigeminovascular system, as well as being under descending control of the hypothalamus, in the pathophysiology of TACs (detailed in Fig. 9.1).

9.3 Animal Models of TACs

The development of an animal model for a disorder requires that it translate at least one aspect of the clinical phenotype, mediated by the same pathophysiology as described in humans. However, the presence of more than one feature would likely improve its translation and reliability. Furthermore, to validate the approach, it would also require a similar response to treatments. With respect to TACs, this includes the combination of lateralisation of trigeminal distribution of pain, and associated cranial autonomic features, and some degree of cyclical recurrence of attacks, likely mediated by hypothalamic manipulation. It should also respond to treatments of proved efficacy in TACs, such as inhaled oxygen and sumatriptan for cluster headache, indomethacin for paroxysmal hemicrania and topiramate, lamotrigine, or gabapentin for SUNCT/SUNA.

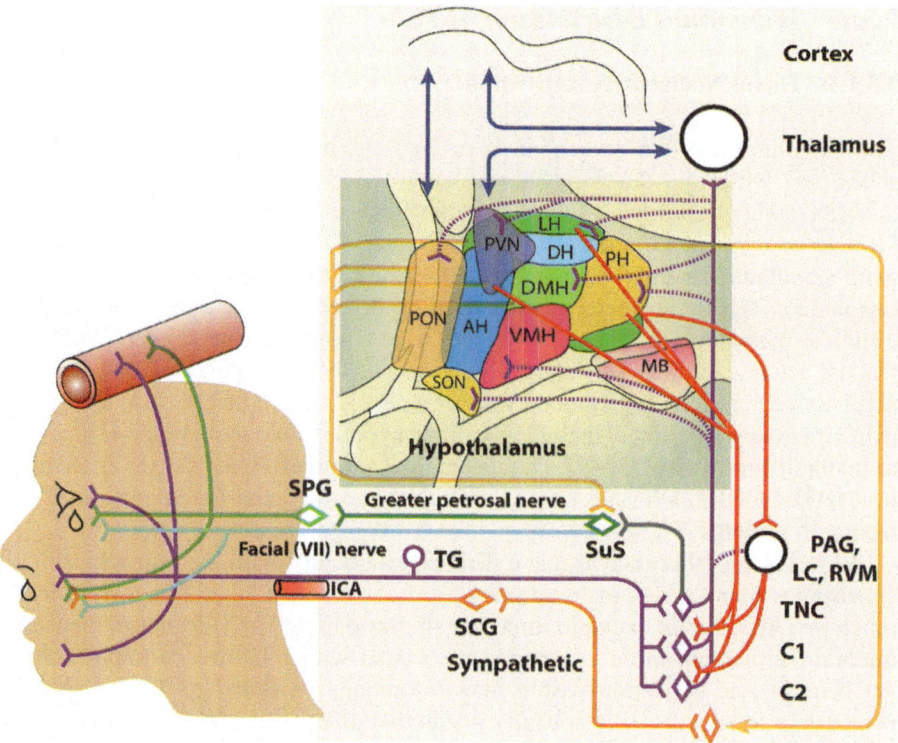

Fig. 9.1 Anatomy and pathophysiology of trigeminal autonomic cephalalgias (TACs). The trigeminal distribution of pain in TACs is likely mediated by activation of the trigeminovascular system. This includes the nociceptive-specific nerve fibres that originate in the trigeminal ganglion (TG) and innervate the peripheral cranial vasculature and its central projection to the trigeminal nucleus caudalis (TNC) and its extension to the cervical spinal cord (*the trigeminocervical complex; TCC*). Nociceptive incoming signals to the TCC ascend to higher brain structures (purple projections) including the midbrain and specific hypothalamic nuclei; the posterior (PH), supraoptic (SON) [40], ventromedial (VMH) and paraventricular hypothalamic nuclei (PVN) [41]; as well as thalamocortical neurons. Dural nociceptive activation also causes neuronal activation in the superior salivatory nucleus (SuS) within the pons [33], through a trigeminal autonomic reflex arc (grey neuron), which is the origin of cells of the autonomic parasympathetic projection to the cranial vasculature [35]. This efferent projection is predominantly through the greater petrosal nerve (green neuron), a branch of the facial (VIIth) cranial nerve (sky blue neuron), and its relay with the sphenopalatine ganglion (SPG). Cranial autonomic symptoms in TACs are believed to result from activation of this trigeminal autonomic reflex arc to the SuS and its projection to the cranial vessels and lacrimal glands. Descending projections (red and yellow neurons) from PH [70], PVN, lateral (LH) [34], dorsomedial (DMH) and preoptic (PON) hypothalamic nuclei to the TCC (red projections), SuS [34–37] and the sympathetic nervous system (both yellow projections) are thought to modulate and control both trigeminovascular nociceptive transmission (purple network of neurons) and parasympathetic (green)/sympathetic (orange) autonomic projections to the cranial vasculature that result indirectly or directly, respectively, in cranial autonomic symptoms ipsilateral to head pain. A third-order sympathetic nerve lesion (orange projection), in part mediated by internal carotid artery (ICA) vasodilation, is thought to result in Horner's syndrome. *AH* anterior hypothalamic area, *DH* dorsal hypothalamus, *MB* mammillary body

9.3.1 Trigeminal Distribution of Pain

9.3.1.1 Dural Nociceptive Activation

The trigeminal distribution of pain is perhaps the most studied in primary headaches, and while the development of many assays was predominantly to study migraine pathophysiology and screen therapeutics, there is considerable overlap for them to be relevant to other primary headaches. Based on the clinical studies of dural vasculature manipulation and pain referral in orbital, peri-orbital or temporal region [26, 27], dural nociceptive activation, driven by electrical stimulation or chemical mediators, is thought to trigger trigeminovascular nociceptive afferents that are activated during headache. This produces dural vasodilation [38] and neuronal activation in the trigeminocervical complex [28, 39], the SuS [33] and higher pain processing structures, including various hypothalamic nuclei [40, 41], as well as midbrain structures [33, 42]. Dural electrical stimulation also causes an increase in levels of CGRP, VIP and PACAP within the extracranial vasculature [43, 44], similar to findings in TACs.

A limitation of this assay is that it perhaps generically maps the neurophysiological changes found across many primary headache disorders that do not specifically relate to TACs. As an example, imaging studies during TACs do not demonstrate midbrain activation, more commonly associated with migraine pathophysiology, yet here we see activation within many structures unrelated to TACs. Also, its response to treatments does not fully match that of TACs. 100% oxygen treatment is known to specifically relieve symptoms of cluster headache, and lamotrigine is used as a preventive for SUNCT/SUNA. Whereas oxygen is unable to inhibit neurogenically mediated dural vasodilation or neuronal activation in the trigeminocervical complex [45], lamotrigine similarly has no effect on dural-nociceptive neuronal responses [46]. In fact only drugs that are effective in treating both migraine and TACs, such as triptans [47–49], non-steroidal anti-inflammatory drugs (NSAIDs) [50, 51] and topiramate [52, 53] are effective in this assay. While nociceptive trigeminovascular activation is very relevant to the pathophysiology of TACs, this model perhaps lends itself more to understanding migraine and screening for migraine therapeutics, rather than TACs. A further limitation is that without a measure of autonomic symptoms, it is difficult to translate this animal model to wider aspects of TAC pathophysiology.

9.3.1.2 Nitrergic Activation of Trigeminovascular Pain Pathways

Nitric oxide (NO) donors, such as nitroglycerin (NTG), are known to provoke cluster headache in patients [54–56] and cause the release of CGRP from the extracerebral vasculature during an attack phase [55]. NTG-provoked cluster headache also physiologically resembles spontaneous cluster headache with craniovascular vasodilation and neuronal activation in the hypothalamus [57]. In preclinical studies, NO donors cause craniovascular vasodilation [58] and activation and sensitization of primary afferent and second-order trigeminovascular neurons [59–62], with increased immunoreactivity for CGRP in the trigeminal ganglion [63] and depletion of CGRP stores in the TNC [64]. Furthermore, some of these nitrergic responses are inhibited by triptans [58], NSAIDs, specifically indomethacin [58, 65], topiramate [52] and also CGRP receptor antagonists [59, 66]. A clear disadvantage to this assay is that when cluster headache patients are in remission, NTG does not trigger a cluster attack or cause the release of CGRP or produce hypothalamic activation [14, 55, 57]. Also, it is assumed that animals are in a 'naïve' state and thus not suffering from cluster headache or another TAC. NTG is also known to trigger migraine [67] and TTH [68] in sufferers of these primary headache types, and the NTG-mediated craniovascular and trigeminovascular neuronal changes are not specific to TACs. It seems NTG in animal models is useful in helping to understand the neurovascular neuronal changes that take place in primary headaches, but it is more difficult to generalise these changes to one specific primary headache. More clues could be derived by the study of the different temporal delay of NTG-induced headache response in cluster headache and migraineurs. The latency of onset of the spontaneous-like attacks is indeed significantly shorter in cluster headache patients [55, 56], as compared with migraine subjects, which suggests possible different activation of pathways/intermediaries.

9.3.2 Trigeminal Distribution of Pain with Cranial Autonomic Features

9.3.2.1 Oral or Nasal Capsaicin Injection

It is perhaps more relevant to demonstrate more than one symptom in a preclinical approach to TACs, such as *trigeminal distribution of pain* and *cranial autonomic symptoms*. Similar to the capsaicin studies in patients, one approach has used oral and intranasal capsaicin in rodents [69]. This caused blood flow changes in dural arteries as a measure of trigeminovascular activation, and lacrimation, measured by placing filter paper to the medial angle of the eye and the change in weight used as an indicator of activation of the autonomic pathway. These responses were reversed by hexamethonium bromide, an autonomic ganglion blocker. The implication is that oral or intranasal capsaicin causes activation of the trigeminal-autonomic reflex to produce cranial vascular changes and lacrimation. While this model demonstrates several symptoms of TACs, there are reservations as to its clinical relevance. In clinical studies, the capsaicin model does not produce the signature hypothalamic activation of TACs but only the craniovascular changes [57]. Also, this approach has not been validated with TAC-specific treatments, such as oxygen or indomethacin. Perhaps this approach is a good example of trigeminal-autonomic activation, but lacking specific hypothalamic activation, it does not fully translate to the pathophysiology of TACs.

9.3.2.2 Superior Salivatory Nucleus Stimulation

To address the necessity for a central component in the mechanism of action under-lying symptoms, with hypothalamic connections, another approach has used SuS activation by means of locally delivered electrical stimuli [45, 50]. Here, dural men-ingeal artery vasodilation and neuronal firing in the trigeminocervical complex were used to measure trigeminal distribution of pain and changes in blood flow in the lacrimal gland/duct as a measure of cranial autonomic activation. SuS stimula-tion caused a modest (3.3%) increase in meningeal diameter [45]. Using electro-physiological methods to record trigeminocervical neurons, two distinct neuronal populations were determined after SuS stimulation: those with short latency of action (between 3 and 20 ms, average 12.1 ms) and those with a much longer latency of action (7–40 ms, average 20.4 ms; Fig. 9.2a, b). Using 100% inhaled oxygen to characterise a specific cluster headache response, only the longer latency neurons

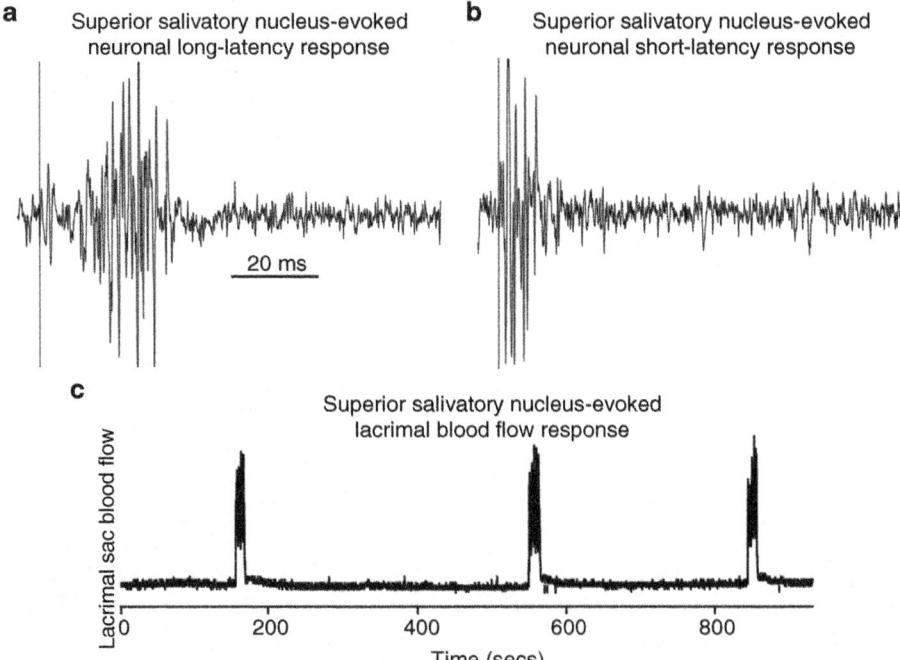

Fig. 9.2 Examples of neuronal and autonomic responses to superior salivatory nucleus (SuS) stimulation. Two populations of neurons are characterised in the trigeminocervical complex in response to SuS stimulation. A long-latency response (**a**) thought to be mediated by activation of the cranial parasympathetic projection, which traverses the dural meninges and subsequently acti-vating central trigeminovascular neurons and (**b**) a short-latency response mediated to antidromic activation of trigeminal-autonomic reflex. Lacrimal blood flow (**c**) also increases concurrent with SuS stimulation, via activation of the cranial parasympathetic projection. (**a**) and (**b**) original fig-ures, (**c**) adapted with permissions from [45]

were inhibited, whereas the shorter latency response was unaffected [45, 50]. Further characterisation with the autonomic ganglion blocker, hexamethonium bromide, determined that again only the longer latency responses were inhibited. These data suggest that the longer latency neuronal response is mediated by activation of the cranial parasympathetic projection and that the locus of action of oxygen is likely via this pathway. The shorter latency response is most likely via antidromic activation of the trigeminal-autonomic reflex. The longer latency response was further validated with TAC treatments. A triptan was significantly more efficacious than a CGRP receptor antagonist, and the cyclooxygenase (COX) inhibitor, indomethacin, was also significantly more efficacious compared to another NSAID, naproxen [50]. These data validate the specificity of the model to TAC treatments and highlight that their mechanism of action may be via the cranial parasympathetic projection.

The cranial autonomic response was determined by measurement of blood flow changes around the lacrimal gland/duct. SuS stimulation caused characteristic changes in flow that were reproducible over 30 min (Fig. 9.2c), indicative of an autonomic response [45]. Both 100% inhaled oxygen and hexamethonium bromide significantly inhibited the responses [45, 50], indicating they are mediated by activation of the cranial parasympathetic projection. Furthermore, both a triptan and indomethacin also inhibited these responses, whereas the CGRP receptor antagonist and naproxen had no effect [50]. These data validate the autonomic changes in this model as similar to those during TACs. Overall this model seems to represent most closely the known pathophysiology of TACs, demonstrating trigeminally mediated pain and autonomic symptoms, as well as responsiveness to treatments. It also uses a central site of origin for the initiation of the symptoms, which receives inputs from the hypothalamus, the likely site of the periodicity of attack. The lack of a dural-vasodilatory response is interesting, but it is now thought that vasodilation during TACs is an epiphenomenon and less relevant to the pathophysiology of the headache symptoms. These data support this, as vasodilation is not necessary to mediate noxious activation of trigeminocervical neurons.

9.3.3 Future Directions and Conclusion

At present perhaps the major failing of these assays is that they do not reproduce hypothalamic activation as a mediator of symptoms and a potential marker of the episodic and seasonal nature of attacks. However, several studies have shown that manipulation of hypothalamic nuclei, including the posterior hypothalamus [70] and the paraventricular hypothalamic nucleus (PVN) [34], can modulate dural-nociceptive trigeminovascular activation, indicative of *trigeminal distribution of pain and hypothalamic mechanisms*. This approach could be readily transferred to the SuS stimulation model to determine if *hypothalamic mechanisms* can alter the *trigeminally mediated pain and cranial autonomic features* observed. Another unexplored aspect of the clinical phenotype is the release of neuropeptides CGRP,

VIP and PACAP. While they have not been studied in patients with TACs, they have in migraine patients. Interestingly both PACAP and VIP mediate profound autonomic symptoms, yet only PACAP triggers migraine-like headache [71]. Similarly, in preclinical studies, PACAP, but not VIP, mediates activation and sensitization of dural-nociceptive central trigeminovascular neurons [72]. Furthermore, PACAP microinjection in the PVN also modulates trigeminovascular neurons [34]. Cranial autonomic features have not been measured in these preclinical studies, but perhaps PACAP and VIP can be used as tools to dissect pathophysiological mechanisms related to TACs in combination with other preclinical approaches mentioned. Another approach is to dissect a common genetic link in patients with TACs, which is likely to have a huge beneficial effect on the development of animal models. Only cluster headache-related studies have been conducted, and they have found there is a far greater risk if a first-degree relative is a sufferer, suggesting a genetic link [5]. However, no definitive link to a specific gene has been identified.

While the current animal models for TACs are far from ideal, not least because a single approach is trying to model all the TACs, rather than one specifically, they do however represent what we currently understand of their pathophysiology and symptomatology. As more time and resources are committed to dissect the mechanisms within these animal approaches, it is likely they will be adapted and finessed to more fully and accurately translate to these primary headache disorders.

References

1. Headache Classification Committee of the International Headache Society. The international classification of headache disorders, 3rd edition (beta version). Cephalalgia. 2013;33(9):629–808.
2. Goadsby PJ. Pathophysiology of cluster headache: a trigeminal autonomic cephalalgia. Lancet Neurol. 2002;1(4):251–7.
3. Lai T-H, Fuh J-L, Wang S-J. Cranial autonomic symptoms in migraine: characteristics and comparison with cluster headache. J Neurol Neurosurg Psychiatry. 2009;80:1116–9.
4. Drummond PD. Autonomic disturbances in cluster headache. Brain. 1988;111(Pt 5):1199–209.
5. Leone M, Bussone G. Pathophysiology of trigeminal autonomic cephalalgias. Lancet Neurol. 2009;8(8):755–64.
6. Robbins MS, Lipton RB. The epidemiology of primary headache disorders. Semin Neurol. 2010;30(2):107–19. https://doi.org/10.1055/s-0030-1249220.
7. Finkel AG. Epidemiology of cluster headache. Curr Pain Headache Rep. 2003;7(2):144–9.
8. Cohen AS, Matharu MS, Goadsby PJ. Trigeminal autonomic cephalalgias: current and future treatments. Headache. 2007;47(6):969–80.
9. May A. Update on the diagnosis and management of trigemino-autonomic headaches. J Neurol. 2006;253(12):1525–32.
10. May A. Cluster headache: pathogenesis, diagnosis, and management. Lancet. 2005;366(9488):843–55.
11. Cittadini E, Matharu MS, Goadsby PJ. Paroxysmal hemicrania: a prospective clinical study of 31 cases. Brain. 2008;131(Pt 4):1142–55.
12. Cohen AS, Matharu MS, Goadsby PJ. Short-lasting Unilateral neuralgiform Headache Attacks with conjunctival injection and Tearing (SUNCT) or cranial Autonomic features (SUNA). A prospective clinical study of SUNCT and SUNA. Brain. 2006;129:2746–60.

13. Cittadini E, Goadsby PJ. Hemicrania continua: a clinical study of 39 patients with diagnostic implications. Brain. 2010;133(Pt 7):1973–86.
14. May A, Bahra A, Buchel C, Frackowiak RS, Goadsby PJ. Hypothalamic activation in cluster headache attacks. Lancet. 1998;352(9124):275–8.
15. Matharu MS, Cohen AS, Frackowiak RS, Goadsby PJ. Posterior hypothalamic activation in paroxysmal hemicrania. Ann Neurol. 2006;59(3):535–45.
16. May A, Bahra A, Buchel C, Turner R, Goadsby PJ. Functional magnetic resonance imaging in spontaneous attacks of SUNCT: short-lasting neuralgiform headache with conjunctival injection and tearing. Ann Neurol. 1999;46(5):791–4.
17. Matharu MS, Cohen AS, McGonigle DJ, Ward N, Frackowiak RSJ, Goadsby PJ. Posterior hypothalamic and brainstem activation in hemicrania continua. Headache. 2004;44:747–61.
18. Leone M, Franzini A, Bussone G. Stereotactic stimulation of posterior hypothalamic gray matter in a patient with intractable cluster headache. N Engl J Med. 2001;345(19):1428–9.
19. Walcott BP, Bamber NI, Anderson DE. Successful treatment of chronic paroxysmal hemicrania with posterior hypothalamic stimulation: technical case report. Neurosurgery. 2009;65(5):E997discussion E. https://doi.org/10.1227/01.NEU.0000345937.05186.73.
20. Bartsch T, Falk D, Knudsen K, Reese R, Raethjen J, Mehdorn HM, et al. Deep brain stimulation of the posterior hypothalamic area in intractable short-lasting unilateral neuralgiform headache with conjunctival injection and tearing (SUNCT). Cephalalgia. 2011;31(13):1405–8. https://doi.org/10.1177/0333102411409070.
21. Leone M, Franzini A, D'Andrea G, Broggi G, Casucci G, Bussone G. Deep brain stimulation to relieve drug-resistant SUNCT. Ann Neurol. 2005;57(6):924–7. https://doi.org/10.1002/ana.20507.
22. May A, Kaube H, Buchel C, Eichten C, Rijntjes M, Juptner M, et al. Experimental cranial pain elicited by capsaicin: a PET study. Pain. 1998;74(1):61–6.
23. Goadsby PJ, Edvinsson L. Human in vivo evidence for trigeminovascular activation in cluster headache. Neuropeptide changes and effects of acute attacks therapies. Brain. 1994;117(Pt 3):427–34.
24. Goadsby PJ, Edvinsson L. Neuropeptide changes in a case of chronic paroxysmal hemicrania—evidence for trigemino-parasympathetic activation. Cephalalgia. 1996;16(6):448–50.
25. Tuka B, Szabo N, Toth E, Kincses ZT, Pardutz A, Szok D, et al. Release of PACAP-38 in episodic cluster headache patients - an exploratory study. J Headache Pain. 2016;17(1):69. https://doi.org/10.1186/s10194-016-0660-7.
26. Penfield W, McNaughton F. Dural headache and innervation of the dura mater. Arch Neurol Psychiatr. 1940;44:43–75.
27. Ray BS, Wolff HG. Experimental studies on headache. Pain sensitive structures of the head and their significance in headache. Arch Surg. 1940;41:813–56.
28. Goadsby PJ, Zagami AS. Stimulation of the superior sagittal sinus increases metabolic activity and blood flow in certain regions of the brainstem and upper cervical spinal cord of the cat. Brain. 1991;114(Pt 2):1001–11.
29. Hoskin KL, Zagami AS, Goadsby PJ. Stimulation of the middle meningeal artery leads to Fos expression in the trigeminocervical nucleus: a comparative study of monkey and cat. J Anat. 1999;194(Pt4):579–88.
30. Bernstein C, Burstein R. Sensitization of the trigeminovascular pathway: perspective and implications to migraine pathophysiology. J Clin Neurol. 2012;8(2):89–99.
31. Goadsby PJ, Lipton RB, Ferrari MD. Migraine—current understanding and treatment. N Engl J Med. 2002;346(4):257–70.
32. Akerman S, Holland PR, Goadsby PJ. Diencephalic and brainstem mechanisms in migraine. Nat Rev Neurosci. 2011;12(10):570–84.
33. Knight YE, Classey JD, Lasalandra MP, Akerman S, Kowacs F, Hoskin KL, et al. Patterns of fos expression in the rostral medulla and caudal pons evoked by noxious craniovascular stimulation and periaqueductal gray stimulation in the cat. Brain Res. 2005;1045(1–2):1–11.
34. Robert C, Bourgeais L, Arreto CD, Condes-Lara M, Noseda R, Jay T, et al. Paraventricular hypothalamic regulation of trigeminovascular mechanisms involved in headaches. J Neurosci. 2013;33(20):8827–40.

35. Spencer SE, Sawyer WB, Wada H, Platt KB, Loewy AD. CNS projections to the pterygo-palatine parasympathetic preganglionic neurons in the rat: a retrograde transneuronal viral cell body labeling study. Brain Res. 1990;534(1–2):149–69.

36. Hosoya Y, Matsushita M, Sugiura Y. A direct hypothalamic projection to the superior saliva-tory nucleus neurons in the rat. A study using anterograde autoradiographic and retrograde HRP methods. Brain Res. 1983;266(2):329–33.

37. Hosoya Y, Sugiura Y, Ito R, Kohno K. Descending projections from the hypothalamic paraven-tricular nucleus to the A5 area, including the superior salivatory nucleus, in the rat. Exp Brain Res. 1990;82(3):513–8.

38. Akerman S, Williamson DJ, Kaube H, Goadsby PJ. Nitric oxide synthase inhibitors can antag-onize neurogenic and calcitonin gene-related peptide induced dilation of dural meningeal ves-sels. Br J Pharmacol. 2002;137(1):62–8.

39. Burstein R, Yamamura H, Malick A, Strassman AM. Chemical stimulation of the intracranial dura induces enhanced responses to facial stimulation in brain stem trigeminal neurons. J Neurophysiol. 1998;79(2):964–82.

40. Benjamin L, Levy MJ, Lasalandra MP, Knight YE, Akerman S, Classey JD, et al. Hypothalamic activation after stimulation of the superior sagittal sinus in the cat: a Fos study. Neurobiol Dis. 2004;16(3):500–5.

41. Malick A, Jakubowski M, Elmquist JK, Saper CB, Burstein R. A neurohistochemical blueprint for pain-induced loss of appetite. Proc Natl Acad Sci U S A. 2001;98(17):9930–5.

42. Hoskin KL, Bulmer DCE, Lasalandra M, Jonkman A, Goadsby PJ. Fos expression in the mid-brain periaqueductal grey after trigeminovascular stimulation. J Anat. 2001;198:29–35.

43. Zagami AS, Goadsby PJ, Edvinsson L. Stimulation of the superior sagittal sinus in the cat causes release of vasoactive peptides. Neuropeptides. 1990;16(2):69–75.

44. Zagami AS, Edvinsson L, Goadsby PJ. Pituitary adenylate cyclase activating polypeptide and migraine. Ann Clin Transl Neurol. 2014;1(12):1036–40. https://doi.org/10.1002/acn3.113.

45. Akerman S, Holland PR, Lasalandra MP, Goadsby PJ. Oxygen inhibits neuronal activation in the trigeminocervical complex after stimulation of trigeminal autonomic reflex, but not during direct dural activation of trigeminal afferents. Headache. 2009;49(8):1131–43.

46. Akerman S, Romero-Reyes M. Targeting the central projection of the dural trigeminovascu-lar system for migraine prophylaxis. J Cereb Blood Flow Metab. 2017.:271678X17729280; https://doi.org/10.1177/0271678X17729280.

47. Burstein R, Jakubowski M. Analgesic triptan action in an animal model of intracranial pain: a race against the development of central sensitization. Ann Neurol. 2004;55(1):27–36.

48. Goadsby PJ, Knight YE. Inhibition of trigeminal neurones after intravenous administration of naratriptan through an action at 5-hydroxy-tryptamine (5-HT(1B/1D)) receptors. Br J Pharmacol. 1997;122(5):918–22.

49. Hoskin KL, Kaube H, Goadsby PJ. Sumatriptan can inhibit trigeminal afferents by an exclu-sively neural mechanism. Brain. 1996;119(Pt 5):1419–28.

50. Akerman S, Holland PR, Summ O, Lasalandra MP, Goadsby PJ. A translational in vivo model of trigeminal autonomic cephalalgias: therapeutic characterization. Brain. 2012;135(Pt 12):3664–75.

51. Jakubowski M, Levy D, Kainz V, Zhang XC, Kosaras B, Burstein R. Sensitization of cen-tral trigeminovascular neurons: blockade by intravenous naproxen infusion. Neuroscience. 2007;148(2):573–83.

52. Akerman S, Goadsby PJ. Topiramate inhibits trigeminovascular activation: an intravital microscopy study. Br J Pharmacol. 2005;146(1):7–14.

53. Storer RJ, Goadsby PJ. Topiramate inhibits trigeminovascular neurons in the cat. Cephalalgia. 2004;24(12):1049–56.

54. Ekbom K. Nitroglycerin as a provocative agent in cluster headache. Arch Neurol. 1968;19(5):487–93.

55. Fanciullacci M, Alessandri M, Figini M, Geppetti P, Michelacci S. Increase in plasma cal-citonin gene-related peptide from the extracerebral circulation during nitroglycerin-induced cluster headache attack. Pain. 1995;60(2):119–23.

56. Sances G, Tassorelli C, Pucci E, Ghiotto N, Sandrini G, Nappi G. Reliability of the nitroglycerin provocative test in the diagnosis of neurovascular headaches. Cephalalgia. 2004;24(2):110–9. https://doi.org/10.1111/j.1468-2982.2004.00639.x.
57. May A, Bahra A, Buchel C, Frackowiak RS, Goadsby PJ. PET and MRA findings in cluster headache and MRA in experimental pain. Neurology. 2000;55(9):1328–35.
58. Akerman S, Williamson DJ, Kaube H, Goadsby PJ. The effect of anti-migraine compounds on nitric oxide-induced dilation of dural meningeal vessels. Eur J Pharmacol. 2002;452(2):223–8.
59. Koulchitsky S, Fischer MJ, Messlinger K. Calcitonin gene-related peptide receptor inhibition reduces neuronal activity induced by prolonged increase in nitric oxide in the rat spinal trigeminal nucleus. Cephalalgia. 2009;29(4):408–17.
60. Lambert GA, Donaldson C, Boers PM, Zagami AS. Activation of trigeminovascular neurons by glyceryl trinitrate. Brain Res. 2000;887(1):203–10.
61. Tassorelli C, Joseph SA. Systemic nitroglycerin induces Fos immunoreactivity in brain-stem and forebrain structures of the rat. Brain Res. 1995;682(1–2):167–81.
62. Zhang X, Kainz V, Zhao J, Strassman AM, Levy D. Vascular extracellular signal-regulated kinase mediates migraine-related sensitization of meningeal nociceptors. Ann Neurol. 2013;73(6):741–50. https://doi.org/10.1002/ana.23873.
63. Dieterle A, Fischer MJ, Link AS, Neuhuber WL, Messlinger K. Increase in CGRP- and nNOS-immunoreactive neurons in the rat trigeminal ganglion after infusion of an NO donor. Cephalalgia. 2011;31(1):31–42.
64. Pardutz A, Multon S, Malgrange B, Parducz A, Vecsei L, Schoenen J. Effect of systemic nitroglycerin on CGRP and 5-HT afferents to rat caudal spinal trigeminal nucleus and its modulation by estrogen. Eur J Neurosci. 2002;15(11):1803–9.
65. Summ O, Andreou AP, Akerman S, Goadsby PJ. A potential nitrergic mechanism of action for indomethacin, but not of other COX inhibitors: relevance to indomethacin-sensitive headaches. J Headache Pain. 2010;11(6):477–83. https://doi.org/10.1007/s10194-010-0263-7.
66. Akerman S, Kaube H, Goadsby PJ. Anandamide is able to inhibit trigeminal neurons using an in vivo model of trigeminovascular-mediated nociception. J Pharmacol Exp Ther. 2004;309:56–63.
67. Iversen HK, Olesen J, Tfelt-hansen P. Intravenous nitroglycerin as an experimental-model of vascular headache—basic characteristics. Pain. 1989;38(1):17–24.
68. Ashina M, Bendtsen L, Jensen R, Olesen J. Nitric oxide-induced headache in patients with chronic tension-type headache. Brain. 2000;123(Pt 9):1830–7.
69. Gottselig R, Messlinger K. Noxious chemical stimulation of rat facial mucosa increases intracranial blood flow through a trigemino-parasympathetic reflex—an experimental model for vascular dysfunctions in cluster headache. Cephalalgia. 2004;24(3):206–14.
70. Bartsch T, Levy MJ, Knight YE, Goadsby PJ. Differential modulation of nociceptive dural input to [hypocretin] orexin A and B receptor activation in the posterior hypothalamic area. Pain. 2004;109(3):367–78.
71. Amin FM, Hougaard A, Schytz HW, Asghar MS, Lundholm E, Parvaiz AI, et al. Investigation of the pathophysiological mechanisms of migraine attacks induced by pituitary adenylate cyclase-activating polypeptide-38. Brain. 2014;137(Pt 3):779–94. https://doi.org/10.1093/brain/awt369.
72. Akerman S, Goadsby PJ. Neuronal PAC1 receptors mediate delayed activation and sensitization of trigeminocervical neurons: relevance to migraine. Sci Transl Med. 2015;7(308):308ra157. https://doi.org/10.1126/scitranslmed.aaa7557.

Chapter 10
The Role of the Sphenopalatine Ganglion in Headache Conditions: New Insights

Erling Tronvik and Rigmor Jensen

10.1 Introduction

For more than 100 years, the sphenopalatine ganglion (SPG) has been targeted for the treatment of headache and facial pain. Several techniques have been used over the years to influence the activity in this neuronal structure, from intranasal cocaine to today's implanted stimulators. Data collected throughout the years point in the direction of an important role of this parasympathetic ganglion in different primary headaches. The aim of the present chapter is to give an overview of the anatomy and physiology of this structure with relation to headache pathophysiology and in particular how it may be targeted to treat headache disorders.

10.2 Anatomy

The SPG is located in the pterygopalatine fossa, a triangular space with a volume between 0.1 and 1 cm^3 [1] (Fig. 10.1). In most individuals (70%), the ganglion is a single, 3–4 mm long (in the craniocaudal direction), conical structure, whereas in around 30% it consists of two separate parts [2]. It contains sensory, sympathetic,

E. Tronvik (✉)
Department of Neuromedicine and Movement Science, NTNU—Norwegian University of Science and Technology, Trondheim, Norway

Department of Neurology and Clinical Neurophysiology, St. Olavs Hospital, Trondheim, Norway
e-mail: erling.tronvik@ntnu.no

R. Jensen
Neurological Clinic, Danish Headache Centre, Rigshospitalet-Glostrup, University of Copenhagen, Copenhagen, Denmark
e-mail: rigmor.jensen@regionh.dk

© Springer Nature Switzerland AG 2020
M. Leone, A. May (eds.), *Cluster Headache and other Trigeminal Autonomic Cephalgias*, Headache, https://doi.org/10.1007/978-3-030-12438-0_10

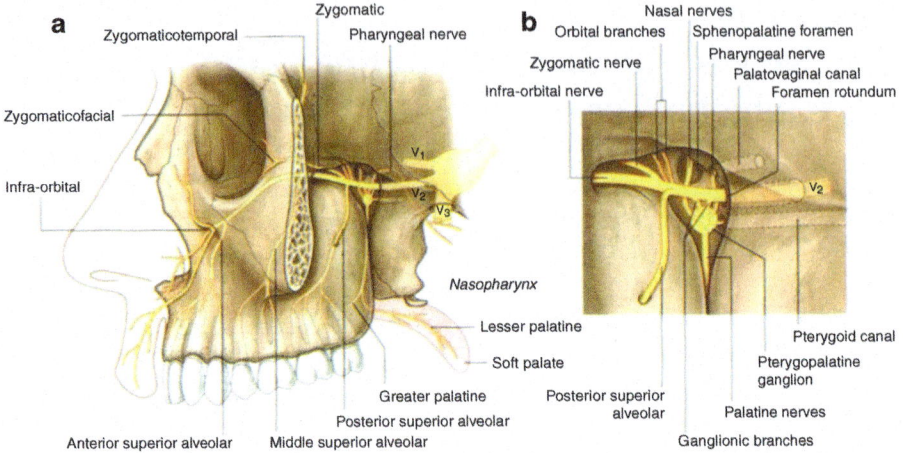

Fig. 10.1 Anatomy of the sphenopalatine ganglion (Gray's Anatomy for Students, 2nd Edition. 2009, ELSEVIER)

and parasympathetic nerve fibers. The sensory fibers enter the ganglion as branches of the maxillary nerve, pass through without synapsing, and exit as the lesser and greater palatine nerves, supplying sensation to the palate and the mucous membrane of the nasal septum [3]. The postganglionic sympathetic fibers from the superior cervical ganglion run through the internal carotid plexus to form the deep petrosal nerve, which merges with the parasympathetic greater petrosal nerve to form the Vidian nerve. The sympathetic fibers of the Vidian nerve, passing through the SPG without synapsing, are distributed to the nose, palate, and lacrimal gland [4]. Preganglionic parasympathetic fibers originating in the superior salivatory nucleus (SSN) in the pons run through the facial nerve and further to the geniculate ganglion from which they exit in the greater petrosal nerve. This nerve merges with the deep petrosal nerve to form the Vidian nerve that enters the SPG where they synapse. The postganglionic fibers coming from the ganglion are distributed to the nose, palate, and lacrimal gland, as well as to cerebral and meningeal vessels [2].

Recent studies have demonstrated that there are small calcitonin gene-related peptide (CGRP) containing neurons in the SPG that most likely originate from the trigeminal ganglion [5], indicating that there may be a direct interaction between the sensory system and the SPG [6].

10.3 Physiology

The trigeminal-parasympathetic reflex center in the brainstem connects trigeminal afferents and the parasympathetic efferents that synapse in the SPG [7, 8]. Activation of the parasympathetic efferent neurons leads to perivascular neurotransmitter release (vasoactive intestinal peptide (VIP), nitric oxide, and acetylcholine), resulting in dilatation of intracerebral blood vessels, plasma protein extravasation, and activation of meningeal trigeminal nociceptors [9, 10]. The current rationale for targeting the SPG in headache conditions is to interrupt parasympathetic outflow and thereby inhibit activation of trigeminal afferents.

10.3.1   Why Are We Targeting the SPG?

Several techniques for disrupting neuronal signaling in the SPG have been used over the years, including application of chemical substances (cocaine, alcohol, local anesthetics, steroids, botulinum toxin) in or near the ganglion, nerve sectioning, radiofrequency ablations, and electrical stimulation of the ganglion. Two case reports on stereotactic neurosurgery on the SPG have also been published [11, 12]. Interruption of parasympathetic outflow is considered the most plausible mechanism of action. Today, one used technique for interrupting neuronal activity in the SPG is high-frequency electrical stimulation. This works possibly by depletion of stored neurotransmitters in parasympathetic efferents, leading to reduced activation of meningeal nociceptors [13, 14]. Other modes of action could include an antidromic inhibitory effect on the SSN or even some degree of nerve conduction block. The latter is considered less likely given the stimulation frequencies used today [15]. Another possibility could be sensory modulation through the sensory (maxillary) fibers in the pterygopalatine fossa, as most techniques targeting the SPG are nonselective as to which types of nerve fibers are influenced (Sect. 10.3.2) [8]. The role of the direct neuronal pathways between the parasympathetic and the sensory system (Sect. 10.2) for the clinical effects is not known but should be further explored.

10.3.2   What in the SPG Are We Targeting?

The SPG is traversed by sympathetic, parasympathetic, and sensory fibers. How do we know which fibers are influenced by current techniques used to target the SPG, and which fibers are most important to target in different headache conditions? These important questions have previously been asked by Narouze [16]. Possibly, it could be more effective to selectively influence one specific type of nerve fiber. Which one, could vary according to the condition we are treating. As an example, targeting of the sensory fibers from the second division of the trigeminal nerve might be more relevant for certain types of orofacial pain than for cluster headache or migraine. In addition to type of fiber to target, it is also important to know *how* the target area responds to the intervention. For instance, what would be the optimal frequency (or dose for chemical agents) for attaining an optimal effect? In a recently published study, low-frequency stimulation of the SPG did not activate Aβ fibers or C fibers when testing for mechanical perception and pain thresholds [17]. High-frequency stimulation, on the other hand, readily elicits sensory symptoms [18]. These data emphasizes the need to determine the thresholds needed (for all types of SPG targeting modalities) to facilitate or inhibit activity in sympathetic, parasympathetic, or sensory fibers.

A main question has been whether parasympathetic activation is involved in the generation or maintenance of pain in different headache conditions, in addition to producing autonomic symptoms. Yarnitsky et al. observed that migraine patients with no parasympathetic symptoms were less likely to experience pain relief after treatment with nasal lidocaine than those with such symptoms [10]. The interpretation was that the parasympathetic pathways could contribute to the pain as well. In cluster headache, further support for the potential importance of the parasympathetic pathways was illustrated by a patient that continued having cluster headache attacks, even after the ipsilateral trigeminal sensory root was excised [19]. Schytz et al. demonstrated that low-frequency (LF) stimulation of the SPG could provoke cluster headache attacks [20]. A recently published study, however, challenges these findings. When the Schytz study was replicated with slightly higher stimulation frequencies and longer duration, LF stimulation did not provoke cluster-like headache significantly more often than sham (35% vs. 25%) [17], although autonomic symptoms *did* appear more frequently with LF stimulation (80% vs. 45%, $p = 0.046$). The role of the parasympathetic efferents in pain generation or maintenance is still unclear.

10.4   Cluster Headache

10.4.1   Intranasal Administration of Topical Agents in Cluster Headache

The first description of intranasal administration of a topical agent (cocaine) toward the SPG ($n = 5$) was made by Sluder in 1908 in "Sluder's neuralgia" (resembling today's cluster headache diagnosis) [21]. The apparent effect of cocaine was seen in other similar cases but had to be applied too often, with risk of negative side effects [22, 23]. The nonaddictive alternative, lidocaine, was found to be just as effective in a couple of case series [24, 25]. Further, 88% phenol applied with cotton swabs intranasally also had a relevant effect over time [26]. However, only one controlled study has been performed ($n = 15$) with intranasal topical agents in cluster headache [27]. Both cocaine and lidocaine showed superiority to saline; with complete cessation of pain after a little more than half an hour for active substances, compared to 1 h for placebo.

10.4.2   Invasive Techniques Targeting the SPG in Cluster Headache

10.4.2.1   Destructive Techniques

Meyer et al. removed the SPG (histologically verified) in 13 patients with cluster headache [28] but with no or only modest clinical effect: seven patients had no effect, four had incomplete relief, and only two had complete relief over the next 12 months. One patient had previously undergone a trigeminal rhizotomy with anesthesia of the maxillary region but no effect on the pain attacks. With the additional SPG resection, there was an initial remission, but later the pain recurred. This demonstrated that even a combined destruction of both the sensory afferent (trigeminal pathways) and the parasympathetic efferent (SPG) was unhelpful. This was in line with previous findings in "sphenopalatine neuralgia" (cluster headache-like symptoms), where stimulation of the greater petrosal nerve provoked pain and sectioning of the nerve in 13 patients provided relief. However, the results obtained were quite variable ("excellent" in 25%, "good to fair" in 50%, and "poor" in 25%) [29].

Later, several other types of irreversible SPG blockades were performed, including supra-zygomatic alcohol injection, relieving pain in 85% of 120 patients with a follow-up time of 6 months to 4 years [30]. However, a disadvantage with this treatment is that the alcohol can spread to the maxillary nerve and cause painful neuritis [31]. The use of radiofrequency techniques has been effective in 60–80% of episodic cluster headache patients and 30–70% of chronic cluster headache patients, in a number of small, uncontrolled studies [31–35]. In order to avoid the more cumbersome fluoroscopy technique, a Chinese group explored the use of CT-guided pulsed radiofrequency treatment in refractory episodic ($n = 13$) and chronic ($n = 3$) cluster headache [34]. Eleven of the former and one of the latter patients showed complete remission within 6 days.

10.4.2.2   Neuromodulatory Techniques

With the use of an endoscopic technique and injecting through the nasal wall, an Italian research group deposited a mixture of local anesthetics and corticosteroids toward the sphenopalatine fossa in 20 patients with refractory chronic cluster headache [36]. The treatment resulted in improvement in 58% of the patients, but the effect was short-lasting, and repeated injections were less efficacious. The same technique was further evaluated in 15 patients with chronic cluster headache, where 60% responded to the treatment [37]. In the latter study, there was a tendency to have a more long-lasting response, possibly owing to the improved injection technique.

One of the problems with using local anesthetics has been their short-lasting effect. Aiming at exploiting the longer-lasting effect of botulinum toxin, a small open-label pilot study on ten patients with refractory chronic cluster headache investigated the efficacy and safety of injecting 25–50 units of botulinum toxin toward the SPG on the symptomatic side [38]. The injection was performed with a new surgical device using an image-guided navigation (MultiGuide®). Five of ten patients responded to the treatment with an average attack frequency reduction (main efficacy outcome) of 77% during the 6 months of follow-up period. The safety profile was considered acceptable by the authors. A physiological basis for the use of botulinum toxin toward the SPG was strengthened when the botulinum toxin receptor, synaptic vesicle glycoprotein 2-A (SV2-A), and the synaptosomal-associated protein 25 (SNAP-25) were found in human SPGs [39]. A randomized controlled trial is currently being planned to confirm the results of this preliminary open-label pilot study.

In 2010 six patients with refractory chronic cluster headache received short-term electrical stimulation of the SPG [15]. The acute treatment response was promising. Later, a multicenter, sham-controlled study using an implantable, on-demand SPG stimulator (Pulsante®) in medically refractory chronic cluster headache (Pathway CH-1 study) demonstrated a clinically significant improvement in 68% of the patients. Among these, 25% were acute responders (i.e., had pain relief at 15 min in >50% of treated attacks), 36% were frequency responders (>50% reduction in attack frequency), and 7% were both acute and frequency responders [13]. The observation that there might be a prophylactic effect of the acute treatment was unexpected, but follow-up data support this finding. An open-label follow-up study at 24 months ($n = 33$) demonstrated a long-term clinical efficacy with 45% acute responders, 33% frequency responders, and 61% either acute responders or frequency responders or both [40]. A recently published open-label study, using the same type of SPG stimulator in 97 cluster headache patients (88 chronic and 9 episodic), investigated efficacy at 12 months [41]. Twelve patients had their stimulators removed due to lack of effect or adverse effects. Of the remaining 85 patients, the mean attack frequency was reduced from 25.2 to 14.4 attacks per week, and 68% were treatment responders (defined as being acute responder or frequency responder or both). Thirty-two percent of all patients were acute responders, and 55% of the chronic patients were frequency responders. The implant procedure requires unique anatomical and surgical skill and is mainly performed by few selected cranio-maxillofacial surgeons in Europe. Therefore, it is recommended that the implants and the follow-up are concentrated to specialized centers with relevant surgical expertise.

A sham-controlled trial testing the Pulsante therapy on 120 patients with chronic cluster headache patients is currently ongoing in the USA (Pathway CH-2 study NCT02168764—ClinicalTrials.gov accessed October 2017).

10.4.3   Clinical Usefulness of SPG-Targeted Treatments in Cluster Headache

- The evidence does not support the widespread clinical use of intranasal local anesthetics in cluster headache.
- Endoscopic injection with local anesthetics and steroids appears to have a relatively short-lasting effect.
- A number of uncontrolled studies have indicated an effect of radiofrequency treatment in cluster headache, but there may be irreversible side effects, and the fluoroscopy method is somewhat cumbersome for widespread clinical use. The use of CT guidance may be an easier technique, but concern about radiation limits the number of repeated injections.
- The use of botulinum toxin injections toward the SPG is currently being further investigated. In theory, the use of botulinum toxin could have a long-term effect. No controlled studies have yet been performed.
- SPG stimulation has increasing evidence for long-term efficacy in chronic cluster headache and is providing interesting new insight into the pathophysiology of cluster headache. Overall, this appears to be a safe therapy with tolerable and transient side effects in most patients. However, confirmation of its role in the treatment of chronic cluster headache awaits the results of the ongoing randomized sham-controlled trial (CH-2). Since the implant procedure is relatively complicated and the eligible number of patients low, patient selection and surgery should be centralized to hospitals with high expertise in headache and dedicated surgeons.

10.5   Migraine

It is firmly established that cranial autonomic symptoms (CAS) indicating activation of the trigemino-parasympathetic reflex can be present in both adult [42–45] and pediatric [46] migraine patients. Yarnitsky et al. showed that migraine patients with parasympathetic symptoms were more likely to experience pain relief 10–30 min after a lidocaine-induced SPG block than those with no parasympathetic symptoms [10]. This could indicate that targeting the SPG in migraine could affect not only parasympathetic symptoms but also influence the pain [8]. In addition, a pathway involving the SPG parasympathetic efferents whereby common migraine triggers activate meningeal nociceptors has been proposed [47]. Stress, lack of sleep, and olfactory stimulation may activate multiple brain areas (hypothalamic, cortical, limbic) with neural connections to the SSN, resulting in activation of postganglionic parasympathetic fibers in the SPG and subsequent activation of meningeal nociceptors [47, 48].

10.5.1 Intranasal Administration of Local Anesthetics in Migraine

The most common way to target the SPG in migraine has been through intranasal application of topical anesthetics, such as lidocaine or bupivacaine. An uncontrolled study on 23 migraine patients in 1995 indicated an effect following application of lidocaine, with 12 patients responding, most within 5 min [49]. Later, five small controlled studies have been performed yielding mixed results:

1. Positive trials:

    (a) 1996 Lidocaine vs. saline with evaluation of effect after 15 min, $n = 81$. Relief in 55% of the lidocaine group compared to 21% in the saline group, $p = 0.04$ [50].
    (b) 1999 Lidocaine vs. saline with evaluation of effect after 15 min, $n = 131$. Relief in 35.8% of the lidocaine group compared to 7.4% in the saline group, $p < 0.001$ [51].
    (c) 2015 Bupivacaine vs. saline with evaluation of effect after 15 min, 30 min, and 24 h, $n = 41$. Relief as early as 15 min with a 20% reduction in numeric rating scale (NRS) scores for the bupivacaine group compared to 7% reduction in the saline group [52]. A follow-up of this study was to continue treating the subjects prophylactically twice per week and compare baseline headache days to number of headache days 1 month posttreatment. A significant decrease was not demonstrated [53].

2. Negative trials:

    (a) 2001 Lidocaine vs. saline with evaluation of relief after 5, 10, 15, 20, and 30 minutes, $n = 49$. No difference between the groups [54]
    (b) 2017 Lidocaine vs. saline with evaluation of relief after 15 and 30 min, $n = 162$. No difference between the groups [55]

10.5.2 Invasive Techniques Targeting the SPG in Migraine

A pilot study on 11 patients with refractory migraine (9 with medication overuse and 2 with episodic migraine) tested the efficacy of inducing migraine attacks and then treating them with electrical stimulation toward the SPG through an infrazygomatic electrode [56]. Two patients experienced complete remission of the attacks, and three reported meaningful pain reduction. Five patients had no effect and one was not stimulated.

A randomized controlled trial (NCT01540799) testing an SPG stimulator in 80 patients with predominantly fixed (no side-shift) episodic migraine is currently ongoing (ClinicalTrials.gov accessed October 2017).

In an uncontrolled pilot study ($n = 10$) using a novel image-guided surgical device, 10 patients with refractory chronic migraine were injected with 25 units botulinum toxin toward the SPG on both sides (total 50 units) [57]. The frequency of moderate or severe headache days in the second month post-injection (primary efficacy measure) was 53% less than at baseline, $p = 0.009$.

10.5.3 Clinical Usefulness of SPG-Targeted Treatments in Migraine

- It has not been proven that intranasal topical local anesthetics blocks the SPG parasympathetic, sensory, or sympathetic fibers.
- Controlled studies on intranasal administration of local anesthetics in migraine report conflicting results. Better data are needed before this method is implemented into routine-clinical practice.
- There are ongoing studies evaluating the efficacy and safety of SPG stimulation in patients with episodic migraine as well as investigation of bilateral injection of botulinum toxin in patients with chronic migraine.

10.6 Other Pain Conditions

A small placebo-controlled crossover study, attempting to target the SPG maxillary nerve fibers in 25 patients with idiopathic second branch trigeminal neuralgia, was performed with 8% lidocaine nasal spray versus saline [58]. Pain recorded on a visual analogue scale (VAS) was reduced from 8.0 at baseline to 1.9 at 15 min after treatment in the lidocaine group ($p < 0.01$). For saline, the numbers were 7.9 at baseline versus 7.6 posttreatment. The effect lasted median 4.3 h (range 0.5–24 h).

Noninvasive management of persistent idiopathic facial pain (PIFP) is the preferred treatment in most cases. A retrospective study on the use of alcohol injections toward the SPG in 42 patients with refractory facial pain showed that 67% of the treatments were deemed as successful with a mean pain relief period of 10.3 months [59]. The patients who were classified as PIFP ($n = 10$) had the highest success rate (85.7% of treatments).

A randomized, placebo-controlled study with intranasal administration of bupivacaine versus saline in 93 patients with acute frontal headache in the emergency department did not detect any difference between active and placebo treatment [60]. The primary endpoint was 50% reduction in pain at 15 min, and this was found in 48.8% of the bupivacaine group and 41.3% of the saline group.

10.7   Cranial Parasympathetic Innervation

The SPG is the main source of parasympathetic innervation to the head. Another cranial parasympathetic ganglion, which has attracted much less attention than the SPG, is the otic ganglion (OTG). There is evidence that postganglionic parasympathetic fibers from the OTG also innervate intracerebral vessels [61–64]. Could there be anything to gain by blocking the OTG or perhaps even a dual block of the SPG and the OTG? Goadsby et al. showed that approximately 50% of the parasympathetic activity to the cranial vessels in cats was conveyed through the OTG and 50% through the SPG [65]. The exact importance of the OTG in humans is not known, but there are data indicating that parasympathetic fibers from the SPG may be more important for the frontal region of the cranium, whereas such fibers from the OTG are more important for the occipital region [10, 66]. Neurochemical studies have demonstrated co-localization of both pituitary adenylate cyclase-activating polypeptide (PACAP) and vasoactive intestinal peptide (VIP) in both the SPG and the OTG [67–69]. Hopefully future studies will shed more light on whether the OTG, which has many similarities with the SPG, has any role in headache pathophysiology and whether it may be a feasible and useful target for therapy.

10.8   Conclusion

The sphenopalatine ganglion appears to have a central role in cluster headache and potentially in other primary headache and idiopathic facial pain disorders. New technology that provides a more accurate technique to target the SPG offers the opportunity to evaluate the efficacy of various treatments that can be more precisely directed toward the SPG. This will also facilitate a better understanding of the role of the SPG in the pathogenesis of a variety of headache and craniofacial pain disorders.

References

1. Stojcev Stajcic L, et al. Anatomical study of the pterygopalatine fossa pertinent to the maxillary nerve block at the foramen rotundum. Int J Oral Maxillofac Surg. 2010;39(5):493–6.
2. Rusu MC, et al. The pterygopalatine ganglion in humans: a morphological study. Ann Anat. 2009;191(2):196–202.
3. Lovasova K, et al. Anatomical study of the roots of cranial parasympathetic ganglia: a contribution to medical education. Ann Anat. 2013;195(3):205–11.
4. Rusu MC, Pop F. The anatomy of the sympathetic pathway through the pterygopalatine fossa in humans. Ann Anat. 2010;192(1):17–22.
5. Ivanusic JJ, et al. 5-HT(1D) receptor immunoreactivity in the sphenopalatine ganglion: implications for the efficacy of triptans in the treatment of autonomic signs associated with cluster headache. Headache. 2011;51(3):392–402.

6. Csati A, et al. Calcitonin gene-related peptide and its receptor components in the human sphenopalatine ganglion—interaction with the sensory system. Brain Res. 2012;1435:29–39.
7. May A, Goadsby PJ. The trigeminovascular system in humans: pathophysiologic implications for primary headache syndromes of the neural influences on the cerebral circulation. J Cereb Blood Flow Metab. 1999;19(2):115–27.
8. Khan S, Schoenen J, Ashina M. Sphenopalatine ganglion neuromodulation in migraine: what is the rationale? Cephalalgia. 2014;34(5):382–91.
9. Noseda R, Burstein R. Migraine pathophysiology: anatomy of the trigeminovascular pathway and associated neurological symptoms, CSD, sensitization and modulation of pain. Pain. 2013;154(Suppl 1):S44–53. https://doi.org/10.1016/j.pain.2013.07.021.
10. Yarnitsky D, et al. 2003 Wolff award: possible parasympathetic contributions to peripheral and central sensitization during migraine. Headache. 2003;43(7):704–14.
11. Lad SP, et al. Cyberknife targeting the pterygopalatine ganglion for the treatment of chronic cluster headaches. Neurosurgery. 2007;60(3):E580–1; discussion E581
12. Tan DY, et al. Frameless linac-based stereotactic radiosurgery treatment for SUNCT syndrome targeting the trigeminal nerve and sphenopalatine ganglion. Cephalalgia. 2013;33(13):1132–6.
13. Schoenen J, et al. Stimulation of the sphenopalatine ganglion (SPG) for cluster headache treatment. Pathway CH-1: a randomized, sham-controlled study. Cephalalgia. 2013;33(10):816–30.
14. Ekstrom J, et al. Depletion of neuropeptides in rat parotid glands and declining atropine-resistant salivary secretion upon continuous parasympathetic nerve stimulation. Regul Pept. 1985;11(4):353–9.
15. Ansarinia M, et al. Electrical stimulation of sphenopalatine ganglion for acute treatment of cluster headaches. Headache. 2010;50(7):1164–74.
16. Narouze S. Neurostimulation at pterygopalatine fossa for cluster headaches and cerebrovascular disorders. Curr Pain Headache Rep. 2014;18(7):432.
17. Guo S, et al. Cranial parasympathetic activation induces autonomic symptoms but no cluster headache attacks. Cephalalgia. 2018;38:1418–28.
18. Assaf AT, et al. Technical and surgical aspects of the sphenopalatine ganglion (SPG) microstimulator insertion procedure. Int J Oral Maxillofac Surg. 2016;45(2):245–54.
19. Matharu MS, Goadsby PJ. Persistence of attacks of cluster headache after trigeminal nerve root section. Brain. 2002;125(Pt 5):976–84.
20. Schytz HW, et al. Experimental activation of the sphenopalatine ganglion provokes cluster-like attacks in humans. Cephalalgia. 2013;33(10):831–41.
21. Sluder G. The role of the sphenopalatine ganglion in nasal headaches. NY State J Med. 1908;27:8–13.
22. Barre F. Cocaine as an abortive agent in cluster headache. Headache. 1982;22(2):69–73.
23. Kittrelle JP, Grouse DS, Seybold ME. Cluster headache. Local anesthetic abortive agents. Arch Neurol. 1985;42(5):496–8.
24. Hardebo JE, Elner A. Nerves and vessels in the pterygopalatine fossa and symptoms of cluster headache. Headache. 1987;27(10):528–32.
25. Robbins L. Intranasal lidocaine for cluster headache. Headache. 1995;35(2):83–4.
26. Puig CM, Driscoll CL, Kern EB. Sluder's sphenopalatine ganglion neuralgia—treatment with 88% phenol. Am J Rhinol. 1998;12(2):113–8.
27. Costa A, et al. The effect of intranasal cocaine and lidocaine on nitroglycerin-induced attacks in cluster headache. Cephalalgia. 2000;20(2):85–91.
28. Meyer JS, et al. Sphenopalatine ganglionectomy for cluster headache. Arch Otolaryngol. 1970;92(5):475–84.
29. Gardner WJ, Stowell A, Dutlinger R. Resection of the greater superficial petrosal nerve in the treatment of unilateral headache. J Neurosurg. 1947;4(2):105–14.
30. Devoghel JC. Cluster headache and sphenopalatine block. Acta Anaesthesiol Belg. 1981;32(1):101–7.
31. Sanders M, Zuurmond WW. Efficacy of sphenopalatine ganglion blockade in 66 patients suffering from cluster headache: a 12- to 70-month follow-up evaluation. J Neurosurg. 1997;87(6):876–80.

32. Narouze S, et al. Sphenopalatine ganglion radiofrequency ablation for the management of chronic cluster headache. Headache. 2009;49(4):571–7.
33. Chua NH, Vissers KC, Wilder-Smith OH. Quantitative sensory testing may predict response to sphenopalatine ganglion pulsed radiofrequency treatment in cluster headaches: a case series. Pain Pract. 2011;11(5):439–45.
34. Fang L, et al. Computerized tomography-guided sphenopalatine ganglion pulsed radiofrequency treatment in 16 patients with refractory cluster headaches: twelve- to 30-month follow-up evaluations. Cephalalgia. 2016;36(2):106–12.
35. Bendersky DC, Hem SM, Yampolsky CG. Unsuccessful pulsed radiofrequency of the sphenopalatine ganglion in patients with chronic cluster headache and subsequent successful thermocoagulation. Pain Pract. 2015;15(5):E40–5.
36. Felisati G, et al. Sphenopalatine endoscopic ganglion block: a revision of a traditional technique for cluster headache. Laryngoscope. 2006;116(8):1447–50.
37. Pipolo C, et al. Sphenopalatine endoscopic ganglion block in cluster headache: a reevaluation of the procedure after 5 years. Neurol Sci. 2010;31(Suppl 1):S197–9.
38. Bratbak DF, et al. Pilot study of sphenopalatine injection of onabotulinumtoxinA for the treatment of intractable chronic cluster headache. Cephalalgia. 2016;36(6):503–9.
39. Steinberg A, et al. Expression of messenger molecules and receptors in rat and human sphenopalatine ganglion indicating therapeutic targets. J Headache Pain. 2016;17(1):78.
40. Jurgens TP, et al. Long-term effectiveness of sphenopalatine ganglion stimulation for cluster headache. Cephalalgia. 2017;37(5):423–34.
41. Jensen R, et al. Sphenopalatine ganglion stimulation for cluster headache, results from a large, open-label European registry. J Headache Pain. 2018;19:6.
42. Lai TH, Fuh JL, Wang SJ. Cranial autonomic symptoms in migraine: characteristics and comparison with cluster headache. J Neurol Neurosurg Psychiatry. 2009;80(10):1116–9.
43. Barbanti P, et al. The phenotype of migraine with unilateral cranial autonomic symptoms documents increased peripheral and central trigeminal sensitization. A case series of 757 patients. Cephalalgia. 2016;36(14):1334–40.
44. Barbanti P, et al. Unilateral cranial autonomic symptoms in migraine. Cephalalgia. 2002;22(4):256–9.
45. Obermann M, et al. Prevalence of trigeminal autonomic symptoms in migraine: a population-based study. Cephalalgia. 2007;27(6):504–9.
46. Gelfand AA, Reider AC, Goadsby PJ. Cranial autonomic symptoms in pediatric migraine are the rule, not the exception. Neurology. 2013;81(5):431–6.
47. Burstein R, Jakubowski M. Unitary hypothesis for multiple triggers of the pain and strain of migraine. J Comp Neurol. 2005;493(1):9–14.
48. Spencer SE, et al. CNS projections to the pterygopalatine parasympathetic preganglionic neurons in the rat: a retrograde transneuronal viral cell body labeling study. Brain Res. 1990;534(1-2):149–69.
49. Kudrow L, Kudrow DB, Sandweiss JH. Rapid and sustained relief of migraine attacks with intranasal lidocaine: preliminary findings. Headache. 1995;35(2):79–82.
50. Maizels M, et al. Intranasal lidocaine for treatment of migraine: a randomized, double-blind, controlled trial. JAMA. 1996;276(4):319–21.
51. Maizels M, Geiger AM. Intranasal lidocaine for migraine: a randomized trial and open-label follow-up. Headache. 1999;39(8):543–51.
52. Cady R, et al. A double-blind, placebo-controlled study of repetitive transnasal sphenopalatine ganglion blockade with tx360® as acute treatment for chronic migraine. Headache. 2015;55(1):101–16.
53. Cady RK, et al. Long-term efficacy of a double-blind, placebo-controlled, randomized study for repetitive sphenopalatine blockade with bupivacaine vs. saline with the Tx360 device for treatment of chronic migraine. Headache. 2015;55(4):529–42.
54. Blanda M, et al. Intranasal lidocaine for the treatment of migraine headache: a randomized, controlled trial. Acad Emerg Med. 2001;8(4):337–42.

55. Avcu N, et al. Intranasal lidocaine in acute treatment of migraine: a randomized controlled trial. Ann Emerg Med. 2017;69(6):743–51.
56. Tepper SJ, et al. Acute treatment of intractable migraine with sphenopalatine ganglion electrical stimulation. Headache. 2009;49(7):983–9.
57. Bratbak DF, et al. Pilot study of sphenopalatine injection of onabotulinumtoxinA for the treatment of intractable chronic migraine. Cephalalgia. 2017;37(4):356–64.
58. Kanai A, et al. Intranasal lidocaine 8% spray for second-division trigeminal neuralgia. Br J Anaesth. 2006;97(4):559–63.
59. Kastler A, et al. Alcohol percutaneous neurolysis of the sphenopalatine ganglion in the management of refractory cranio-facial pain. Neuroradiology. 2014;56(7):589–96.
60. Schaffer JT, et al. Noninvasive sphenopalatine ganglion block for acute headache in the emergency department: a randomized placebo-controlled trial. Ann Emerg Med. 2015;65(5):503–10.
61. Walters BB, Gillespie SA, Moskowitz MA. Cerebrovascular projections from the sphenopalatine and otic ganglia to the middle cerebral artery of the cat. Stroke. 1986;17(3):488–94.
62. Suzuki N, Hardebo JE, Owman C. Origins and pathways of cerebrovascular vasoactive intestinal polypeptide-positive nerves in rat. J Cereb Blood Flow Metab. 1988;8(5):697–712.
63. Uddman R, Hara H, Edvinsson L. Neuronal pathways to the rat middle meningeal artery revealed by retrograde tracing and immunocytochemistry. J Auton Nerv Syst. 1989;26(1):69–75.
64. Suzuki N, Hardebo JE. Anatomical basis for a parasympathetic and sensory innervation of the intracranial segment of the internal carotid artery in man. Possible implication for vascular headache. J Neurol Sci. 1991;104(1):19–31.
65. Goadsby PJ, Lambert GA, Lance JW. The peripheral pathway for extracranial vasodilatation in the cat. J Auton Nerv Syst. 1984;10(2):145–55.
66. Suzuki N, Hardebo JE, Owman C. Origins and pathways of choline acetyltransferase-positive parasympathetic nerve fibers to cerebral vessels in rat. J Cereb Blood Flow Metab. 1990;10(3):399–408.
67. Uddman R, et al. Neuronal messengers and peptide receptors in the human sphenopalatine and otic ganglia. Brain Res. 1999;826(2):193–9.
68. Tuka B, et al. Release of PACAP-38 in episodic cluster headache patients—an exploratory study. J Headache Pain. 2016;17(1):69.
69. Edvinsson L, Uddman R. Neurobiology in primary headaches. Brain Res Brain Res Rev. 2005;48(3):438–56.

Chapter 11
Acute Treatment of Cluster Headache Attacks

Stefan Evers

11.1 Introduction

The treatment of acute cluster headache attacks is based on clinical trials and on empirical data. In the last decades, we also learnt more about the pathophysiology of cluster headache leading to new substances for both acute and prophylactic treatment. Although cluster headache is a very impressive somatic disorder, it has to be considered that drug treatment in cluster headache shows a placebo rate similar to that observed in migraine treatment [1]. There are treatment guidelines available published for different parts of the world [2, 3], and the superiority of guideline-adherent treatment over purely intuitive treatment in cluster headache has been shown [4].

11.2 Attack Treatment

After the first published report on the use of oxygen to abort cluster headache attacks [5], the use of oxygen in cluster headache has been proposed for decades. The first controlled clinical trial was published in the 1980s [6]. The most recent trial showed that inhalation of pure (100%) oxygen with a flow of at least 12 L/min is effective in abortion of acute cluster headache attacks [7]. Oxygen should be inhaled for 15 min in a sitting, upright position by demand valve oxygen (full facial mask) [8]. There are no contraindications known for the use of oxygen. It is safe and without side effects. More than 70% of all cluster headache patients respond to this treatment with a significant pain reduction within 30 min.

In double-blind, placebo-controlled trials, the $5\text{-}HT1_{B/D}$ agonist sumatriptan injected subcutaneously was effective in about 75% of all cluster headache patients (i.e., pain free

S. Evers (✉)
Department of Neurology, Krankenhaus Lindenbrunn, Coppenbrügge, Germany
e-mail: everss@uni-muenster.de

© Springer Nature Switzerland AG 2020   131
M. Leone, A. May (eds.), *Cluster Headache and other Trigeminal Autonomic Cephalgias*, Headache, https://doi.org/10.1007/978-3-030-12438-0_11

within 20 min) [9, 10]. It is safe and without side effects in most of the patients even if it is taken nearly daily as some cluster headache patients do off-label [11]. Contraindications are cardio- and cerebrovascular disorders and untreated arterial hypertension. The most unpleasant side effects are chest pain and distal paraesthesia. Even 3 mg subcutaneous sumatriptan is effective in the majority of patients [12]. Zolmitriptan 5 mg nasal spray has also been shown to be effective in two placebo-controlled trials and has been approved by the EMA for the acute treatment of cluster headache [13, 14]. In one single open and one double-blind, placebo-controlled trial, sumatriptan nasal spray 20 mg was also effective in the abortion of attacks [15, 16]. These triptan nasal sprays should be installed into the contralateral nostril as ipsilateral rhinorrhea might hamper the uptake of the drug by the nasal mucosa. Finally, oral zolmitriptan 10 mg was also effective within 30 min [17]. However, oral use of triptans in the approved dose is not recommended for cluster headache attacks, since the onset of efficacy is too late.

Oral and intranasal ergotamine tartrate has been used in the treatment of acute cluster headache attacks for more than 60 years [18] and is probably effective when given very early in the attack. However, placebo-controlled trials are missing. Short-term prophylaxis with ergotamine is not recommended anymore because of severe side effects. The intranasal application of dihydroergotamine in cluster headache attacks was not superior to placebo in a single trial [19]. The intravenous application of 1 mg dihydroergotamine over 3 days has been shown to be effective in the abortion of severe cluster attacks in an open retrospective trial [20].

The nasal installation of lidocaine into the ipsilateral nostril (1 mL with a concentration of 4–10%; the head should be reclined by 45° and rotated to the affected side by 30–40°) is effective in at least one third of the patients [21–23].

One hundred microgramme subcutaneous octreotide has been shown to be effective in the treatment of acute cluster headache attacks in a double-blind, placebo-controlled trial [24].

The use of the so-called peripheral analgesics and of opioids is not recommended in the treatment of cluster headache attacks [2]. Although controlled trials on these substances in cluster headache are lacking, there is expert consensus that they are ineffective or show much lower efficacy than the substances discussed above.

Although the (nearly) daily intake of acute drugs to abort cluster headache attacks is safe and without further complications in most cluster headache patients, the induction of medication overuse headache cannot be excluded, in particular in those patients with concomitant migraine or migraine in their family [25]. Therefore, the intake of acute drugs should be restricted to 10 days per month which is possible in nearly all patients with successful prophylactic treatment.

11.3   Future Developments

New drugs affecting the CGRP pathways are under development for the treatment of cluster headache. The so-called CGRP antagonists (class group of gepants), which are given orally, might be an option for long-lasting cluster headache attacks; however, no clinical trials have been performed so far. The class of CGRP antibodies is mainly investigated for the prevention of cluster headache attacks; however, for very severe cluster attacks, a parenteral application could be efficacious.

Stimulation techniques to treat cluster headache focus on the prevention of attacks. However, the acute treatment of attacks has also been investigated. In a first unblinded, but sham-controlled pilot study on sphenopalatine ganglion stimulation in the acute attack, 67% of 28 patients showed significant pain relief by this stimulation [26]. However, in the largest trial on this stimulation technique, there was no significant difference in the primary endpoint (responder rates) between verum and sham stimulation with only maximal 26.7% responders, and patients with episodic cluster headache responded significantly better [27]. Another technique under development for acute attack treatment is the transdermal vagal nerve stimulation [28], suggesting an efficacy also for the acute attack abortion. However, further trials with a real sham control have to follow, before these techniques can be recommended.

References

1. Nilsson-Remahl AI, Laudon Meyer E, Cordonnier C, Goadsby PJ. Placebo response in cluster headache trials: a review. Cephalalgia. 2003;23:504–10.
2. May A, Leone M, Afra J, Linde M, Sandor PS, Evers S, Goadsby PJ. EFNS guidelines on the treatment of cluster headache and other trigeminal-autonomic cephalalgias. Eur J Neurol. 2006;13:1066–77.
3. Robbins MS, Starling AJ, Pringsheim TM, Becker WJ, Schwedt TJ. Treatment of cluster headache: The American Headache Society evidence-based guidelines. Headache. 2016;56:1093–106.
4. Lademann V, Jansen JP, Evers S, Frese A. Evaluation of guideline-adherent treatment in cluster headache. Cephalalgia. 2016;36:760–4.
5. Janks JF. Oxygen for cluster headaches. JAMA. 1978;239:191.
6. Fogan L. Treatment of cluster headache. A double-blind comparison of oxygen v air inhalation. Arch Neurol. 1985;42:362–3.
7. Cohen AS, Burns B, Goadsby PJ. High-flow oxygen for treatment of cluster headache: a randomized trial. JAMA. 2009;302:2451–7.
8. Petersen AS, Barloese MC, Lund NL, Jensen RH. Oxygen therapy for cluster headache. A mask comparison trial. A single-blinded, placebo-controlled, crossover study. Cephalalgia. 2017;37:214–24.
9. Ekbom K, Monstad I, Prusinski A, Cole JA, Pilgrim AJ, Noronha D. Subcutaneous sumatriptan in the acute treatment of cluster headache: a dose comparison study. The Sumatriptan Cluster Headache Study Group. Acta Neurol Scand. 1993;88:63–9.
10. The Sumatriptan Cluster Headache Study Group. Treatment of acute cluster headache with sumatriptan. N Engl J Med. 1991;325:322–6.
11. Leone M, Proietti Cecchini A. Long-term use of daily sumatriptan injections in severe drug-resistant chronic cluster headache. Neurology. 2016;86:194–5.
12. Gregor N, Schlesiger C, Akova-Oztürk E, Kraemer C, Husstedt IW, Evers S. Treatment of cluster headache attacks with less than 6 mg subcutaneous sumatriptan. Headache. 2005;45:1069–72.
13. Cittadini E, May A, Straube A, Evers S, Bussone G, Goadsby PJ. Effectiveness of intranasal zolmitriptan in acute cluster headache: a randomized, placebo-controlled, double-blind crossover study. Arch Neurol. 2006;63:1537–42.

14. Rapoport AM, Mathew NT, Silberstein SD, Dodick D, Tepper SJ, Sheftell FD, Bigal ME. Zolmitriptan nasal spray in the acute treatment of cluster headache: a double-blind study. Neurology. 2007;69:821–6.
15. Schuh-Hofer S, Reuter U, Kinze S, Einhaupl KM, Arnold G. Treatment of acute cluster headache with 20 mg sumatriptan nasal spray - an open pilot study. J Neurol. 2002;249:94–9.
16. Van Vliet JA, Bahra A, Martin V, Ramadan N, Aurora SK, Mathew NT, Ferrari MD, Goadsby PJ. Intranasal sumatriptan in cluster headache: randomized placebo-controlled double-blind study. Neurology. 2003;60:630–3.
17. Bahra A, Gawel MJ, Hardebo JE, Millson D, Breen SA, Goadsby PJ. Oral zolmitriptan is effective in the acute treatment of cluster headache. Neurology. 2000;54:1832–9.
18. Graham JR, Malvea BP, Gramm HF. Aerosol ergotamine tartrate for migraine and Horton's syndrome. N Engl J Med. 1960;263:802–4.
19. Andersson PG, Jespersen LT. Dihydroergotamine nasal spray in the treatment of attacks of cluster headache. Cephalalgia. 1986;6:51–4.
20. Magnoux E, Zlotnik G. Outpatient intravenous dihydroergotamine for refractory cluster headache. Headache. 2004;44:249–55.
21. Costa A, Pucci E, Antonaci F, Sances G, Granella F, Broich G, Nappi G. The effect of intranasal cocaine and lidocaine on nitroglycerin-induced attacks in cluster headache. Cephalalgia. 2000;20:85–91.
22. Mills TM, Scoggin JA. Intranasal lidocaine for migraine and cluster headaches. Ann Pharmacother. 1997;31:914–5.
23. Robbins L. Intranasal lidocaine for cluster headache. Headache. 1995;35:83–4.
24. Matharu MS, Levy MJ, Meeran K, Goadsby PJ. Subcutaneous octreotide in cluster headache: randomized placebo-controlled double-blind crossover study. Ann Neurol. 2004;56:488–94.
25. Paemeleire K, Bahra A, Evers S, Matharu MS, Goadsby PJ. Medication-overuse headache in patients with cluster headache. Neurology. 2006;67:109–13.
26. Schoenen J, Jensen RH, Lantéri-Minet M, Láinez MJ, Gaul C, Goodman AM, Caparso A, May A. Stimulation of the sphenopalatine ganglion (SPG) for cluster headache treatment. Pathway CH-1: a randomized, sham-controlled study. Cephalalgia. 2013;33:816–30.
27. Silberstein SD, Mechtler LL, Kudrow DB, Calhoun AH, McClure C, Saper JR, Liebler EJ, Rubenstein Engel E, Tepper SJ, ACT1 Study Group. Non-invasive vagus nerve stimulation for the ACute Treatment of cluster headache: findings from the randomized, double-blind, sham-controlled ACT1 study. Headache. 2016;56:1317–32.
28. Gaul C, Diener HC, Silver N, Magis D, Reuter U, Andersson A, Liebler EJ, Straube A, PREVA Study Group. Non-invasive vagus nerve stimulation for PREVention and Acute treatment of chronic cluster headache (PREVA): a randomised controlled study. Cephalalgia. 2016;36:534–46.

Chapter 12
Prophylactic Drugs

Andrea Negro and Paolo Martelletti

12.1 Introduction

Prophylactic treatment is the mainstay in the management for both episodic and chronic cluster headache (CH). The typical CH patient may suffer one to eight attacks a day requiring abortive therapy with risk of medication overuse and drug toxicity.

The primary goal of prophylactic treatment is to shorten cluster episodes, reduce the number of attacks during the bouts, and maintain the patient attack-free for all the expected duration of the cluster period. An appropriate prophylactic medication can reduce triptans use, save medical resources, and improve quality of life of CH patients.

Prophylactic therapy often becomes effective quite rapidly, but unfortunately total attack suppression is not always achievable, and patients need to wait the natural ending of the bouts. Patients with active CH require close follow-up both to monitor the efficacy and the toxicity of maintenance treatments. Moreover, patients with chronic CH (CCH) often need periodic tailoring of medications, and some of them may become refractory to prophylactic treatments [1].

There are fundamental principles in the pharmacological prevention of CH [2]:

- Medications should be selected on the basis of CH course (episodic or chronic), attack frequency and duration, pain intensity, contraindications, and patients comorbidities.
- Prophylaxis should begin at the first signals of the start of a new cluster bout with caution to find the lowest effective dose, maintained during the cluster period and then discontinued by slowly tapering the doses after full remission.

A. Negro (✉) · P. Martelletti
Department of Clinical and Molecular Medicine, Regional Referral Headache Centre,
Sant'Andrea Hospital, Sapienza University of Rome, Rome, Italy
e-mail: andrea.negro@uniroma1.it

© Springer Nature Switzerland AG 2020
M. Leone, A. May (eds.), *Cluster Headache and other Trigeminal Autonomic
Cephalgias*, Headache, https://doi.org/10.1007/978-3-030-12438-0_12

- Treatments for CCH may need to be continued long-term without reduce mainte-
  nance medications and sometimes patients may require prophylaxis indefinitely.
- Combinations of prophylactic medications are often required, particularly for
  CCH patients, although the high potential for toxicity.

Only few randomized clinical trials (RCTs) investigated efficacy of preventive
drugs in CH, and drugs employed as prophylactic treatments for the disease have
been introduced on empirical bases rather than full knowledge of pathophysiological mechanisms [3].

Another issue is for how long prophylaxis should be maintained after the patient has
no more attacks. It is helpful to know the average length of a patient's cluster period to
estimate if attacks were stopped due to treatment or to the natural history of the disease.
Once cluster attacks stopped, it is recommended to continue prophylaxis for a period
of time that is at least the half of the duration of previous cluster periods, but also tapering in shorter periods can be done [4]. In the case of prolonged cluster that lasts
≥3 months, prophylaxis may need to be maintained for at least the same period.

In 2006 a Task Force of the European Federation of Neurological Societies
(EFNS) published comprehensive guidelines on the treatment of cluster headache
(Table 12.1) [4].

12.2 First-Line Medications

12.2.1 Verapamil

Verapamil, a calcium channel blocker, is considered the first choice for the prophylaxis
of both episodic and chronic CH [2–9]. The prophylactic efficacy has been established
by clinical evidence and by two RCTs [8, 9]. In a double-blind placebo-controlled trial
of verapamil 360 mg daily, 80% of patients receiving verapamil had a ≥50% reduction
in headache frequency with half of responders improving in the 1st week and the rest
responding in the 2nd week of therapy [8]. A double-blind, crossover study compared
verapamil (360 mg daily) for 8 weeks to lithium (900 mg daily) for CCH prophylaxis.
Both substances provided similar reductions in analgesic consumption and headache
index, but verapamil showed more rapid action and better tolerability [9].

Although there is no evidence for an optimal dosage, for CH prophylaxis a daily
dosage of 240–960 mg of verapamil is typically used [5, 6, 10, 11]. Most patients
will improve at 240–480 mg/day [12], but in some cases, a daily dose of >720 mg
can be necessary [6, 7, 13], up to 1200 mg/day in rare refractory cases [4]. Only
experienced physicians should give higher dosages.

Given the short half-life of verapamil (3–7 h), the daily dose is divided into three
administration, and regular release tablets are preferred to slow release preparations
because they are more reliable in maintaining drug blood levels.

A baseline electrocardiogram (EKG) is mandatory before initiating verapamil
therapy and should be repeated with each dosage increase to monitor atrioventricular

Table 12.1 Prophylactic and transitional therapies for cluster headache (modified from [4])

	Therapy	Dose	Monitoring	Comment	Common AEs	Advice (EFNS)
First-line medications	Verapamil	240–960 mg	Baseline and periodic EKGs	Starting dose is 80 mg or 120 mg three times daily and increase the dosage by 80 or 120 mg every week up to a dose of 480 mg a day CCH patients may need higher doses	Constipation, gastrointestinal discomfort, dizziness, distal edema, hypotension, fatigue, bradycardia, cardiac conduction impairment (AV blockade), gingival hyperplasia, dull headache	A
Second line medications	Lithium carbonate	600–1800 mg	Lithium levels, CBC, thyroid function, renal function	Starting dose is 300 mg twice a day Increase to 300 mg three times a day after 1 week if no response, and increase further if necessary Usual therapeutic range 0.4–0.8 mEq/L	Tremor, insomnia, nausea, diarrhea, slurred speech, blurred vision, polyuria, polydipsia, arrhythmias, thyroid dysfunction	B
	Methysergide	4–12 mg	Laboratory controls, chest X-ray, EKG, abdominal MRI	Starting dose is 1 mg/day and then increase of 1 mg every 3–5 days up to maximum of 12 mg/day Usage interrupted for at least 1 month in every 6 months Not recommended to be used concomitantly with sumatriptan (synergistic vasoconstrictive effects)	Nausea, dizziness, abdominal pain, and peripheral edema, retroperitoneal, pulmonary, pleural, and cardiac fibrosis	B
	Topiramate	50–200 mg	Serum bicarbonate	Starting dose is 25 mg that should be slowly increased by 25 mg to reach at least 100 mg/day Drink at least 2 L of water per day (to prevent nephrolithiasis)	Paresthesias, cognitive symptoms, fatigue, insomnia, nausea, alteration in taste, loss of appetite, weight loss, anxiety, dizziness, taste alteration, glaucoma, nephrolithiasis	B

(continued)

Table 12.1 (continued)

Therapy	Dose	Monitoring	Comment	Common AEs	Advice (EFNS)
Third-line medications					
Valproic acid	500–2000 mg	CBC, liver function	Contraindicated in females in their childbearing years because of the risk of fatal birth defects	Weight gain, fatigue, tremor, hair loss, nausea	C
Melatonin	10 mg	None	Preferably in the late evening before going to sleep	Fatigue, sedation	C
Baclofen	15–30 mg	None	Starting at low dosage, increased slowly, and slowly decreased when stopping	Drowsiness, dizziness, ataxia, muscle weakness	C
Pizotifen	1.5–3 mg	None	Preferably in the late evening before going to sleep	Sedation, dry mouth, drowsiness, increased appetite, weight gain	Not rated
Capsaicin	0.025% cream	None	Applied twice daily	Burning, itching, dryness, pain, redness, swelling, or soreness at the application site	Not rated
Civamide	100 mL of 0.025%	None	In each nostril daily	Burning, lacrimation, pharyngitis, rhinorrhea	Not rated
Gabapentin	800–3600 mg	CBC	–	Somnolence, fatigue, dizziness, weight gain, peripheral edema, ataxia	Not rated
Clonidine	5–7.5 mg	None	Transdermal patch	Tiredness, hypotension	Not rated
Botulinum toxin A	155–195 U	None	–	Weakness of injected muscles, pain at injection sites	Not rated

Transitional therapies			Laboratory controls		AEs	
	Corticosteroids	Prednisone and prednisolone: 60–100 mg Methylprednisolone: i.v. 500 mg Dexamethasone: 4 mg		Prednisone: starting dose for 5–7 days and then tapered every 2–3 days by 10 mg down to zero Methylprednisolone: sometimes followed by oral steroids Dexamethasone: starting dose for 2 weeks followed by 4 mg/day for the subsequent weeks Possible CH relapse during dose reduction	Blood glucose imbalance, hypertension, sleep disturbance, aseptic bone necroses	A
	Ergotamine and DHE	2–4 mg	Liver function	IV, IM, SC, or IN Repeated two or three times a day for a week if tolerated and may be continued Once or twice a day for another week—longer if necessary and tolerated Not recommended to be used concomitantly with sumatriptan (synergistic vasoconstrictive effects)	Nausea, diarrhea, muscle cramps, cold numb hands and feet, chest tightness, unpleasant taste (IN)	B
	Occipital nerve block	Methylprednisolone (slow release): 40–80 mg (or equivalent)	None	Is usually done in combination with lidocaine Repeated injections can be used	Abscess, hair loss, procedural risks of injection	Not rated

AEs adverse effects, *AV* atrioventricular, *CBC* complete blood count, *CH* cluster headache, *CCH* chronic cluster headache, *DHE* dihydroergotamine, *EFNS* European Federation of Neurological Societies, *EKG* electrocardiogram, *IM* intramuscular, *IV* intravenous, *NS* nasal spray, *SC* subcutaneous conduction. The dosages required for CH prophylaxis are considerably higher than those used for cardiovascular indications (240–480 mg/day) [11]. Consequently, PR interval prolongation, bradycardia, hypotension, syncope, dizziness, crural edema, constipation, and impotence are more likely to occur [14, 15]. Nearly 20% of patients receiving verapamil develop EKG abnormalities, the great majority of these consisting of prolonged PR intervals. Moreover, 5% of patients develop complete heart block with junctional rhythms, in particular those taking higher doses (720 mg or more) [16, 17]. Blockade of atrioventricular conduction can be caused not only by verapamil but also by some of its metabolites such as norverapamil [18]. Because of this, slow titration up to the target dose has been recommended to reduce the AEs.

Long-term verapamil administration can reduce its clearance and increase the plasmatic availability through the CYP3A enzymes auto inhibition [19]. Verapamil metabolism could be affected also by xenobiotics. Patients should be warned to avoid grapefruit and related fruit as limes and pomelos, which contain furanocoumarins that cause irreversible inactivation of CYP3A4 resulting in increased verapamil levels [20, 21]. An excess of coffee and/or tea consumption may enhance both the excretion of verapamil and its first-pass metabolism by CYP1A2 [22].

There are no evidence-based guidelines suggesting the optimal way of dosing verapamil, and the recommendations are based on effectiveness and tolerability. Slow dosage escalation is questionable considering the severity of CH attacks and the additional risks of prolonged use of bridging medications, but on the other hand, faster dosage escalation (80–160 mg every 2 or 3 days) increases the risk of cardiac AEs. An acceptable compromise would be to start verapamil at 80 mg or 120 mg three times daily and then increase the dosage by 80 mg every week up to a dose of 480 mg a day. However, verapamil is generally well tolerated and can be co-administered with sumatriptan, ergotamine, corticosteroids, and other preventive substances with less concern about drug interactions and then with other prophylactic treatment (e.g., lithium carbonate). Lithium and verapamil should be co-administered with great caution in elderly: profound bradycardia developed was reported on two elderly manic patients taking the combination and was followed by a fatal myocardial infarction in one case [23].

The full efficacy of verapamil can be expected within 1–3 weeks in episodic CH at doses of 240–360 mg/day, while CCH patients may need higher doses and up to 4–5 weeks to manifest a response. In the first 2 weeks of verapamil administration, some clinicians also administer corticosteroids as transitional therapy (see after).

12.3 Second-Line Medications

12.3.1 Lithium

Lithium (lithium carbonate), a mood stabilizer medication, has been studied in CH prophylaxis in more than 20 open trials [24]. It was noted that patients suffering from psychiatric disorders improved their cluster headaches while on lithium therapy [25].

Lithium is considered a second-line treatment for maintenance prophylaxis of CH because of its narrow therapeutic window, the need for periodical blood test monitoring during therapy, frequent adverse events (AEs), and several drug interactions.

As mentioned above, a RCT compared lithium (900 mg daily) to verapamil (360 mg daily) for 8 weeks in patients with CCH; the efficacy was similar, but lithium acted more slowly and had more AEs [9]. A recent placebo-controlled trial comparing lithium to placebo in patients with episodic CH found no difference in the primary outcome (cessation of attacks within 1 week) [26]. Even if this study did not reproduce the beneficial effect found in CCH, the dose used (800 mg) was too low and the treatment period (1 week) too short for an adequate efficacy assessment.

Common dosage to obtain benefit is 900 mg (600–1200 mg) per day usually corresponding to 0.4–0.8 mEq/L lithium serum levels [27]. Higher daily dosages can be required in non-responders; it is important to consider that above 1.2 mEq/L lithium serum levels, the risk to develop AEs is high [28]. The drug should be started considering both age and severity of CH, usually a single dose of 300 mg bedtime, then increased after 3–4 days. Lithium plasma level should be measured after 10 days. The dose can be increased to 300 mg three times a day and increased even more in steps of 150–300 mg/day if necessary. Some patients may require 1200 mg/day. In general, if the subject improves or headaches stop at a given dosage, there is no need to further increase the dose. The dosage increase should be stopped if AEs appear.

Baseline thyroid, renal, and liver function tests, as well as electrolytes, should be done prior to start lithium and regularly monitored thereafter. Long-term use can induce hypothyroidism, polymorphonuclear leukocytosis, and renal dysfunction leading to polyuria due to diabetes insipidus [29]. The probability of drug-induced AEs is increased by dehydration; thus patients have to be warned of the importance of an appropriate water intake.

Special caution is again needed when lithium is administered in the elderly particularly because lithium effects and drug interactions on renal function, diuretics, and nonsteroidal anti-inflammatory drugs (NSAIDs) can reduce lithium renal clearance [22, 30], and angiotensin-converting enzyme (ACE) inhibitors can increase the steady-state serum lithium levels up to threefold [31]. Also prokinetic drugs as metoclopramide accelerating gastrointestinal motility may increase lithium absorption and blood concentration [32]. Verapamil metabolites (especially when verapamil is given at >560 mg daily) can reduce renal clearance of lithium; in such patients lithium dosage has to be reduced to prevent AEs [33]. Alcohol should be avoided, and caffeine intake controlled because it increases lithium excretion [29]. Conversely, caffeine discontinuation reduces lithium excretion, and lithium dosage should be decreased as well.

12.3.2 Methysergide

Federigo Sicuteri introduced methysergide, an ergotamine alkaloid derivative as effective headache treatment more than 50 years ago [34]. It has been used as effective CH preventative also in CH [4]. However, no placebo-controlled, double-blind studies are available. Open-label studies showed that between 20% and 73% of patients improve at dosages ranging from 4 to 16 mg daily particularly patients with chronic CH [33].

Usually, methysergide is administered at a daily dose of 4–8 mg starting from 1 mg/day and then increasing 1 mg every 3–5 days up to maximum of 12 mg/day.

Methysergide is indicated for patients with short cluster periods (less than 4 months) [13] as prolonged treatment has been reported to cause retroperitoneal, pulmonary, pleural, and cardiac fibrosis [35, 36]. Laboratory controls including renal function, chest X-ray, electrocardiogram, and abdominal MRI should be undertaken after 4–6 months of treatment.

Methysergide is used much less now because of concerns due to side effects, and its prescription has also been prohibited in several countries (e.g., USA). Methysergide is contraindicated in patients with coronary or peripheral arterial insufficiency and should not be co-administered with triptans because of the synergistic vasoconstrictive effects. Because of the problematic safety profile, methysergide should be used only by experienced practitioners and only as third-line pharmacotherapy.

12.3.3 Topiramate

Topiramate is considered a second-line therapy for CH prophylaxis.

Open-label studies suggest that topiramate in doses ranging from 50 to 200 mg/day is effective in the 70% of patients [37], although one study showed only a minor, if at all, topiramate effect [38].

The recommended starting dose is 25 mg that should be slowly increased by 25 mg every week to minimize adverse effects, to reach at least 100 mg/day. However some authors consider topiramate effective only at higher daily dosages (>100–150 mg/day) or in combination with verapamil and/or lithium.

AEs occur in about 40% of patients, and even if rarely severe, they are a major cause of treatment discontinuation. Topiramate is contraindicated with a history of nephrolithiasis because it may increase the risk of recurrent stones. To prevent nephrolithiasis, patients should be warned to drink at least 2 L of water per day, particularly in warm periods.

Topiramate binding to proteins is quite variable (9–41%) and inversely correlated to its plasmatic concentration [39]. Among 55–97% of administered dose is excreted unchanged in urine. Topiramate may induce the CYP3A4 enzyme leading to a reduction of plasmatic concentrations of oral contraceptive steroids (e.g., ethinylestradiol) [40]. The maintenance of an effective contraception may require higher estrogen doses. Topiramate can have other drug-drug interactions through inhibition of the CYP2C19 enzyme, with consequent decreased clearance of drugs like omeprazole, diazepam, or mephenytoin [41].

12.4 Third-Line Medications

12.4.1 Ergotamine Tartrate

Oral ergotamine has been found to be effective in CH prophylaxis, but its use is limited by the vasoconstrictive properties, variable gastrointestinal absorption, and the potentially threatening AEs associated with ergotism. Ergotism is suggested when limb paresthesia start; in this case the drug must be stopped. Ergot derivatives can be prescribed to hypertensive patients only if arterial blood pressure values are fully controlled.

It is recommended to use this drug category only for short-term treatment courses. Ergotamine tartrate 2 mg per rectum taken at bedtime may help to prevent nocturnal attacks, while 3–4 mg daily in divided doses may be administered for 2–3 weeks as transitional prophylaxis [42].

Dihydroergotamine (DHE) also seems an alternative in CCH patients not responding to other prophylactic drugs. In an open-label study, repeated intravenous (i.v) DHE administration induced remission lasting 12 months in 83% of patients with intractable episodic CH and in 39% of patients with intractable CCH [43].

Because of synergistic side effects, ergot derivatives cannot be administered simultaneously with triptans as for methysergide.

12.4.2 Valproic Acid

Valproic acid has been studied in three small-sample open-label trials that showed efficacy in 54–73% of CH patients, both episodic and chronic [44–46]. A randomized controlled double-blind study did not confirm its efficacy; however, this may have been due to an exceedingly high response rate of 62% in the placebo group, most likely due to spontaneous remission [47].

The clinical experience is that valproic acid is generally ineffective in CH but can be tried as drug of third choice in doses ranging from 500 to 2000 mg daily used alone or in combination with ergots and possibly lithium. Valproic acid may be more effective in CH patients with migrainous features, such as nausea, vomiting, and photo and phonophobia [2]. Regular evaluation of hemogram and liver and pancreatic function are necessary to monitor AEs [19].

Valproic acid is contraindicated in female potentially childbearing patients because of the risk of fatal birth defects [48].

12.4.3 Melatonin

Melatonin is a natural sleep hormone. Cluster patients have reduced serum melatonin levels, and this has the potential to favor CH attacks particularly during the night [49]. This and other observations prompted its use as a CH preventive agent.

In a double-blind, placebo-controlled trial, melatonin 10 mg in regular release tablets was effective to induce cluster remission in five of ten subjects within 5 days while none of the ten subjects randomized to placebo went into remission [50]. A subsequent study that used a 2 mg slow release tablet investigated melatonin efficacy as adjunctive therapy in CH prophylaxis but failed to show benefits [51]. However melatonin can be used with other cluster medications at a starting dose of 10 mg, titrated quickly to 25 mg, and given in the late evening before going to sleep [27].

12.4.4 Pizotifen

One old controlled trial showed that pizotifen exerts some effect [52, 53]. It can be used in one dose of 1.5–3 mg before retiring. Its use is limited by side effects, and it should be used in rare cases as third-line drug [27].

12.4.5 Capsaicin

The effect of repeated capsaicin application to the nasal mucosa in cluster headache has been evaluated in two open [54, 55] and one double-blind, placebo-controlled [56] trial that showed an efficacy in about two-third of the patients. Results from the double-blind study are questionable because of the irritating properties of the active drug [56].

12.4.6 Baclofen

A small open-label study evaluated the efficacy of baclofen 15–30 mg in three divided doses in nine CH patients [57]. Six patients went into remission within a week, and one additional patient improved with cessation of attacks at week 2 [57]. Baclofen should be started at low dosage, increased slowly, and slowly decreased until stopped.

12.4.7 Civamide

A randomized double-blind, placebo-controlled study evaluated the efficacy of intranasal application of civamide for 7 days in 28 CH patients [58]. The primary endpoint was change in frequency of CH attacks per week during posttreatment period (20 days). During the 1st week of the study, civamide was significantly better than placebo in decreasing number of attacks (55.5% vs. 25.9%); a similar trend was present for the entire posttreatment period but did reach statistical significance (61.4% vs. 30.9%; p 0.054). As for capsaicin, blindness is difficult to achieve because of the irritating nature of the nasally applied substance.

12.4.8 Gabapentin

Gabapentin was used in two open-label studies. In the first, 900 mg/day induced remission in eight episodic and four CCH patients within 8 days, with a bout duration reduction ranging from 16 to 40% compared to previous bouts (in episodic cluster headache patients) [59]. In the second study, gabapentin was used as add-on drug in eight patients suffering from CCH refractory to first-line treatment [60]. Six of them responded to treatment, and the longest remission under gabapentin treatment was 18 months.

12.4.9 Clonidine

Clonidine 5–7.5 mg transdermal patch has been studied in two small open-label studies [61, 62]. The first included eight episodic and five chronic CH patients, and all had significant reduction in frequency, intensity, and duration of the attacks [61]. The second study included 16 episodic CH patients but failed to confirm the previous positive results [62].

12.4.10 Botulinum Toxin Type A

Botulinum toxin type A has been tested as add-on therapy in a small open-label study that gave mixed results [63]. Patients with CH (three episodic and nine chronic) received 50 units injected ipsilateral to the headache. One chronic CH patient had remission, other two chronic patients had improvement in attack frequency and severity, and another chronic CH patient had his continuous headache improved but no change in cluster headache attacks. The remaining eight patients had no benefit.

12.4.11 Calcitonin Gene-Related Peptide (CGRP)-Targeted Therapies

Calcitonin gene-related peptide (CGRP)-targeted therapies represent the new frontiers in migraine and CH treatment. At this time, two monoclonal antibodies, galcanezumab (LY2951742 by Eli Lilly) and fremanezumab (TEV-48125 by TEVA), are under evaluation in Phase 3 clinical trials.

Galcanezumab is being studied for both episodic (NCT02397473) [64] and chronic CH (NCT02438826) [65]. The drug is administered subcutaneously every 30 days for 8 weeks and 12 months (in episodic and chronic trial, respectively). In both studies the primary outcome is the mean change in number of weekly attacks, and the secondary outcome is the proportion of participants with ≥30 or ≥50% reduction in number of weekly attacks. Both studies estimate to enroll 162 patients. The estimated completion date for the episodic study is June 2018 and for the chronic one is July 2019. Patients that complete those trials will be invited to participate to a long-term safety and tolerability study [NCT02797951] estimated to be completed in August 2020 [66].

Similarly, fremanezumab in two dose regimens (intravenous/subcutaneous and subcutaneous) is under evaluation for both episodic [NCT02945046] [67] and chronic [NCT02964338] [68] CH prophylaxis. The primary outcome is the mean change in the weekly average number of attacks during the 4-week (for episodic) and the 12-week period (for chronic) after administration of the first dose. The secondary outcomes are the mean change from baseline in the number of CH attacks during the 4-week (for episodic) and the 12-week period (for chronic) after the first dose and the proportion of participants with ≥50% reduction in number of weekly attacks during same period. Both studies estimate to enroll 300 patients. The estimated completion date for the episodic study is June 2018 and for the chronic one is November 2018. Patients that complete those trials will be invited to participate to a 68 weeks study to evaluate the long-term safety of fremanezumab [NCT03107052] estimated to be completed in August 2020 [69].

12.5 Transitional Therapies

The transitional medications are usually administered initially together with CH prophylactic treatment until prophylactic treatment effectiveness begins. Transitional therapies are indicated primarily in episodic CH patients with relatively high attacks frequency (>2 attacks/day). This approach aims to quickly stop CH attacks to prevent pain and reduce disability, also reducing use of acute medications. In the meantime dosage of prophylactic medication can be gradually increased up to therapeutic range. Transitional therapies are generally used for 1–3 weeks depending on the prophylactic drug titration and cluster period severity. Occipital nerve blockade with steroids and/or local anesthetics can require only one injection.

12.5.1 Corticosteroids

Corticosteroids as prednisolone, prednisone, and dexamethasone are rapidly effective drugs for CH and are considered the most effective transitional treatment [27]. About 70–80% of all CH patients report headache-free or near headache-free states within 24–48 h from steroid administration, but some patients require prolonged administration as headaches recur once steroid is tapered/stopped [70]. Because of the high risk for side effects, steroids should be used for short-term courses only trying to limit their use as long-term treatment [2].

CH is very likely to relapse when transitional steroid treatment is reduced and stopped unless a nonsteroidal prophylactic therapy as verapamil or lithium has been initiated in the meantime. A steroid course lasting 15–18 days provides time to increase the dose of the prophylactic drug to the expected therapeutic dosage.

There are no adequate randomized, placebo-controlled trials available for the use of corticosteroids in CH. Common dosage of oral prednisone or prednisolone is 60–100 mg given once a day for 5–7 days; the dose should then be tapered every 2–3 days by 10 mg down to zero. The tapering could be slower in CCH because of relapse occurrence. Intravenous corticosteroids (methylprednisolone i.v. 500 mg), sometimes followed by oral steroids, may also be effective [71, 72]. Also dexamethasone, a synthetic corticosteroid used mainly to manage cerebral edema, resulted in a clinical positive response when administered intramuscularly or orally as 4 mg twice a day for 2 weeks followed by 4 mg/day for the subsequent week [71].

12.5.2   Ergot Derivatives

Even though controlled trial data supporting their use are lacking, ergotamine tartrate and DHE may be used for CH transitional prophylaxis. Ergotamine tartrate (3–4 mg/day in divided doses) may be administered for 2–3 weeks [42]. Repetitive intravenous DHE administrations (two or three times a day) stop the attacks within 3 days from initiating therapy in more than 90% of patients [73]. The most practical method of administration for use at home is by SC or intramuscular self-injection. DHE given subcutaneously as 1 mg twice a day or just 1 mg at bedtime can be continued beyond 1 week [74]. DHE nasal spray could theoretically also be used, but not all the medication is absorbed [75], and consequently a higher dose of 2 mg is recommended [76].

12.5.3   Occipital Nerve Block

An effective alternative to steroid oral administration is occipital nerve block injecting local anesthetic and corticosteroid or corticosteroid alone; compared to oral administration, this route has the advantage of not inducing the rebound effect [77].

Blockade of greater occipital nerve (GON) was investigated as CH treatment in several studies, with the majority showing positive results. In a small open-label trial, GON block ipsilateral to the head pain using lidocaine 1% in combination with triamcinolone 40 mg was associated with good or moderate response in 64% of patients [78]. However, triamcinolone should be avoided because of reported risk of cutaneous atrophy and localized alopecia [79]. A prospective open-label study showed a positive response to GON blockade in 57% of CCH patients: 42% of responders were pain free and 15% having a partial benefit [80]. Duration of improvement was 3 weeks (median); efficacy, overall rate, and average duration of response remained consistent with repeated quarterly injections.

Also, suboccipital injection of steroids was effective in a double-blind, placebo-controlled trial [81]. A single injection of a mixture of short- and long-acting beta-methasone (12.46 mg betamethasone dipropionate and 5.26 mg betamethasone disodium phosphate mixed with 0.5 mL lidocaine 2%) suppressed cluster attacks in 85% of patients (both episodic and chronic) with 61% remaining attack-free for at least 4 weeks. In another randomized, double-blind, placebo-controlled trial, three suboccipital injections (48–72 h apart) of cortivazol 3.75 mg reduced the number of attacks during the first 15 days after the first injections in both episodic and chronic CH patients [75].

Long-acting preparation of steroids may be more useful for occipital nerve block, and based on the two controlled trials, a relatively high dose can be used [75, 81]. Betamethasone has a five times higher potency than methylprednisolone, so methylprednisolone dosages between 40 and 80 mg in a slow release preparation would be appropriate in case of several repeated injections. In the case of only a single injection, 80 mg of methylprednisolone might be more appropriate than 40 mg.

References

1. Mitsikostas DD, Edvinsson L, Jensen RH, Katsarava Z, Lampl C, Negro A, Osipova V, Paemeleire K, Siva A, Valade D, Martelletti P. Refractory chronic cluster headache: a consensus statement on clinical definition from the European Headache Federation. J Headache Pain. 2014;15:79.
2. Tfelt-Hansen PC, Jensen RH. Management of cluster headache. CNS Drugs. 2012;26:571–80.
3. Martelletti P, Curto M. Headache: cluster headache treatment—RCTs versus real-world evidence. Nat Rev Neurol. 2016;12:557–8.
4. May A, Leone M, Afra J, Linde M, Sándor PS, Evers S, Goadsby PJ, EFNS Task Force. EFNS guidelines on the treatment of cluster headache and other trigeminal-autonomic cephalalgias. Eur J Neurol. 2006;13:1066–77.
5. May A. Headaches with (ipsilateral) autonomic symptoms. J Neurol. 2003;250:1273–8.
6. Matharu MS, Boes CJ, Goadsby PJ. Management of trigeminal autonomic cephalgias and hemicrania continua. Drugs. 2003;63:1637–77.
7. Gabai IJ, Spierings EL. Prophylactic treatment of cluster headache with verapamil. Headache. 1989;29:167–8.
8. Leone M, D'Amico D, Frediani F, Moschiano F, Grazzi L, Attanasio A, Bussone G. Verapamil in the prophylaxis of episodic cluster headache: a double-blind study versus placebo. Neurology. 2000;54:1382–5.
9. Bussone G, Leone M, Peccarisi C, Micieli G, Granella F, Magri M, Manzoni GC, Nappi G. Double blind comparison of lithium and verapamil in cluster headache prophylaxis. Headache. 1990;30(7):411–7.
10. Weaver-Agostoni J. Cluster headache. Am Fam Physician. 2013;88:122–8.
11. Tfelt-Hansen P, Tfelt-Hansen J. Verapamil for cluster headache. Clinical pharmacology and possible mode of action. Headache. 2009;49:117–25.

12. Blau JN, Engel HO. Individualizing treatment with verapamil for cluster headache patients. Headache. 2004;44:1013–8.
13. Francis GJ, Becker WJ, Pringsheim TM. Acute and preventive pharmacologic treatment of cluster headache. Neurology. 2010;75:463–73.
14. Kivistö KT, Neuvonen PJ, Tarssanen L. Pharmacokinetics of verapamil in overdose. Hum Exp Toxicol. 1997;16:35–7.
15. Busse D, Templin S, Mikus G, Schwab M, Hofmann U, Eichelbaum M, Kivistö KT. Cardiovascular effects of (R)- and (S)-verapamil and racemic verapamil in humans: a placebo-controlled study. Eur J Clin Pharmacol. 2006;62:613–9.
16. Cohen AS, Matharu MS, Goadsby PJ. Electrocardiographic abnormalities in patients with cluster headache on verapamil therapy. Neurology. 2007;69:668–75.
17. Lanteri-Minet M, Silhol F, Piano V, Donnet A. Cardiac safety in cluster headache patients using the very high dose of verapamil (≥720 mg/day). J Headache Pain. 2011;12:173–6.
18. Abernethy DR, Wainer IW, Anacleto AI. Verapamil metabolite exposure in older and younger men during steady-state oral verapamil administration. Drug Metab Dispos. 2000;28:760–5.
19. de Andrés F, Lionetto L, Curto M, Capi M, Cipolla F, Negro A, Martelletti P. Acute, transitional and long-term cluster headache treatment: pharmacokinetic issues. Expert Opin Drug Metab Toxicol. 2016;129:1011–20.
20. Pillai U, Muzaffar J, Sen S, Yancey A. Grapefruit juice and verapamil: a toxic cocktail. South Med J. 2009;102:308–9.
21. Bailey DG, Dresser G, Arnold JM. Grapefruit-medication interactions: Forbidden fruit or avoidable consequences? CMAJ. 2013;185:309–16.
22. Wishart DS, Knox C, Guo AC, Shrivastava S, Hassanali M, Stothard P, Chang Z, Woolsey J. DrugBank: a comprehensive resource for in silico drug discovery and exploration. Nucleic Acids Res. 2006;34:D668–72.
23. Dubovsky SL, Franks RD, Allen S. Verapamil: a new antimanic drug with potential interactions with lithium. J Clin Psychiatry. 1987;48:371–2.
24. Ekbom K. Lithium for cluster headache: review of the literature and preliminary results of long-term treatment. Headache. 1981;21:132–9.
25. Kudrow L. Lithium prophylaxis for chronic cluster headache. Headache. 1977;17:15–8.
26. Steiner TJ, Hering R, Couturier EGM, Davies PTG, Whitmarsh TE. Double-blind placebo-controlled trial of lithium in episodic cluster headache. Cephalalgia. 1997;17:673–5.
27. Ashkenazi A, Schwedt T. Cluster headache-acute and prophylactic therapy. Headache. 2011;51:272–86.
28. Becker WJ. Cluster headache: conventional pharmacological management. Headache. 2013;53:1191–6.
29. Shine B, McKnight RF, Leaver L, Geddes JR. Long-term effects of lithium on renal, thyroid, and parathyroid function: a retrospective analysis of laboratory data. Lancet. 2015;386:461–8.
30. Sternieri E, Coccia CP, Pinetti D, Guerzoni S, Ferrari A. Pharmacokinetics and interactions of headache medications, part II: prophylactic treatments. Expert Opin Drug Metab Toxicol. 2006;2:981–1007.
31. Juurlink DN, Mamdani MM, Kopp A, Rochon PA, Shulman KI, Redelmeier DA. Drug-induced lithium toxicity in the elderly: a population-based study. J Am Geriatr Soc. 2004;52:794–8.
32. Finley PR, Warner MD, Peabody CA. Clinical relevance of drug interactions with lithium. Clin Pharmacokinet. 1995;29:172–91.
33. Krabbe AA. Cluster headache: a review. Acta Neurol Scand. 1986;74:1–9.
34. Sicuteri F. Prophylactic and therapeutic properties of 1-methyl-lysergic acid butanolamide in migraine. Int Arch Allergy Appl Immunol. 1959;15:300–7.
35. Graham JR, Suby HI, LeCompte PR, Sadowsky NL. Fibrotic disorders associated with methysergide therapy for headache. N Engl J Med. 1966;274:359–68.
36. Müller R, Weller P, Chemaissani A. Pleural fibrosis as a side effect of years-long methysergide therapy. Dtsch Med Wochenschr. 1991;116(38):1433–6.
37. Pascual J, Láinez MJ, Dodick D, Hering-Hanit R. Antiepileptic drugs for the treatment of chronic and episodic cluster headache: a review. Headache. 2007;47:81–9.

38. Leone M, Dodick D, Rigamonti A, D'Amico D, Grazzi L, Mea E, Bussone G. Topiramate in cluster headache prophylaxis: an open trial. Cephalalgia. 2003;23:1001–2.
39. Perucca E, Bialer M. The clinical pharmacokinetics of the newer antiepileptic drugs. Focus on topiramate, zonisamide and tiagabine. Clin Pharmacokinet. 1996;31:29–46.
40. Rosenfeld WE, Doose DR, Walker SA, Nayak RK. Effect of topiramate on the pharmacokinetics of an oral contraceptive containing norethindrone and ethinyl estradiol in patients with epilepsy. Epilepsia. 1997;38:317–23.
41. Benedetti MS. Enzyme induction and inhibition by new antiepileptic drugs: a review of human studies. Fundam Clin Pharmacol. 2000;14:301–19.
42. Halker R, Vargas B, Dodick DW. Cluster headache: diagnosis and treatment. Semin Neurol. 2010;30:175–85.
43. Silberstein SD, Schulman EA, Hopkins MM. Repetitive intravenous DHE in the treatment of refractory headache. Headache. 1990;30:334–9.
44. Hering R, Kuritzky A. Sodium valproate in the treatment of cluster headache: an open clinical trial. Cephalalgia. 1989;9(3):195–8.
45. Freitag FG, Diamond S, Diamond ML, Urban GJ. Divalproex in the long-term treatment of chronic daily headache. Headache. 2001;41:271–8.
46. Gallagher RM, Mueller LL, Freitag FG. Divalproex sodium in the treatment of migraine and cluster headaches. J Am Osteopath Assoc. 2002;102:92–4.
47. El Amrani M, Massiou H, Bousser MG. A negative trial of sodium valproate in cluster headache: methodological issues. Cephalalgia. 2002;22:205–8.
48. Negro A, Delaruelle Z, Ivanova TA, Khan S, Ornello R, Raffaelli B, Terrin A, Reuter U, Mitsikostas DD, European Headache Federation School of Advanced Studies (EHF-SAS). Headache and pregnancy: a systematic review. J Headache Pain. 2017;18:106.
49. Bruera O, Sances G, Leston J, Levin G, Cristina S, Medina C, Barontini M, Nappi G, Figuerola MA. Plasma melatonin pattern in chronic and episodic headaches: evaluation during sleep and waking. Funct Neurol. 2008;23:77–81.
50. Leone M, D'Amico D, Moschiano F, Fraschini F, Bussone G. Melatonin versus placebo in the prophylaxis of cluster headache: a double-blind pilot study with parallel groups. Cephalalgia. 1996;16:494–6.
51. Pringsheim T, Magnoux E, Dobson CF, Hamel E, Aubé M. Melatonin as adjunctive therapy in the prophylaxis of cluster headache: a pilot study. Headache. 2002;42(8):787–92.
52. Ekbom K. Prophylactic treatment of cluster headache with a new serotonin antagonist, BC 105. Acta Neurol Scand. 1969;45:601–10.
53. Sicuteri F, Fusco BM, Marabini S, Campagnolo V, Maggi CA, Geppetti P, Fanciullacci M. Beneficial effect of capsaicin application to the nasal mucosa in cluster headache. Clin J Pain. 1989;5:49–53.
54. Fusco BM, Marabini S, Maggi CA, Fiore G, Geppetti P. Preventative effect of repeated nasal applications of capsaicin in cluster headache. Pain. 1994;59:321–5.
55. Marks DR, Rapoport A, Padla D, Weeks R, Rosum R, Sheftell F, Arrowsmith F. A double-blind placebo-controlled trial of intranasal capsaicin for cluster headache. Cephalalgia. 1993;13:114–6.
56. Hering-Hanit R, Gadoth N. Baclofen in cluster headache. Headache. 2000;40:48–51.
57. Saper JR, Klapper J, Mathew NT, Rapoport A, Phillips SB, Bernstein JE. Intranasal civamide for the treatment of episodic cluster headaches. Arch Neurol. 2002;59:990–4.
58. Leandri M, Luzzani M, Cruccu G, Gottlieb A. Drug-resistant cluster headache responding to gabapentin: a pilot study. Cephalalgia. 2001;21:744–6.
59. Schuh-Hofer S, Israel H, Neeb L, Reuter U, Arnold G. The use of gabapentin in chronic cluster headache patients refractory to first-line therapy. Eur J Neurol. 2007;14:694–6.
60. D'Andrea G, Perini F, Granella F, Cananzi A, Sergi A. Efficacy of transdermal clonidine in short-term treatment of cluster headache: a pilot study. Cephalalgia. 1995;155:430–3.
61. Leone M, Attanasio A, Grazzi L, Libro G, D'Amico D, Moschiano F, Bussone G. Transdermal clonidine in the prophylaxis of episodic cluster headache: an open study. Headache. 1997;379:559–60.

62. Sostak P, Krause P, Förderreuther S, Reinisch V, Straube A. Botulinum toxin type-A therapy in cluster headache: an open study. J Headache Pain. 2007;84:236–41.
63. US National Library of Medicine. ClinicalTrials.gov. https://clinicaltrials.gov/ct2/show/NCT02397473. Accessed 11 Dec 2017.
64. US National Library of Medicine. ClinicalTrials.gov. https://clinicaltrials.gov/ct2/show/NCT02438826. Accessed 11 Dec 2017.
65. US National Library of Medicine. ClinicalTrials.gov. https://clinicaltrials.gov/ct2/show/NCT02576951. Accessed 11 Dec 2017.
66. US National Library of Medicine. ClinicalTrials.gov. https://clinicaltrials.gov/ct2/show/NCT02945046. Accessed 11 Dec 2017.
67. US National Library of Medicine. ClinicalTrials.gov. https://clinicaltrials.gov/ct2/show/NCT02964338. Accessed 11 Dec 2017.
68. US National Library of Medicine. ClinicalTrials.gov. https://clinicaltrials.gov/ct2/show/NCT03107052. Accessed 11 Dec 2017.
69. Couch JR Jr, Ziegler DK. Prednisone therapy for cluster headache. Headache. 1978;18:219–21.
70. Antonaci F, Costa A, Candeloro E, Sjaastad O, Nappi G. Single high-dose steroid treatment in episodic cluster headache. Cephalalgia. 2005;254:290–5.
71. Mir P, Alberca R, Navarro A, Montes E, Martínez E, Franco E, Cayuela A, Lozano P. Prophylactic treatment of episodic cluster headache with intravenous bolus of methylprednisolone. Neurol Sci. 2003;245:318–21.
72. Mather PJ, Silberstein SD, Schulman EA, Hopkins MM. The treatment of cluster headache with repetitive intravenous dihydroergotamine. Headache. 1991;318:525–32.
73. Magnoux E, Zlotnik G. Outpatient intravenous dihydroergotamine for refractory cluster headache. Headache. 2004;443:249–55.
74. Mathew NT. Dosing and administration of ergotamine tartrate and dihydroergotamine. Headache. 1997;37(Suppl 1):S26–32.
75. Ekbom K, Krabbe AE, Paalzow G, Paalzow L, Tfelt-Hansen P, Waldenlind E. Optimal routes of administration of ergotamine tartrate in cluster headache patients. A pharmacokinetic study. Cephalalgia. 1983;3:15–20.
76. Martelletti P, Giamberardino MA, Mitsikostas DD. Greater occipital nerve as target for refractory chronic headaches: from corticosteroid block to invasive neurostimulation and back. Expert Rev Neurother. 2016;16:865–6.
77. Peres MF, Stiles MA, Siow HC, Rozen TD, Young WB, Silberstein SD. Greater occipital nerve blockade for cluster headache. Cephalalgia. 2002;22:520–2.
78. Lambru G, Lagrata S, Matharu MS. Cutaneous atrophy and alopecia after greater occipital nerve injection using triamcinolone. Headache. 2012;52:1596–9.
79. Lambru G, Abu Bakar N, Stahlhut L, McCulloch S, Miller S, Shanahan P, Matharu MS. Greater occipital nerve blocks in chronic cluster headache: a prospective open-label study. Eur J Neurol. 2014;21:338–43.
80. Ambrosini A, Vandenheede M, Rossi P, Aloj F, Sauli E, Pierelli F, Schoenen J. Suboccipital injection with a mixture of rapid- and long-acting steroids in cluster headache: a double-blind placebo-controlled study. Pain. 2005;118(1–2):92–6.
81. Leroux E, Valade D, Taifas I, Vicaut E, Chagnon M, Roos C, Ducros A. Suboccipital steroid injections for transitional treatment of patients with more than two cluster headache attacks per day: a randomised, double-blind, placebo-controlled trial. Lancet Neurol. 2011;10:891–7.

Chapter 13
Neurostimulation: Why, When, and Which One?

Michel Lantéri-Minet, Denys Fontaine, and Delphine Magis

Neuromodulation has been proposed for more than a decade to treat primary headaches including cluster headache. Neuromodulation can be separated into invasive techniques, that is, with a surgical procedure to implant the stimulation device, and noninvasive techniques (transcutaneous or transcranial stimulation). For the treatment of cluster headache (CH), the only noninvasive neuromodulation technique studied up to now is vagus nerve stimulation (cervical portion), while invasive neuromodulation has been applied to target the posteroinferior hypothalamic area, the great occipital nerve, or the sphenopalatine ganglion. For each target, we will review key elements in terms of background, efficacy evidence, limits, and mechanisms of action.

13.1 Vagus Nerve Stimulation

13.1.1 Background

Vagus nerve stimulation has been considered as a promising treatment of primary headaches following migraine improvement in epileptic patients with a migraine comorbidity, while their epilepsy was treated by implanted vagus nerve stimulation [1]. Recent devices allowing a noninvasive stimulation of the vagus nerve (nVNS)

M. Lantéri-Minet (✉)
Pain Department and FHU InovPain, CHU Nice and Côte Azur University, Nice, France
e-mail: lanteri-minet.m@chu-nice.fr

D. Fontaine
Neurosurgical Department FHU InovPain, CHU Nice and Côte Azur University, Nice, France

D. Magis
Headache Research Unit, University Department of Neurology CHR, Liege, Belgium

© Springer Nature Switzerland AG 2020
M. Leone, A. May (eds.), *Cluster Headache and other Trigeminal Autonomic Cephalgias*, Headache, https://doi.org/10.1007/978-3-030-12438-0_13

have increased interest for this target, the gammaCore® device having been mean-while specifically developed for the treatment of headache by noninvasive stimulation of the cervical branch of the vagus nerve.

13.1.2 Evidence

PREVA study is an *open* randomized controlled trial (RCT) in which nVNS was examined as adjunctive prophylactic treatment of chronic CH [2]. The PREVA study compared adjunctive prophylactic nVNS ($n = 48$) with standard of care (SoC), i.e., medications alone as a control ($n = 49$). A 2-week baseline phase was followed by a 4-week randomized phase (SoC plus nVNS vs. SoC alone) and a 4-week extension phase (SoC plus nVNS). The primary endpoint was the reduction in the mean number of CH attacks per week. During the randomized phase, individuals in intent-to-treat population treated with SoC plus nVNS ($n = 45$) had a significantly greater reduction in the number of attacks per week compared to those receiving SoC alone ($n = 48$) (-5.9 vs. -2.1, respectively) for a mean therapeutic gain of 3.9 fewer attacks per week (95% CI: 0.5–7.2; $p = 0.02$). This preventive effect was maintained during the 4-week extension phase during which all patients benefited from nVNS [3]. Using PREVA study data, a pharmacoeconomic model from the German statutory health insurance perspective showed cost-effectiveness of nVNS, suggesting that adjunctive nVNS provides economic benefits in the treatment of chronic CH [4].

The PREVA study did not show any evidence of nVNS efficacy for the acute treatment of CH in patients with chronic CH [5]. Conversely, nVNS showed its efficacy to abort or relieve attacks of episodic CH in two large sham-controlled trials (ACT1 and ACT2, ref.). ACT2 study is a RCT that compared nVNS with a sham (placebo) device for acute treatment in patients suffering from episodic or chronic CH [6]. After completing a 1-week run-in period, subjects were randomly assigned to receive nVNS or sham stimulation during a 2-week double-blind period. The primary efficacy endpoint was the proportion of all treated attacks that achieved pain-free status within 15 min after treatment initiation, without rescue medication. The Full Analysis Set comprised 48 nVNS-treated (14 episodic CH, 34 chronic CH) and 44 sham-treated patients (13 episodic CH, 31 chronic CH). From the primary endpoint, nVNS (14%) and sham (12%) treatments were not significantly different for the entire CH population. No significant differences were seen between nVNS (5%) and sham (13%) in the chronic CH subgroup. By contrast, nVNS (48%) was superior to sham (6%; $p < 0.01$) in the episodic CH subgroup. Efficacy of nVNS for the acute treatment of episodic CH was also supported by the ACT1 study [7]. ACT1 study is a RCT similar to ACT2, but the primary endpoint was the response rate, defined as the proportion of subjects who achieved pain relief at 15 min after treatment initiation for the first attack without any rescue medication use through 60 min. The intent-to-treat population comprised 133 subjects: 60 nVNS-treated (episodic CH, $n = 38$;

chronic CH, $n = 22$) and 73 sham-treated (episodic CH, $n = 47$; chronic CH, $n = 26$). Again, response rates were overall not significantly different between nVNS-treated and sham-treated patients (26.7% vs. 15.1% $p = 0.1$), but were significantly higher with nVNS than with sham when the episodic CH subgroup was considered (34.2% vs. 10.6%; $p = 0.008$).

13.1.3 Limits

Evidence supports the use of nVNS as an acute treatment of episodic CH and as a prophylactic treatment of chronic CH. Nevertheless, based on clinical experience, therapeutic benefit from prophylactic treatment would be more convincing than from acute treatment especially in chronic CH [8]. Acute nVNS use requires the self-application of three stimulation sessions of 2 min each separated by 1 min from the beginning of the attack. For preventive use, the administration of a stimulation period of 2 min three times a day is necessary and must be evaluated over 3 months. The gammaCore® device has only one nVNS program. The subject can use the device on the right or left sides of the neck by putting it next to his/her carotid pulse (usually alternate sessions are recommended). Intensity is raised until the subject feels a tingling sensation deep in the neck, and the device is well positioned when the subject feels a tightness of its lower lip (due to platysma muscle contraction). Safety and tolerability of nVNS with gammaCore® was confirmed by the three RCTs (PREVA, ACT1, ACT2) performed in CH. In these trials, the side effects (voice change, skin irritation, muscle contraction, dysesthesia) were mild to moderate and all transient [2, 6, 7]. The manufacturer of gammaCore® advises not to use it in pregnancy and in the following situations: cervical atheroma, implanted stimulator, high blood pressure, hypotension, tachycardia, bradycardia, cervical vagotomy, and metallic device implanted in the cephalic segment. This device has a CE mark, but it is not reimbursed by all health insurance systems. It is available, on prescription, on the manufacturer's website (https://gammacore.com) at a rate of 260 €. Although comparable to the triptan budget, this price might therefore represent a limit to nVNS use, especially as this device allows a limited number of stimulations (or "doses," up to 300) but its battery cannot be recharged. Thus, a new device must be purchased at the end of the battery.

13.1.4 Mechanism of Action

The precise mechanism of action of nVNS in primary headaches is not known, but corpus of data is available and allows certain assumptions [9]. The reality of vagus nerve stimulation by gammaCore® has been confirmed using a neurophysiological approach in healthy volunteers, which showed that cervical nVNS induced evoked nerve potentials similar to those induced by invasive vagus nerve stimulation devices [10]. Similarly, a functional magnetic resonance imaging study, also performed in healthy controls stimulated by gammaCore®, highlighted an activation of the solitary tract nucleus, which is the main central relay of vagal afferences [11]. The therapeutic effect of nVNS is probably mediated by the stimulation of large myelinated fibers as argued by magnetic resonance-based model predicting the properties of the induced electric field in different anatomical planes [12]. The lack of C fibers recruitment suggested by this model accounts for the absence of pain and parasympathetic signs with nVNS using gammaCore®. Experimental works have also tried to specify the mechanism of the therapeutic effect of gammaCore® in primary headaches. Centered on migraine, a first experimental work has shown an inhibition of cortical spreading depression (CSD) support of the migraine aura and possible trigger of migraine headache [13]. Another study, focused on trigeminal pain and performed on a murine model of trigeminal allodynia induced by dural inflammation, has shown a significant reduction in periorbital skin sensitivity for more than 3.5 h after nVNS, this reduction being associated with a reduction of extracellular glutamate concentration in the trigemino-cervical complex [14]. A neuroimaging study showed an activation of the solitary tract nucleus that was associated to changes in the pain matrix (parabrachial nucleus, primary somatosensory cortex, and the insula) and the trigemino-cervical complex [11]. Finally, an experimental electrophysiological work demonstrated the ability of implanted vagus nerve stimulation to reduce dose-dependent nociceptive activation of neurons of the trigemino-cervical complex and the superior salivary nucleus which are the two essential relays of the trigemino-autonomic pathway supporting primary headaches like migraine and cluster headache [15].

13.2 Deep Brain Stimulation of Posteroinferior Hypothalamic Area

13.2.1 Background

Deep brain stimulation (DBS) of the posteroinferior hypothalamus has been the first neuromodulation technique to be proposed in drug-refractory chronic CH. The initial concept was to inhibit the presumed CH attack generator [16, 17] identified in this area shortly before, by neuroimaging studies. Indeed, positron emission tomography (PET) imaging during CH attacks showed a specific activation of an area located at the diencephalo-mesencephalic region, close to the floor of the third ventricle [18]. Based on its projection on the Talairach grid, this region has been called posteroinferior hypothalamus.

13.2.2 Evidence

Preventive treatment with high-frequency (130 Hz) DBS of the posteroinferior hypothalamus area has been reported in the literature in about 80 patients up to now (Table 13.1) [16, 17, 19–27] with an overall 50% responders' rate (≥50% decrease of attack frequency) of 62.8%, including 30% of patients being almost pain-free at longer follow-up. This approach has been evaluated in controlled conditions by a single study [22]. However due to methodological issues, including the too short duration (1 month) of the randomized periods, this RCT failed to demonstrate a significant decrease of CH attacks with DBS (ON) compared to control (OFF) conditions. As a matter of fact, retro-hypothalamic DBS therapeutic effect may be delayed, and a clinically significant headache decrease can be observed in an interval ranging from 1 to 86 days. Several studies reported that some patients with a long follow-up showed few bouts of attacks per year, like episodic CH.

13.2.3 Limits

DBS is the last-line preventive treatment of the most severe chronic CH patients and should only be practiced by medico-surgical teams combining headache expertise and functional neurosurgery expertise with a strict respect of patient selection criteria (at least 2 years of disease duration, at least one attack per day, resistance to pharmacotherapy including verapamil and lithium, headache "locked" to the same side, normal neurological examination, and absence of psychiatric comorbidity) [28, 29]. This position as a last-line treatment is justified by the invasiveness and the

Table 13.1 Open series and RCT related to DBS in chronic CH

Study	Patients (n)	Country	Mono/ multi centric	Mean follow-up (years)	At least 50% improvement (n)
Leone et al. [17, 23], and Franzini et al. [16]	17	Italy	Mono	8.7	12
Schoenen et al. [25]	6	Belgium	Mono	4	3
Starr et al. [27]	4	USA	Mono	1	2
Owen et al. [24]	1	GB	Mono	0.7	1
Bartsch et al. [20]	6	Germany	Mono	1.4	3
Fontaine et al. [22] (RCT)	11	France	Multi	1	6
Seijo et al. [26]	5	Spain	Mono	2.8	5
Akram et al. [19]	21	GB	Mono	1.5	11
Chabardès et al. [21]	7	France	Mono	1	6
Total	78				49 (62.8%)

risks of this therapeutic approach. If few side effects are related to the stimulation itself (essentially gaze disturbances), the implantation of the electrode can be associated to brain hemorrhages which can be fatal [25]. This risk can be reduced by endoventricular stimulation of the hypothalamus using a floating DBS electrode laid on the floor of the third ventricle [21].

13.2.4 Mechanisms of Action

The common target used for posteroinferior hypothalamic DBS is located 5 mm below the mid-commissural point (MCP), 2 mm lateral to the midline, and 3 mm posterior to the MCP [16], although stimulation delivered from an electrode located on the floor of the third ventricle is also effective [21]. The neural structure corresponding to these coordinates and whose stimulation induces the therapeutic effect is still debated. Fontaine and colleagues studied the anatomical locations of the DBS electrodes and identified several candidates [30], including the mesencephalic gray substance, the ventral tegmental area, and several tracts connecting the hypothalamus with autonomic nuclei of the brain stem. Recently, a more precise modeling of volume of cerebral tissue activated by DBS in responders and non-responders was used to identify the region associated with the highest improvement [19]. The spot that correlated with better outcome was located 6 mm lateral, 2 mm posterior, and 1 mm inferior to MCP, in an area between the red nucleus and the mammillothalamic tract, encompassing the ventral tegmental area and mesencephalic gray and the lateral wall of the floor of the third ventricle (explaining the efficacy of DBS lead implanted in the V3). An additional tractography study showed that this area was crossed by a so-called trigemino-hypothalamic tract, connecting the trigeminal system (and other brain stem nuclei associated with nociception and pain modulation) with the hypothalamus, the prefrontal, and the mesio-temporal area. However, as the electrodes' coordinates are usually similar in DBS responders and non-responders, failure of DBS in CH may be caused by factors other than electrode misplacement, likely related to the disease itself.

Very few neuroimaging studies have explored brain activity changes following retro-hypothalamic DBS. May et al. studied the acute (60 s) effects of DBS by positron emission tomography. They reported cerebral blood flow changes induced by stimulation in the ipsilateral posterior hypothalamic gray (site of electrode implantation), the ipsilateral thalamus, the somatosensory cortex and precuneus, the anterior cingulate cortex, and the ipsilateral trigeminal nucleus and ganglion [31]. A magnetoencephalography study in a single patient reported short-term (10 min) retro-hypothalamic DBS-induced activity changes in the orbitofrontal cortices and in the periaqueductal gray [32]. No study explored long-term effect of DBS in chronic CH patients. Together, these data suggest two alleged mechanisms of action for DBS in CCH. First is the inhibition of a CH generator located in the hypothalamus via stimulation of afferent fibers located in the retro-hypothalamic area. This mechanism might be specific to CH. Second is the modulation of non-specific antinociceptive systems, including the mesencephalic gray substance, and the orexinergic system [33] leading to modulation of regions belonging to the "pain matrix."

13.3 Occipital Nerve Stimulation

13.3.1 Background

Occipital nerve stimulation (ONS) is characterized by the application of a continuous electrical stimulation over the great and/or lesser occipital nerves (respectively, GON and LON), using a subcutaneous chronically implanted electrode that is placed close to the nerve and connected to a battery. This procedure was originally described by Weiner and Reed [34] and has been first proposed to treat occipital neuralgia and then primary headaches, including CH.

13.3.2 Evidence

The demonstration of ONS efficacy in controlled conditions is challenging because its clinical effect is conditioned by the induction of paresthesia within the GON territory, which limits the double-blind. The ICON study was set up with a methodology aiming to maintain as much as possible this double-blind [35]. This RCT, comparing high-amplitude (100%) and low-amplitude (30%) ONS, is ongoing (NCT01151631, as for March 2018), and, pending its results, the use of ONS in the preventive treatment of chronic CH is only supported by data obtained under uncontrolled conditions [26, 36–46] (Table 13.2).

ONS was first experimented by Schwedt and colleagues with beneficial effect on headache frequency, duration, and intensity in one patient with refractory chronic CH [47]. Subsequently, Magis and colleagues suggested the interest of ONS in the preventive treatment of refractory chronic CH by reporting an attack frequency reduction of more than 50% in five out of eight subjects treated in a prospective pilot study [42]. These results were duplicated by Burns and colleagues who reported a similar percentage of responders in another open pilot study including eight patients [36]. These two teams confirmed their preliminary results in larger longer-term trials [37, 43], and other European centers proposed ONS in a compassionate use to patients with refractory chronic CH and reported results in larger series. Thus, Leone and colleagues reported a 50% attack frequency reduction in 20 (66.7%) out of 35 patients with a median follow-up of more than 6 years [41]. A lower (46.1%) 50% responders' rate was reported by Miller and colleagues, but 19 of the 51 included patients presented another primary headache associated with their chronic CH. Considering the subpopulation of patients with chronic CH alone, the 50% responders' rate was 53.1% [44]. In a prospective multicenter series including

Table 13.2 Open series related to ONS in chronic CH

Study	Patients (n)	Country	Mono/ multi centric	Mean follow-up (months)	At least 50% improvement (n)
Magis et al. [42, 43, 53]	15	Belgium	Mono	36.8	12
Burns et al. [36, 37]	14	GB	Mono	17.5	5
de Quintana-Schmidt et al. [38]	4	Spain	Mono	6	4
Mueller et al. [46]	24	Germany	Mono	20	21
Fontaine et al. [39]	13	France	Multi	14.6	10
Strand et al. [61]	3	USA	Mono	10	2
Fontaine et al. [40]	44[a]	France	Multi	12	26
Miller et al. [44]	32[b]	GB	Mono	42.6	17
Leone et al. [41]	35	Italy	Mono	73.2	20
Total	184				117 (63.6%)

[a]Only patients with complete after 12 months follow-up
[b]Only patients with CH alone

44 chronic CH sufferers treated by ONS with 1-year follow-up, the French ONS registry has reported a 30% attack frequency reduction and a 50% attack frequency reduction in 28 (64%) and 26 (59%) of patients, respectively, whereas near half of patients were considered as excellent responders according to a composite criterion associating a 30% attack frequency reduction, a high level of satisfaction, and a stability or a reduction in preventive pharmacological treatment [40].

Overall, ONS procedure presents a 66% success rate (improvement >50%) (Table 13.2). An obvious limitation is the lack of controlled conditions. This is of particular concern as a significant placebo effect is seen in CH like in other primary headaches; and the natural history of CH is often characterized by fluctuations and spontaneous remissions. Nevertheless, two main elements in collected data suggest more than a placebo effect or a natural history: the preceding very long duration of the chronic phase in the implanted patients and the rapid worsening and recovery after technical failures which appears as consistent finding across the series.

Beyond the preventive effect of ONS, analysis of the collected data provided important additional informations for the clinical practice. Some patients found that ONS helped abort acute attacks but acute use of ONS is not supported by the literature. Similarly, the available data do not suggest that ONS reduces the duration and the intensity of CH attacks. Retrospective evaluation of time to improvement in individual cases appears to show two groups, the first being patients with quick improvement in few weeks and the second being those gradually improving over months. Burns and colleagues stated that the group with delayed improvement has a lesser ONS benefit than the group with quick improvement [37] but such a difference in benefit was not confirmed later.

13.3.3 Limits

The European Headache Federation considers ONS as a valuable therapeutic alternative in drug-refractory chronic CH [29] with a statement supported by evidence and the benefit/risk ratio of this approach sometimes considered as "minimally invasive." Nevertheless, ONS is not devoid of side effects. As any invasive neuromodulation technique, ONS exposes to a risk of immediate or delayed infections. On the other hand, ONS is associated with two adverse events of its own. The first one is a fast battery depletion (mean life from 1 to 2 years) due to high current consumption related to high intensity and duration (daytime and nighttime) of the stimulation. This depletion requires battery replacement in up to 100% of patients at long term and increases the cost of this treatment, especially in countries where rechargeable batteries are not allowed in first-line use. The second adverse event limiting ONS is the lead migration due to neck movements. Migration, like the other complications concerning leads (fracture, skin erosion), is partly related to surgical implantation technique. Multiple surgical techniques have been reported in the literature, using percutaneous cylindrical or surgical paddle leads, approach from the midline or from retro-mastoid incision(s) [48], but no evidence is available claiming the superiority of one technique over others in terms of complication incidence. One of the main important technical aspects to limit the risk of migration is a firm anchorage of the lead. This point has been considered by manufacturers, and, in order to limit the risk of migration, Medtronic has developed a new electrode specifically dedicated to the ONS (Ankerstim®), which has just obtained its CE marking but will need to demonstrate its superiority in CH therapy.

Bilateral stimulation is recommended to treat CH to avoid headache side-shift, which has been reported in up to one third of the patients stimulated unilaterally [36, 37]. Trial stimulation is not useful because some patients can improve after several months of continuous stimulation [39]. Response to occipital nerve block is not useful in selecting patient for ONS treatment [49], but a recent retrospective study showed that prior response to greater occipital nerve block was associated with increased likelihood of ONS response [5].

13.3.4 Mechanisms of Action

If several hypotheses have been proposed to understand how ONS improves CH patients, its exact mechanism of action remains unknown. ONS could act through the modulation of the convergent nociceptive inputs in the trigemino-cervical complex [50, 51], by a "gate control theory-like" mechanism [52]. Nevertheless, the latency of the effect appearance in many patients with CH benefiting from ONS makes one consider a more complex mechanism. This mechanism would be generic and imply structures involved in pain modulation. Two arguments suggest that ONS might act through a non-specific regulation of the central pain control systems rather than modulation of a central CH generator. Firstly, some successfully ONS-treated chronic CH patients still report autonomic attacks without pain [36, 37, 47]. Secondly, a functional imaging study has described ONS-induced metabolic changes in the "pain matrix," especially in the perigenual anterior cingulate cortex in ONS responders, but no change in the ipsilateral hypothalamic [53]. These results should be duplicated to confirm the absence of hypothalamic change in ONS responders and the symptomatic character of this treatment. MET-ONS study, a similar functional imaging study performed by the French ONS registry, included 18 patients with chronic CH treated with ONS, and its results are being analyzed (NCT02081482/clinicaltrials.gov).

13.4 Stimulation of the Sphenopalatine Ganglion

13.4.1 Background

The sphenopalatine ganglion has been chosen as a valuable target of neuromodulation due to the involvement of the parasympathetic system in the pathophysiology of trigeminal autonomic cephalalgias. This background justified a proof-of-concept study with five patients with CH in which the majority of attacks could be controlled by a sphenopalatine ganglion stimulation (SPGS) via an electrode connected to an external stimulator [54]. This neuromodulation approach could be considered in a practical perspective through the development of Pulsante® (Autonomic Technologies, USA) which is an original implantable SPG microstimulator allowing to abort CH attacks on demand. Specifically designed for acute SPGS, the device is implanted along the posterior wall of the maxillary bone in the pterygopalatine fossa (PPF), fixed with a screwed plate to the zygomatic process, and the lead is in contact with the sphenopalatine ganglion. No battery is contained in the neurostimulator, so power and activation are initiated transcutaneously by a remote controller using radio-frequency energy.

13.4.2 Evidence

Evidence supporting SPGS by Pulsante® is limited to CH with the PATHWAY CH-1 study which is a RCT promoted by ATI to evaluate this device in the treatment of cluster headache attacks [55]. This multicenter randomized sham-controlled study tested the safety and efficacy of the Pulsante® device. Thirty-two patients suffering from refractory chronic CH were enrolled and 28 completed the randomized experimental period. Optimal, suboptimal, or sham stimulation were randomly used to treat each CH attack, and pain relief 15 min after the start of the SPGS was the main criterion. Pain relief was achieved in 67.1% of optimal stimulation-treated attacks compared to 7.4% of sham-treated and 7.3% of suboptimal-treated attacks ($p < 0.0001$). Absence of pain was achieved in 34.1% and 1.5% of attacks after optimal stimulation and sham stimulation, respectively ($p < 0.0001$). Nineteen of 28 (68%) patients experienced a clinically significant improvement, but only 32% achieved a pain relief in more than 50% of the treated attacks.

Results of the long-term (24 months) open extension phase of PATHWAY CH-1 study have been recently published [56]. This open extension phase involved 33 patients who were initially included in the PATHWAY CH-1 study, although 11 of them were not included in the first analysis for time reasons. Moreover, ten patients included in the initial study were excluded from this long-term analysis, because they no longer had the stimulator implanted or due to previous protocol noncompliance. Across all 33 patients, a total of 5956 attacks were treated. Effective treatment (pain relief and/or absence of pain) was achieved in 65% of CH attacks, with a delay of 11.2 min on average, including 50% becoming pain-free. Fifteen out of 33 patients (45%) were considered as acute responders (at least 50% of attacks were successfully treated). In 79% of the attacks, patients did not report the use of acute medication.

In PATHWAY CH-1 study, there was also an unexpected reduction in attack frequency noted with repetitive attack stimulation in 12 of 28 (43%) patients who experienced a reduction in attack frequency of at least 50% (average 88%). This reduction was confirmed in the open extension phase and suggested that repeated use of SPG stimulation might act as a CH preventive treatment. Nevertheless, this study was not designed to demonstrate a preventive effect, and spontaneous transformation from chronic to episodic forms of the disease cannot be excluded.

13.4.3 Limits

According to available evidence, SPGS with Pulsante® should be dedicated to the acute treatment of chronic CH. This device is indicated for patients with strictly lateralized attacks and, intuitively, mostly indicated in those with no response to oxygen inhalation and subcutaneous sumatriptan administration and those with a high daily number of attacks since the system allows a 5-min stimulation that can be repeated as many times as needed. The place of SPGS is also to be determined in patients who suffer from an episodic CH form with painful bouts of long duration and the same attack characteristics. Finally, implanted patients with Pulsante® will likely try to use this device as a preventive treatment by administering one or two stimulations of 15 min per day outside their attacks [57]. Immediately after implantation, use of Pulsante® requires a learning phase to allow patients to find the stimulation parameters producing paresthesia in the soft palate [57].

The implantation of the Pulsante® often requires the expertise of a maxillofacial surgeon because of the approach. It remains a minimally invasive surgery, but it exposes to damage of maxillary branch of the trigeminal nerve with a risk of sensory disturbances and possibly neuropathic pain. In the PATHWAY CH-1 study, 81% of patients experienced transient, mild-to-moderate hypoesthesia within the maxillary (V2) nerve territory, resolving within 3 months in most of the cases [55]. More recently, the safety of the surgical implantation procedure has been evaluated in a cohort of 99 patients, including 43 patients of the PATHWAY CH-1 study and 56 patients from the Pathway-R1 registry [58]. Eighty-one percent of the patients experienced at least one adverse event, most of them being transient. Sensory disturbances were the most frequent complications, observed in 67% of the patients, 46% of them resolving within a mean delay of 104 days. Transient allodynia was rare (3%). Pain and/or swelling was reported by 47% of the patients, resolving in 80% of the cases with a mean delay of 68 days. Dry eye (3%, resolving in 40% of cases), transient trismus (8%), and limited jaw movements (6%) were also reported. Infection rate was 5%. Device revision procedures were performed in 13 cases due to inappropriate initial placement of the stimulating electrode within the PPF. Five devices were explanted. Although frequent, most (92%) of the adverse events were transient and evaluated as mild or moderate. The authors concluded that Pulsante® insertion procedure has sequelae comparable to other oral cavity surgical procedures. Moreover, the technique is recent, and the rate of surgical complications will likely decrease with progression of the learning curve, further refinement of the surgical procedure and tools, and the use of neuronavigation systems [59].

13.4.4   Mechanisms of Action

The mechanism of action of the SPGS by Pulsante® is supposed to be the parasympathetic inhibition. This inhibition appears secondary to the high-frequency stimulation generated by the Pulsante®, and it has been shown that, conversely, the SPGS using a low-frequency stimulation was likely to trigger attacks in subjects with CH [60].

13.5   Conclusion

Substantial progress has been achieved in invasive and noninvasive neuromodulation techniques to treat cluster headache, but evidence for using such approaches was relatively sparse. This weak evidence had been outlined by the European Headache Federation in a consensus statement [28]. According to this international consensus, the application of an invasive neuromodulation, either in a trial or on the basis of a CE mark treatment, should be considered only once all alternative therapies as recommended by international guidelines have failed. This implies that the patients have been evaluated in a tertiary care headache center. When invasive neuromodulation technique is indicated for a refractory chronic CH patient, it is advisable to use ONS and SPGS before considering DBS. nVNS is an attractive treatment option with excellent safety profile, and, if its efficacy is confirmed, it should be used prior to surgical implantation of a neurostimulator in refractory chronic CH and eventually considered as an adjunctive treatment in less severe CH.

References

1. Lenaerts ME, Oommen KJ, Couch JR, Skaggs V. Can vagus nerve stimulation help migraine? Cephalalgia. 2008;28:392–5.
2. Gaul C, Diener HC, Silver N, Magis D, Reuter U, Andersson A, et al. Non-invasive vagus nerve stimulation for prevention and acute treatment of chronic cluster headache (PREVA): a randomized controlled study. Cephalalgia. 2016;36:534–46.
3. Gaul C, Magis D, Liebler E, Straube A. Effects of non-invasive vagus nerve stimulation on attack frequency over time and expended response rates in patients with chronic cluster headache: a post hoc analysis of the randomized, controlled PREVA study. Headache Pain. 2017;18(1):22.
4. Morris J, Straube A, Diener HC, Ahmed F, Silver N, Walker S, et al. Cost-effectiveness analysis of non-invasive vagus nerve stimulation for the treatment of chronic cluster headache. J Headache Pain. 2016;17:43.
5. Miller S, Watkins L, Matharu M. Predictors of response to occipital nerve stimulation in refractory chronic headache. Cephalalgia. 2018;38:1267–75. https://doi.org/10.1177/0333102417728747.
6. Goadsby PJ, de Coo IF, Silver N, Tyagi A, Ahmed F, Gaul C, et al. Non invasive vagus nerve stimulation for the acute treatment of episodic and chronic cluster headache: a randomized, double-blind, sham-controlled ACT2 study. Cephalalgia. 2018;38:959–69. https://doi.org/10.1177/0333102417744362.
7. Silberstein SD, Mechtler LL, Kudrow DB, Calhoun AH, McClure C, Saper JR, et al. Non-invasive vagus nerve stimulation for the acute treatment of cluster headache: findings from the randomized, double-blind, sham-controlled ACT1 study. Headache. 2016;56:1317–32.
8. Holle-Lee D, Gaul C. Noninvasive vagus nerve stimulation in the management of cluster headache: clinical evidence and practical experience. Adv Neurol Disord. 2016;9:230–4.
9. Simon B, Blake J. Mechanism of action of non-invasive cervical vagus nerve stimulation for the treatment of primary headaches. Am J Manag Care. 2017;23(Suppl. 17):S312–6.
10. Nonis R, D'Ostilio K, Schoenen J, Magis D. Evidence of activation of vagal afferents by non-invasive vagus nerve stimulation: an electrophysiological study in healthy volunteers. Cephalalgia. 2017;37:1285–93.
11. Frangos E, Komisaruk BR. Access to vagal projections via cutaneous stimulation of the neck: fMRI evidence in healthy humans. Brain Stimul. 2017;10:19–27.
12. Mourdoukoutas AP, Truong DQ, Adair DK, Simon BJ, Bikson M. High-resolution multiscale computational model for non-invasive cervical vagus nerve stimulation. Neuromodulation. 2018;21:261–8. https://doi.org/10.1111/ner.12706.
13. Chen SP, Ay I, de Morais AL, Qin T, Zheng Y, Sadeghian H, et al. Vagus nerve stimulation inhibits cortical spreading depression. Pain. 2016;157:797–805.
14. Oshinsky ML, Murphy AL, Hekierski H, Cooper M, Simon B. Non-invasive vagus nerve stimulation as treatment for trigeminal allodynia. Pain. 2014;155:1037–42.
15. Akerman S, Simon B, Romero-Reyes M. Vagus nerve stimulation suppresses acute noxious activation of trigeminocervical neurons in animals models of primary headache. Neurobiol Dis. 2017;102:96–104.
16. Franzini A, Ferroli P, Leone M, Broggi G. Stimulation of the posterior hypothalamus for the treatment of chronic intractable cluster headache. Neurosurgery. 2003;52:1095–9.
17. Leone M, Franzini A, Bussone G. Stereotactic stimulation of posterior hypothalamic grey matter for intractable cluster headache. N Engl J Med. 2001;345:1428–9.
18. May A, Bahra A, Buchel C, Frackowiak R, Goadsby P. Hypothalamic activation in cluster headache attacks. Lancet Neurol. 1998;352:275–8.
19. Akram H, Miller S, Lagrata S, HYam J, Jahanshari M, Hariz M, et al. Ventral tegmental area deep brain stimulation for refractory chronic cluster headache. Neurology. 2016;86:1676–82.
20. Bartsch T, Pinsker M, Rasche D, Kinfe T, Hertel F, Diener H, et al. Hypothalamic deep brain stimulation for cluster headache: experience from a new multicase series. Cephalalgia. 2008;28:285–95.

21. Chabardès S, Carron R, Seigneuret E, Torres N, Goetz L, Krainik A, et al. Endoventricular deep brain stimulation of the third ventricle: proof of concept and application to cluster headache. Neurosurgery. 2016;79:806–15.
22. Fontaine D, Lazorthes Y, Mertens P, Blond S, Géraud G, Fabre N, et al. Safety and efficacy of deep brain stimulation in refractory cluster headache: a randomized placebo-controlled double-blind trial followed by a one-year open extension. J Headache Pain. 2010;11:23–31.
23. Leone M, Franzini A, Proietti Cecchini A, Bussone G. Success, failure, and putative mechanisms in hypothalamic stimulation for drug-resistant chronic cluster headache. Pain. 2013;154:89–94.
24. Owen S, Green A, Davies P, Stein J, Aziz T, Behrens T, Voets N, et al. Connectivity of an effective hypothalamic surgical target for cluster headache. J Clin Neurosci. 2007;14:955–60.
25. Schoenen J, Di Clemente L, Vandenheede M, Fumal A, De Pasqua V, Mouchamps M, et al. Hypothalamic stimulation in chronic cluster headache: a pilot study of efficacy and mode of action. Brain. 2005;128:940–7.
26. Seijo F, Saiz A, Lozano B, Santamarta E, Alvarez-Vega M, Seijo E, et al. Neuromodulation of the posterolateral hypothalamus for the treatment of chronic refractory cluster headache: experience in five patients with a modified anatomic target. Cephalalgia. 2011;31:1634–41.
27. Starr P, Barbaro N, Raskin N, Ostrem J. Chronic stimulation of the posterior hypothalamic region for cluster headache: technique and 1-year results in four patients. J Neurosurg. 2007;106:999–1005.
28. Leone M, May A, Franzini A, Broggi G, Dodick D, Rapoport A, Goadsby P, Schoenen J, Bonavita V, Bussone G. Deep brain stimulation for intractable chronic cluster headache: proposals for patient selection. Cephalalgia. 2004;24:934–7.
29. Marteletti P, Jensen RH, Antal A, Arcioni R, Brighina F, de Tommaso M, et al. Neuromodulation of chronic headache from the European Headache Federation. J Headache Pain. 2013;14:86.
30. Fontaine D, Lanteri-Minet M, Ouchchane L, Lazorthes Y, Mertens P, Blond S, et al. Anatomical location of effective deep brain stimulation electrodes in chronic cluster headache. Brain. 2010;133:1214–23.
31. May A, Leone M, Boecker H, Sprenger T, Juergens T, Bussone G, Tolle T. Hypothalamic deep brain stimulation in positron emission tomography. J Neurosci. 2006;26:3589–93.
32. Ray NJ, Kringembach M, Jenkinson N, Owen S, Davies P, Wang S, et al. Using magnetoencephalography to investigate brain activity during high frequency deep brain stimulation in a cluster headache patient. Biomed Imaging Interv J. 2007;3:e25.
33. Goadsby HP. The hypothalamic orexinergic system: pain and primary headaches. Headache. 2007;47:951–62.
34. Weiner R, Reed K. Peripheral neurostimulation for control of intractable occipital neuralgia. Neuromodulation. 1999;2:217–22.
35. Wilbrink LA, Teemstra OP, Haan J, van Zwet EW, Evers SM, Spincemaille GH, et al. Occipital nerve stimulation in medically intractable, chronic cluster headache. The ICON study: rationale and protocol of a randomized trial. Cephalalgia. 2013;33(15):1238–47.
36. Burns B, Watkins L, Goadsby PJ. Treatment of medically intractable cluster headache by occipital nerve stimulation: long-term follow-up of eight patients. Lancet. 2007;369:1099–106.
37. Burns B, Watkins L, Goadsby PJ. Treatment of intractable chronic cluster headache by occipital nerve stimulation in 14 patients. Neurology. 2009;72:341–5.
38. de Quintana-Schmidt C, Casajuana Garreta E, Mollet-Teixido J, Garcia-Bach M, Roig C, Clavel-Laria P, Rodriguez-Rodriguez R, Oliver-Abadal B, Batumeus-Jené F. Stimulation of the occipital nerve in the treatment of drug-resistant cluster headache. Rev Neurol. 2010;51:19–26.
39. Fontaine D, Sol JC, Raoul S, Fabre N, Geraud G, Magne C, et al. Treatment of refractory chronic cluster headache by chronic occipital nerve stimulation. Cephalalgia. 2011;31:1101–5.
40. Fontaine D, Blond S, Lucas C, Regis J, Donnet A, Derrey S, et al. Occipital nerve stimulation improve the quality of life in medically-intractable chronic cluster headache: results of an observational prospective study. Cephalalgia. 2017;37:1173–9.
41. Leone M, Proietti Cecchini A, Messina G, Franzini A. Long-term occipital nerve stimulation for drug-resistant chronic cluster headache. Cephalalgia. 2017;37:756–63.

42. Magis D, Allena M, Bolla M, De Pasqua V, Remacle JM, Schoenen J. Occipital nerve stimulation for drug-resistant chronic cluster headache: a prospective pilot study. Lancet Neurol. 2007;6:314–21.
43. Magis D, Gerardy PY, Remacle JM, Schoenen J. Sustained effectiveness of occipital nerve stimulation in drug-resistant chronic cluster headache. Headache. 2011;51:1191–201.
44. Miller S, Watkins L, Matharu M. Treatment of intractable chronic cluster headache by occipital nerve stimulation: a cohort of 51 patients. Eur J Neurol. 2017;24:381–90.
45. Müeller O, Gaul C, Katsarava Z, Diener H, Sure U, Gasser T. Occipital nerve stimulation for the treatment of chronic cluster headache—lessons learned from 18 months experience. Cen Eur Neurosurg. 2011;72:84–9.
46. Mueller O, Diener HC, Dammann P, Rabe K, Hagel V, Sure U, et al. Occipital nerve stimulation for intractable chronic cluster headache or migraine: a critical analysis of direct treatment costs and complications. Cephalalgia. 2013;33(16):1283–91.
47. Schwedt TJ, Dodick DW, Trentman TL, Zimmerman RS. Occipital nerve stimulation for chronic cluster headache and hemicrania continua: pain relief and persistence of autonomic features. Cephalalgia. 2006;26(8):1025–7.
48. Fontaine D, Vandersteen C, Magis D, Lanteri-Minet M. Neuromodulation of cluster headache. Adv Tech Stand Neurosurg. 2015;42:3–21.
49. Schwedt TJ, Dodick DW, Trentman TL, Zimmerman RS. Response to occipital nerve block is not useful in predicting efficacy of occipital nerve stimulation. Cephalalgia. 2007;27:271–4.
50. Bartsch T, Goadsby PJ. Stimulation of the greater occipital nerve induces increased central excitability of dural afferent input. Brain. 2002;125:1496–509.
51. Bartsch T, Goadsby PJ. Increased responses in trigeminocervical nociceptive neurons to cervical input after stimulation of the dura mater. Brain. 2003;126:1801–13.
52. Goadsby P, Bartsch T, Dodick D. Occipital nerve stimulation for headache: mechanisms and efficacy. Headache. 2008;48:313–8.
53. Magis D, Bruno MA, Fumal A, Gerardy PY, Hustinx R, Laureys S, et al. Central modulation in cluster headache patients treated with occipital nerve stimulation: an FDG-PET study. BMC Neurol. 2011;11:25.
54. Ansarinia M, Rezai A, Tepper SJ, Steiner CP, Stump J, Stanton-Hicks M, et al. Electrical stimulation of sphenopalatine ganglion for acute treatment of cluster headaches. Headache. 2010;50:1164–74.
55. Schoenen J, Jensen RH, Lantéri-Minet M, Láinez MJ, Gaul C, Goodman AM, et al. Stimulation of the sphenopalatine ganglion (SPG) for cluster headache treatment. Pathway CH-1: a randomized, sham-controlled study. Cephalalgia. 2013;33:816–30.
56. Jürgens TP, Barloese M, May A, Láinez JM, Schoenen J, Gaul C, et al. Long-term effectiveness of sphenopalatine ganglion stimulation for cluster headache. Cephalalgia. 2017;37(5):423–34.
57. Miller S, Sinclaire AJ, Davies B, Matharu M. Neurostimulation in the treatment of primary headaches. Pract Neurol. 2016;16:362–75.
58. Assaf A, Hillerup S, Rostgaard J, et al. Technical and surgical aspects of the sphenopalatine ganglion (SPG) microstimulator insertion procedure. Int J Oral Maxillofac Surg. 2016;45(2):245–54.
59. Kohlmeier C, Behrens P, Böger A, et al. Improved surgical procedure using intraoperative navigation for the implantation of the SPG microstimulator in patients with chronic cluster headache. Int J Comput Assist Radiol Surg. 2017;12(12):2119–28.
60. Schytz HW, Barlose M, Guo S, Selb J, Caparso A, Jensen R, et al. Experimental activation of the sphenopalatine ganglion provokes cluster like attacks in humans. Cephalalgia. 2013;33:831–41.
61. Strand N, Trentman T, Vargas B, Dodick D. Occipital nerve stimulation with the Bion microstimulator for the treatment of medically refractory chronic cluster headache. Pain Physician. 2011;14:435–40.

Chapter 14
Behavioral and Psychological Aspects, Quality of Life, and Disability and Impact of Cluster Headache

Lauren Ashley-Marie Schenck, Alberto Raggi, Domenico D'Amico, Alberto Proietti Cecchini, and Frank Andrasik

14.1 Introduction

Cluster headache (CH) is among the most severe and disabling primary headache disorders. A bout of CH results in excruciating unilateral pain occurring several times daily, with each episode lasting up to 3 hours and being accompanied by prominent ipsilateral cranial autonomic features [1]. Extreme restlessness, explosive anger, and even self-injury often occur during full-blown attacks, something rarely if ever seen in other acute pain conditions. Although first coined by Horton in 1952 as the "suicide headache" [2], it may be more appropriately characterized as the "aggressive headache," as violent behaviors are much more commonly reported than actual suicide attempts or completions [3]. Dr. Lee Kudrow, a seminal investigator on CH, early on provided the following personal account of a cluster headache attack: "I am stuck with the additional fear that the pain will never end, but I dismiss it as impossible. Even if it were the case, I would surely kill myself" [4]. No matter what descriptor is used, it is clear the pain experienced during these attacks is most often unbearable.

Between 2000 and 2017, more than 200 literature reviews addressing CH were published: the most cited—and oldest—ones dealt with diagnostic and pathophysiological issues, as well as with treatment options [5–8], and the same is true for

L. A.-M. Schenck · F. Andrasik (✉)
Department of Psychology, University of Memphis, Memphis, TN, USA
e-mail: ladahlke@memphis.edu; fndrasik@memphis.edu

A. Raggi
Neurology, Public Health and Disability Unit, Neurological Institute C. Besta IRCCS Foundation, Milan, Italy
e-mail: alberto.raggi@istituto-besta.it

D. D'Amico · A. P. Cecchini
Division of Neuroalgology, Neurological Institute C. Besta IRCCS Foundation, Milan, Italy
e-mail: domenico.damico@istituto-besta.it; alberto.proietti@istituto-besta.it

© Springer Nature Switzerland AG 2020
M. Leone, A. May (eds.), *Cluster Headache and other Trigeminal Autonomic Cephalgias*, Headache, https://doi.org/10.1007/978-3-030-12438-0_14

reviews published in the last 2 years [9–12]. That said, the potential role of behavioral and psychological factors in this disorder remains uncertain, as psychopathological assessment results have been variable, due in part to the complexity of this disorder as well as methodological shortcomings (i.e., uncontrolled clinical interviews, small sample sizes, absence of appropriate control or comparison groups, non-standardized assessment procedures or measures, etc. [13]). Given the widely acknowledged pronounced impact of CH, it is surprising that this aspect has been relatively ignored in the literature. During CH attacks, patients are typically unable to function as desired, which in turn leads to adverse psychosocial sequelae, marked impairments in daily activities, and reduced quality of life (QoL) also outside the CH bouts. In this chapter, we examine what is currently known about psychological and behavioral factors related to CH, how CH impacts disability and QoL, and, in brief, how what is known may help inform management of CH.

14.2   Psychological and Behavioral Aspects

Unlike other pain disorders, CH is more prevalent in men than women, although this ratio appears to have decreased from a high of 6.2:1 in the 1960s to 2.1:1 in the 1990s [14]. Early characterizations of psychological profiles of individuals with cluster headache (such as those described by Friedman and Graham in the 1950s–1970s [15, 16]) were "hypermasculinized" and framed as ambitious, hardworking, rugged in appearance, heavy smokers and drinkers, yet internally passive. Much of the literature produced during this time was driven by psychoanalytic perspectives and lacked methodological rigor [17].

Since then, more rigorous attempts, incorporating objective, validated measures, with a focus on multiple headache disorders as well as matched non-headache samples, have been pursued, but, again, with limited convergence. In one of the earliest controlled investigations, 12 patients with episodic cluster were compared to 26 migraineurs, 39 tension-type (TTH; then termed "muscle contraction"), 22 combined migraine and TTH, and 30 non-headache controls (who were asked to assist in recruiting a friend or relative of the same sex, approximate age and marital status, and presumably similar socioeconomic status) on a comprehensive battery of psychometrically validated measures: Minnesota Multiphasic Personality Inventory (MMPI), modified Hostility Scale derived from the MMPI, Beck Depression Inventory, State-Trait Anxiety Inventory, Autonomic Perception Questionnaire, Rathus Assertiveness Schedule, Social Readjustment Rating Scale, Psychosomatic Symptom Checklist, Schalling-Sifneos Scale, Need for Achievement, and Hostile Press [18]. On the MMPI scales of most interest, patients with CH were rarely significantly different from controls (and incidentally most similar to the profiles for migraineurs). The only scale where differences emerged between controls and CH patients was scale 3, which reflects tendencies toward somatization during periods of stress. It is important to point out that the slight differences in elevations did not reach the level reflecting clinical significance. The remaining tests in the battery yielded 16 separate scores, none of which revealed significant differences between controls and CH patients (although two scales showed some slight, but again clinically nonsignificant elevations). Prior to this more comprehensive investigation, Kudrow and Sutkus [19] had researched whether the main clinical scales of the MMPI alone could reliably distinguish six different headache types: migraine, TTH (then termed chronic scalp muscle contraction), combined migraine and TTH, cluster, post-traumatic cephalalgia, and conversion cephalalgia. For males and females alike, CH and migraine shared a similar profile, with no clinically elevated scales (with the other groupings showing increased scores). These findings for CH and migraine were soon thereafter replicated with the MMPI for males and females [13]. A subsequent investigation incorporating the MMPI, with larger sample sizes (160 migraineurs, 95 TTH, 149 migraine combined with TTH, and 30 CH) yielded similar findings, showing no major differences between different types of headache [20]. Although slight elevations were noted overall, none fell into the clinically significant range, and, as non-headache controls were not included, it is not possible to determine if the slight elevations would have exceeded those for individuals absent of headache. A more recent investigation of 120 patients with CH, which included a like number of age- and gender-matched controls (case-control study), revealed no significant elevations or differences in MMPI scores between the two groups [21]. Additionally, no visible differences in appearance were found as well when neurologists performed a series of blind ratings of pictures for a subset of both groups.

Yet even more recently, however, investigations using different broad-spectrum personality measures have produced markedly different findings. In a small sample of 26 CH "in-ward" patients, 92% were reported as evidencing pathological levels of personality disorders, particularly obsessive-compulsive and histrionic, when assessed by the Millon Clinical Multiaxial Inventory-III questionnaire [22]. How the obtained profiles might have compared to other headache types on the inpatient unit or to non-headache controls is unknown. A larger study, comparing outpatients with CH ($n = 80$) to migraineurs ($n = 164$), reported a higher percentage of negative personality traits among patients with CH compared to migraineurs [23]. Specifically, paranoid and schizoid traits were significantly more prevalent among CH patients (30% and 42.5%, respectively) than migraineurs (11.6% and 25.6%, respectively), as assessed by the Salamanca screening test. Again, comparisons to non-headache controls were lacking.

All studies here-to-date have failed to consider the role that having a pain condition, such as CH, may play in how individuals respond to and are evaluated by personality tests and psychological measures. Nearly all such tests are aimed at capturing traits that are presumed to be relatively stable throughout the lifetime, and many have not been normed among medical populations. With this in mind, it could well be the case that what appears to be psychopathological traits or disorders are more aptly viewed as a reflection of pain state. Indeed, in a broad review of 32 studies on personality characteristics evidenced before and after treatment of chronic pain, 90% of studies using the MMPI showed an improvement in MMPI scores after treatment [24]. One study, specifically focused on headache and craniofacial pain, showed MMPI scores improved after treatment for women, but not men [25]. Overall, these traits were not predictive of treatment outcome.

So, what can be made of this? Although some research advances have been made over the years, significant methodological problems remain—differences in sampling strategies, sample sizes, and settings where data are collected; quality and type of measures used; adequacy of comparison groups selected, with non-headache controls often omitted and other recurring pain conditions rarely included; and, perhaps of most importance, is the failure to take into account the headache *status* of patients at the time of assessment, distinguish episodic (ECH) from chronic forms (CCH) of CH, and track changes over time. Hence, debates surrounding the "cluster headache personality" continue [3, 26]. Although individual personality characteristics may be informative for how patients may respond to treatment, the conflicting evidence steers us away from using personality as a diagnostic indicator of headache type.

Even though a typical personality profile does not seem to exist *in general* for CH patients, some findings point to other possible reliable behavioral correlates. Pain disorders in general are largely known to have high co-occurrence with psychological symptoms, particularly anxiety and depression, especially when the condition is chronic [27–29]. Although evidence bearing on this topic is more limited for CH than for migraine, available findings to date suggest the patterns are similar. One particular study of interest was able to examine US insurance claims for individuals diagnosed with CH (both ECH and CCH) and compare them to patients without a headache diagnosis [30]. Claims due to depressive disorders, sleep disturbance, anxiety disorders, and suicidal ideation were around twice as likely in the CH group than controls. Using an insurance claims database allows for large sample sizes (7,589 CH patients and 30,341 controls in this instance), but it is only representative of select individuals with insurance coverage that perceived their condition so burdensome to require some kind of compensation. Additionally, claims and diagnoses could not be cross-verified; thus, results should be interpreted with caution. A more well-controlled study included patients with CCH and ECH (both in and out of active cluster bouts), migraine patients, and healthy controls who were screened for psychiatric co-occurrence using the Mini-DIPS, a validated structured clinical interview [31]. These researchers found that CCH patients fared the worst, with over half the group endorsing depressive symptoms compared to 27% of active ECH patients, 36% of inactive ECH patients, 29% of migraine patients, and 19% of controls. Suicidal tendencies and symptoms of agoraphobia were also higher in this group. It is important to note that these findings are based only on screener items and that few symptoms were endorsed across groups overall, such that only descriptive statistics could be provided. It could be the case that the chronicity, rather than CH itself, is the more salient linkage to these elevated symptoms (consistent with a point made earlier).

Taken altogether, it appears that those who have CH do not experience much psychological distress during times of remission, suggesting the experience of pain itself leads to any psychological sequelae noted. This is consistent with the findings of Liang and colleagues [32] who were able to analyze 673 patients with CH residing within a Taiwan National Health Insurance database over an extensive time period (2005–2009) and compare findings from this group to two large age-, sex-, and comorbidity-matched cohort comparison groups (2,692 patients with migraine only versus 2,692 patients absent migraine or CH; comorbidity matching was based on scores derived from the Charlson Comorbidity Index). Over an extensive follow-up period (median of 2.5 years), the patients with CH were 5.6 times more likely to develop depression when compared to pure controls. However, rates of depression were similar when compared to the migraineurs.

The early descriptor based on observations of the CH patient as a heavy smoker may not be far off, however. Govare's review [33] found a higher prevalence of reported licit and illicit drug use in CH compared to the general population, particularly for tobacco and cannabis. In the more recent study conducted by Choong and colleagues [30] using an insurance claim database, those diagnosed with CH were three times more likely to have a tobacco use disorder than controls. What is not clear is the nature of this relation. Does it represent a linked predisposition to addiction and CH pathologies, or might substance use contribute to CH onset? An interesting note to consider is that as the gender gap for CH prevalence has closed, so too has the gap for smoking habits, lowering from nearly 9:1 (male to female) in the 1960s to around 2:1 in the 1990s [14], alongside a general decrease in smoking habits in the USA [34] and EU [35]. More longitudinal research in this area may help to further inform our understanding of behavioral precipitants to CH.

Sleep, too, is closely tied to CH pathology [36]. Nocturnal sleeping is often a trigger for cluster headaches, and patients with CH show much poorer sleep compared to controls. Attacks often occur during rapid eye movement (REM) sleep, though they are not limited to this phase. Heightened activity in emotional arousal brain centers, namely, amygdala and medial prefrontal cortex, suggests these areas are key to regulating REM sleep [37]. Interestingly, one study showed abnormal metabolism in the amygdala in ECH during an active phase [38]. This could cause a derangement in the crosstalk between the amygdala and hypothalamus, with a putative role to generate a permissive state of the brain leading to the activation of the cluster circuit [39]. As with substance use and abuse, the full picture of the relationship between sleep dysregulation and CH is not yet clear.

14.3   Quality of Life, Disability, and Impact

Although psychological and behavioral factors related to the onset and maintenance of CH can be informative, what is equally important to consider is how CH affects the lives of these individuals. The socioeconomic burden of CH patients was evaluated in 2007 in a Danish survey using a telephone interview [40]. Data showed that 78% reported restrictions in daily living (13% also outside of cluster periods) and 25% reported a major decrease in their ability to participate in social activities, family life, and housework. Furthermore, the absenteeism rate was 30%, which was significantly higher than 12% among the general population.

In this section, we review studies in which standard tools were used to assess QoL and disability in CH patients, aiming to highlight the main results and discuss possible research developments bearing on these topics. We have limited our focus to manuscripts published between 2000 and 2017. A summary of included studies is provided in Table 14.1.

14.3.1   Evaluation of QoL

QoL was evaluated in six studies relying on generic tools: in five studies, the Medical Outcome Study Short Form (MOS-SF-36) was used [41–45] and in one case with the 12-item version [41], while three studies used the EuroQoL-VAS [41, 42, 46]. Parallel to this, the Migraine Specific Quality of Life Questionnaire (MSQ) was used in only one study [44]. Table 14.2 summarizes cross-sectional and longitudinal data evaluating QoL. On average, the Physical Composite Summary (PCS) of MOS-SF scored 37.5, the Mental Composite Summary (MCS) scored 35.2, and the EuroQol-VAS scored around 50. The SF-36 and the EuroQoL are generic instruments and, thus, not intended to specifically measure QoL in headache populations. The SF-36 [47] comprises eight scales that can be summed to yield two composite scores: the first addresses physical health issues (e.g., pain, general health, or ability to undertake physical activities), while the second addresses mental health issues (e.g., vitality, emotional state, and mental health). The EuroQoL [48] covers five domains (mobility, self-care, usual activities, pain/discomfort, and depression/anxiety) that comprise a single composite score and also includes a visual analog scale addressing "current health state." The MSQ [49] is a migraine-specific QoL tool, which has not been formally validated in patients with CH. For all of the three instruments, higher scores indicate higher QoL.

We note that some of these studies were performed on intractable and/or refractory CH patients [41–43]. For example, interesting data were obtained in two studies on consecutive patients, not "selected" for their particular severe forms, but who were experiencing daily attacks when assessed. In the study by Ertsey and colleagues [44], patients with ECH had lower scores in all domains of the MOS-SF-36 when compared to those obtained in controls as well as in patients with migraine, with a significant difference occurring for the MOS-SF-36 domains evaluating bodily pain and social functioning. With regard to the MSQ, patients reported the following scores: Role-Restriction (RR) = 39.6, Role-Prevention (RP) = 52.2, and Emotional Function (EF) = 51.0. These scores are slightly lower compared to those reported by episodic migraineurs, and by those observed by Bagley and colleagues (respectively, RR = 44.4, RP = 61.4, EF = 48.3) [50] and Rendas-Baums and colleagues (respectively, RR = 44.6, RP = 62.2, EF = 59.7) [51], but are in line with those reported by Raggi and colleagues (respectively, RR = 33.2, RP = 52.2, EF = 51.0) [52] found for samples of patients with chronic migraine. In the study by D'Amico and colleagues [45], both ECH and CCH patients had lower scores on the MOS-SF-36, with a significant difference noticed when comparing these findings to

Table 14.1 Description of included studies evaluating QoL and disability in patients with CH

Author, year	Design	Sample size	No. women	Mean age	ECH/CCH	CH duration	Weekly attacks	Pain intensity (0–10)	Paper's main results
Miller et al. (2017)	Long	51	16	47.8	0/51	7.9	25.9	8.4	ONS reduced attacks frequency, intensity, duration, disability, impact, and mental components of QoL
Jürgens et al. (2017)	Long	33	5	41.5	0/33	10.5	17	–	SPGS produced, in responders (35% of patients), a significant improvement in CCH frequency. At the group level, HIT-6 was significantly reduced
Akram et al. (2016)	Long	21	4	52	0/21	15	35	10	VTA-DBS reduced attacks frequency, intensity, headache load, disability, impact
Torkamani et al. (2015)	Cross	22	5	45	11/11	12.7	–	–	Compared to healthy controls, patients with CH show poorer QoL. Minor differences were found between CCH and ECH
Gaul et al. (2011)	Cross	179	43	44.7	107/72	12.9	24.5	–	CCH had higher HIT-6 compared to ECH. HIT-6 was correlated to direct costs and to attacks frequency
Hakim (2011)	Long	27	6	44.6	0/27	7	21	9	12-week treatment with warfarin reduced attacks frequency, duration, and intensity; also reduced impact measured with HIT-6
Jürgens et al. (2011)	Cross	75	18	41.4	48/27	12	–	–	Patients with CCH report higher HDI than those with ECH (those in active > non-active); higher than migraineurs and higher than healthy controls
Fontaine et al. (2010)	Long	11	3	44.1	0/11	12.1	14	6	Following HY-DBS, patients with CCH underwent a nonsignificant improvement in CH frequency and intensity and in PCS-MCS components of QoL
Narouze et al. (2009)	Long	15	–	–	0/15	–	17	8.6	Patients with CCH undergoing SPG-RFA underwent a significant reduction in CH frequency, pain intensity and PDI

(continued)

Table 14.1 (continued)

Author, year	Design	Sample size	No. women	Mean age	ECH/CCH	CH duration	Weekly attacks	Pain intensity (0–10)	Paper's main results
Ertsey et al. (2004)	Cross	35	10	44.7	35/0	12.7	12.2	–	Patients with CH show worse QoL compared to healthy controls
D'Amico et al. (2002)	Cross	56	16	45	34/22	12.7	–	–	Patients with CH show worse QoL compared to normative scores
Summary	–	525	126	44.6	235	11.8	22.6	8.6	ONS reduced attacks frequency, intensity, duration, disability, impact, and mental components of QoL

Notes: *ECH* episodic cluster headache, *CCH* chronic cluster headache, *ONS* occipital nerve stimulation, *SPGS* sphenopalatine ganglion stimulation, *VTA-DBS* ventral tegmental area deep brain stimulation, *HY-DBS* hypothalamic stimulation, *SPG-RFA* sphenopalatine ganglion radiofrequency ablation, *QoL* quality of life, *HIT-6* 6-item headache impact test, *PCS* physical composite score, *MCS* mental composite score, *HDI* headache disability inventory, *PDI* pain disability index

Table 14.2 Studies addressing quality of life

Ref. no. Author, year	Design	Sample size	Weekly attacks	Attacks intensity	EQ-VAS	PCS	MCS	Intervention	Follow-up (months)	Weekly attacks	Attacks intensity	EQ-VAS	PCS	MCS
Miller et al. (2017) [41]	Long	51	25.9	8.4	49.7	32.1	34.1	ONS	39.2	14.7* (−43%)	6.2* (−26%)	52.4 (+5%)	33.8 (+5%)	38.3* (+12%)
Akram et al. (2016) [42]	Long	21	35	10	49	32	32	VTA-DBS	12	14* (−60%)	7* (−30%)	45 (−8%)	35 (+9%)	34 (+6%)
Fontaine et al. (2010) [43]	Long	11	14	6	–	33.2	32.7	HY-DBS	12	8* (−49%)	4.5 (−25%)	–	37 (+11%)	39.7 (+21%)
Ertsey et al. (2004) [44]	Cross-sectional	35	12.2	–	–	38.2	37.7	–	–	–	–	–	–	–
D'Amico et al. (2002) [45]	Cross-sectional	56	–	–	–	45.0	36.5	–	–	–	–	–	–	–
Torkamani et al. (2015) [46]	Cross-sectional	22	–	–	50.5	–	–	–	–	–	–	–	–	–

Notes: *ONS* occipital nerve stimulation, *VTA-DBS* ventral tegmental area deep brain stimulation, *HY-DBS* hypothalamic stimulation, *PCS* physical composite score, *MCS* mental composite score, *EQ-VAS* EuroQoL Visual Analogue Scale

*$P < 0.05$

those in the general population for most QoL domains (i.e., those exploring physical, emotional, and social dimensions) and also for those dedicated to the personal evaluation of health status. No significant differences, however, were found between patients with ECH and CCH in this study.

In three studies, a longitudinal evaluations of change in QoL were addressed. Miller and colleagues [41] found a 12% significant improvement for the MOS-SF-36 MCS over 39 months in patients with intractable CCH that underwent occipital nerve stimulation, but no significant improvements were obtained for the EuroQol-VAS or MOS-SF-36 PCS. Akram and colleagues [42] and Fontaine and colleagues [43] failed to demonstrate any significant change in QoL measures in refractory patients treated with ventral tegmental area deep brain stimulation (DBS) and hypothalamic DBS, respectively.

In sum, data on QoL in regard to CH show a marked reduction compared to normative values, controls, and migraineurs. However, on the few occasions when QoL was reassessed following successful surgical procedures that positively impacted CH attack frequency, no appreciable improvements have been found.

14.3.2   Evaluation of Disability and Impact

Disability and impact of CH have been evaluated in seven studies, and cross-sectional and longitudinal data pertaining to disability or impact evaluation are reported in Table 14.3. The 6-item Headache Impact Test (HIT-6) was used in four longitudinal studies on refractory CH patients [41, 42, 53, 54] and in two cross-sectional studies [46, 55]; the Migraine Disability Assessment (MIDAS) was used in two longitudinal [41, 42] and one cross-sectional study [46]; the Headache Disability Inventory (HDI) was used in one cross-sectional study [31]; and the Pain Disability Index (PDI) was used in another longitudinal study [56]. HIT-6 [57] and MIDAS [58] are brief questionnaires, comprising six and five items, respectively, that specifically address the impact of headaches on patients' daily lives. Although they are largely used in headache disorders in general, both have been separately validated for migraine. The HDI [59] is a headache-specific disability inventory composed of 25 items that yield two composite scores and an overall score: the emotion score measures the influence of headaches on mood, while the function score assesses restrictions in daily tasks. The PDI [60] is a pain-specific disability index composed of seven items that has been validated in different groups of patients with pain-related conditions, but it, too, is not headache-specific. For all of these questionnaires, higher scores indicate greater levels of disability or impact.

Average HIT-6 scores are generally indicative of a very relevant impact of CH on patients' lives with mean scores >60 in refractory patients [41, 42, 53, 55] and >50 in two cross-sectional studies on consecutive patients; not "selected" for their particular severe forms [46, 55]. A moderate improvement after study treatments was suggested: in fact, with the exception of trial on warfarin [54]—which basically produced an almost complete short-term remission—follow-up scores were still

Table 14.3 Studies addressing disability and impact

Ref. no. Author, year	Design	Sample size	Weekly attacks	Attacks intensity	MIDAS	HIT-6	Intervention	Follow-up (months)	Weekly attacks	Attacks intensity	MIDAS	HIT-6
Miller et al. (2017) [41]	Long	51	25.9	8.4	149.8	67.7	ONS	39.2	14.7* (−43%)	6.2* (−26%)	114.9* (−23%)	60.7* (−10%)
Akram et al. (2016) [42]	Long	21	35	10	137	69	VTA-DBS	12	14* (−60%)	7* (−30%)	29* (−79%)	64* (−7%)
Torkamani et al. (2015) [46]	Cross-sectional	22	–	–	62.3	64.6	–	–	–	–	–	–
Jürgens et al. (2017) [53]	Long	33	17	–	–	67.7	SPGS	24	17 (0%)	–	–	62.9* (−7%)
Hakim (2011) [54]	Long	27	21	9	–	64	Warfarin	3	0* (−100%)	3* (−60%)	–	38* (−41%)
Gaul et al. (2011) [55]	Cross-sectional	179	24.5	–	–	56.7	–	–	–	–	–	–

Notes: *ONS* occipital nerve stimulation, *SPGS* sphenopalatine ganglion stimulation, *VTA-DBS* ventral tegmental area deep brain stimulation, *MIDAS* migraine disability assessment, *HIT-6* 6-item headache impact test

*$P < 0.05$

suggestive of a significant deleterious impact. Average MIDAS scores are also suggestive of a significant disability level [41, 42]. In fact, all baseline scores were far higher than the threshold of 21, which is considered indicative of significant problems as a result of headache [58]. This threshold was not reached even with a reduction of 79% of baseline scores in the study by Akram and colleagues [42].

Jürgens and colleagues [53] addressed disability as measured by the HDI and found that patients with CCH or ECH in the active phase had higher disability scores (HDI totals were 62.5 and 59.4, respectively) when compared to patients with ECH outside of the active period and to patients with migraine (HDI totals were 45.3 and 42.0, respectively). To the best of our knowledge, this is the only published paper in which the HDI was used in patients with CH. The above scores are suggestive of significant disability in patients with CH, and all were minimally comparable to or more elevated than those reported in other large samples of patients with different forms of headache: 32.5 in a sample of 492 persons with headache in a nonclinical setting [61], 45.7 in a sample of 225 patients with chronic migraine and comorbid depression and anxiety [62], and 18.8 in a sample of 197 patients with TTH [63].

Finally, Narouze and colleagues used the PDI to assess disability in a sample of 15 patients with refractory CCH that underwent sphenopalatine ganglion radiofrequency ablation [56]. Twelve months following the intervention, the frequency of attacks per week decreased from 17 to 8.6 (49% reduction) and the PDI decreased from 55 to 25.6 (53% reduction), both significant.

14.4 Discussion and Conclusions

The results of our review point out a few simple messages: (a) patients with CH, at least when not experiencing a bout of headaches, reveal few signs of psychological distress; (b) patients with CCH or ECH experience a strong reduction of their QoL and report considerable disability levels; (c) reduced QoL and increased disability observed in patients with CH is much greater than that of patients with other headache disorders. This conclusion, however (and unfortunately), is based on a limited amount of research and on a relatively small number of patients, who are often among the most severely affected (i.e., with refractoriness to standard pharmacological therapies), thus receiving invasive surgical treatments. In a sense it is puzzling that so little data are available, considering the severity profile of CH, a condition where pain is excruciating, often leading to suicidal ideation as a possible means of terminating the pain (reported in 55% of patients in a large cohort study [63]). Fortunately, reported suicide attempts were fairly low (2%) [63]. It is even more puzzling when considering the position taken by regulatory agencies that explicitly requires patients' perspectives to be taken into account in research [64–66].

Of further note, differences do exist between the two outcomes (QoL versus Disability) with regard to the detection of significant longitudinal changes. The three studies that addressed the impact of surgical procedures and improvements in

QoL [41–43] found reductions of weekly attacks between 40% and 60% and improvements in pain severity between 25% and 30%. However, improvements in QoL were nonsignificant and ranged between 5% and 21%. On the contrary, studies incorporating measures of disability and impact found improvements that, although smaller in terms of percentage reduction, were generally significant. We presume that QoL items, which typically address general and affective components related to "having a disease," may be less sensitive to change as patients continue to be affected by the fact of "still having CH" after receiving invasive treatment. Alternatively, some individuals may perceive QoL differences while others do not, resulting in mean differences that reveal no or minimal longitudinal change when findings are combined for groups. Percentage of patients deriving various levels of improvement in QoL is one way to examine if the present state of affairs is yet another case where mean values are not all that representative of the typical individual patterns of improvement.

On the contrary, evaluations of disability or impact are based on the *amount of times* during which a patient was unable to do something (the case for MIDAS ratings) or the *degree to which* he or she was unable to do something desired (the case for HDI ratings). Clearly, an instrument addressing this type of construct is likely to be more sensitive to the main goal of interventions aimed to reduce the frequency and intensity of CH attacks. Based on this logic, one might conclude that disability measures may be more appropriate than QoL measures for capturing a patient's experience of living with CH. However, we note that the most commonly used tools (HIT-6 and MIDAS) were developed to address migraine headaches and, thus, they have not been validated for use with patients with CH. MIDAS questions in particular are based on patient recall for the prior 3 months, with respondents being asked to report the number of days with missed work, household, and leisure time activities [58]. Consequently, the MIDAS does not distinguish between having a single attack per day or four to five attacks per day (as reported by Miller et al. [41] and Akram et al. [42]). This aspect alone questions whether the MIDAS is appropriate for addressing the impact of CH, wherein the number of days with headaches in a given period, frequency, intensity, and duration of single attacks, as well as time until relief, constitutes the primary clinical outcomes of interest [67–73]. Similar concerns arise for the other existing measures.

At this juncture, the need for "cluster"-specific measures of QoL, disability, and impact is readily apparent. To date, we could find only one such scale—the Cluster Headache Quality of Life Scale (CHQ)—that was published in 2016 [74]. It is composed of 28 items, grouped into four subscales: (1) restriction of activities of daily living (i.e., being unable to leave the house, complete work duties, or being involved in leisure activities); (2) impact on mood and interpersonal relationships (i.e., feeling unrespected by others, aggressive, impatient, or less tolerant, and having problems with relationships); (3) pain and anxiety; and (4) lack of vitality. Preliminary data reveal good construct validity, internal consistency, convergent validity, and test-retest reliability, while sensitivity to change has yet to be examined. Most of the explained variance is due to the first factor that, rather than QoL, seems to more appropriately reflect disability issues.

We conclude our summary of QoL and disability by pointing out the hetero-geneity in the studies available for this review, as this suggests caution on the part of the reader in extrapolating the findings reported. To list a few, the sample sizes ranged from 11 to 175, with a third of the entire number of subjects being included in a single study; although the distribution of ECH and CCH was simi-lar (235 and 290 cases, respectively), 6 of the 13 studies focused on CCH patients alone; and the follow-up duration varied greatly as well, ranging from 3 to 39 months.

A final point that merits discussion concerns what role, if any, might psychologi-cal science play in managing symptoms of CH. Evidence-based guidelines and comprehensive reviews of high flow oxygen and various pharmacological agents and stimulation techniques show steady progress at developing efficacious interven-tions for acute and prophylactic treatment [9, 67, 68, 75–78]. Existing guidelines, however, rarely, if ever, mention behavioral or non-drug approaches for CH.

Based on scattered early case reports of some success with applying varied forms of biofeedback and relaxation for CH (11 total, 5 retrospective recall) [79–81], Blanchard and colleagues [82] embarked on a single-group, uncontrolled outcome investigation of the potential benefits of an intensive, standardized course of pro-gressive muscle relaxation training (10 sessions over 8 weeks) followed by 12 ses-sions of thermal biofeedback administered over 6 to 9 weeks for CH. The later component was supplemented with aspects of autogenic training, and patients were provided with temperature-sensitive bands to help guide and evaluate home practice at temperature warming. Eleven patients with ECH (7 male, 4 female) began treat-ment when headache-free, with four ceasing participation during baseline headache monitoring. Three of the patients completing the trial reported some reductions in distress and overall debilitation over follow-up periods ranging from 5 months to 3 years, time points well beyond the point at which their headache bouts were pre-dicted to reoccur based on their prior history. One patient evolved from episodic to chronic CH, with us being unable to assess whether this was at all related to treatment.

While the role that psychological aspects have in CH is not well-recognized, it appears from the abovementioned review of cases that relaxation-based approaches may be of value for some patients and that targeting some behavioral factors known to affect CH, such as smoking and sleep, may be of further incremental value. Indeed, a decrease in the CH gender ratio has coincided with a decrease in the gen-der ratio for smoking [14] and an overall decrease in smoking habits [34, 35], mak-ing this a prime area to consider targeting. It is also important to take note that pain and emotion processing are closely linked in the brain [83]—pain is a subjective experience that influences and is influenced by emotional and cognitive processing, which is especially so for CH. In Blanchard et al. [82], all but one patients were seen at varying points during their headache-free periods. For some, by history, the next expected bout was predicted to occur many months or even years later. Having mas-tered the coping skills provided, the very likely possibility of skill decay during the intervening period was not considered. When patients with ECH now seek behavioral treatment, in addition to helping them find appropriate medical care and upon explaining the experimental nature of procedures, we recommend delaying pursuit of behavioral adjunctive procedures until a few months before the next bout is expected to occur (when such predictions are possible) to maximize readiness to employ learned coping skills. We offer, as well, to train during existing bouts if conditions permit this. Whether implementation of supplemental "just-in-time" behavioral coping training is of measurable value for CH awaits more rigorous evaluation. Finally, the findings of Jensen and colleagues [84], who provided outcomes from their comprehensive multidisciplinary treatment of over 1000 patients, approximately 50 of whom were diagnosed as CH, support this call for further investigations.

References

1. Headache Classification Committee of the International Headache Society (IHS). The International Classification of Headache Disorders, 3rd edition (beta version). Cephalalgia. 2013;33:629–808.
2. Horton BT. Histamine cephalgia. Lancet. 1952;72:92–8.
3. Markley HG, Buse DC. Cluster headache: myths and the evidence. Curr Pain Headache Rep. 2006;10:137–41.
4. Kudrow L. Cluster headache: mechanisms and management. New York: Oxford University Press; 1980.
5. Bahra A, May A, Goadsby PJ. Cluster headache: a prospective clinical study with diagnostic implications. Neurology. 2002;58:354–61.
6. Goadsby PJ. Pathophysiology of cluster headache: a trigeminal autonomic cephalgia. Lancet Neurol. 2002;1:251–7.
7. Dodick DW, Rozen TD, Goadsby PJ, Silberstein SD. Cluster headache. Cephalalgia. 2000;20:787–803.
8. Dodick DW, Capobianco DJ. Treatment and management of cluster headache. Curr Pain Headache Rep. 2001;5:83–91.
9. Leone M, Proietti Cecchini A. Advances in the understanding of cluster headache. Expert Rev Neurother. 2017;17:165–72.
10. Láinez MJA, Marti AS. Sphenopalatine ganglion stimulation in cluster headache and other types of headache. Cephalalgia. 2016;36:1149–55.
11. Oude Nijhuis JC, Haane DYP, Koehler PJ. A review of the current and potential oxygen delivery systems and techniques utilized in cluster headache attacks. Cephalalgia. 2016;36:970–9.
12. VanderPluym J. Cluster headache: special considerations for treatment of female patients of reproductive age and pediatric patients. Curr Neurol Neurosci Rep. 2016;16:5.
13. Andrasik F, Blanchard EB, Arena JG, Teders SJ, Rodichok LD. Cross-validation of the Kudrow-Sutkus MMPI classification system for diagnosing headache type. Headache. 1982;22:2–5.
14. Manzoni GC. Gender ratio of cluster headache over the years: a possible role of changes in lifestyle. Cephalalgia. 1998;18:138–42.
15. Friedman AP. Cluster headaches. Neurology. 1958;8:653–63.
16. Graham JR. Cluster headache. Headache. 1972;11:175–85.
17. Kempner J. Uncovering the man in medicine: lessons learned from a case study of cluster headache. Gend Soc. 2006;20:632–56.
18. Andrasik F, Blanchard EB, Arena JG, Teders SJ, Teevan RC, Rodichok LD. Psychological functioning in headache sufferers. Psychosom Med. 1982;44:171–82.
19. Kudrow L, Sutkus BJ. MMPI pattern specificity in primary headache disorders. Headache. 1979;19:18–24.

20. Pfaffenrath V, Hummelsberger J, Pöllmann W, Kaube H, Rath M. MMPI personality profiles in patients with primary headache syndromes. Cephalalgia. 1991;11:263–8.
21. Italian Cooperative Study Group on the Epidemiology of Cluster Headache (ICECH). Case-control study on the epidemiology of cluster headache. II: anthropometric data and personality profile. Funct Neurol. 2000;15:215–23.
22. Piacentini SHMJ, Draghi L, Cecchini AP, Leone M. Personality disorders in cluster headache: a study using the Millon clinical multiaxial inventory-III. Neurol Sci. 2017;38:S181–4.
23. Muñoz I, Hernández MS, Santos S, Jurado C, Ruiz L, Toribio E, Sotelo EM, Guerrero AL, Molina V, Uribe F, Cuadrado ML. Personality traits in patients with cluster headache: a comparison with migraine patients. J Headache Pain. 2016;17:25. https://doi.org/10.1186/s10194-016-0618-9.
24. Fishbain DA, Cole B, Cutler RB, Lewis J, Rosomoff HL, Rosomoff RS. Chronic pain and the measurement of personality: do states influence traits? Pain Med. 2006;7:509–29.
25. Mongini F, Ilbertis F, Ferla E. Personality characteristics before and after treatment of different head pain syndromes. Cephalalgia. 1994;14:368–73.
26. Bertolotti G, Vidotto G, Sanavio E, Frediani F. Psychological and emotional aspects of pain. Neurol Sci. 2003;24(Suppl 2):S71–S5.
27. Tunks ER, Crook J, Weir R. Epidemiology of chronic pain with psychological comorbidity: prevalence, risk, course, and prognosis. Can J Psychiatr. 2008;53:224–34.
28. Bair MJ, Wu J, Damush TM, Sutherland JM, Kroenke K. Association of depression and anxiety alone and in combination with chronic musculoskeletal pain in primary care patients. Psychosom Med. 2008;70:890–7.
29. Antonaci F, Nappi G, Galli F, Manzoni GC, Calabresi P, Costa A. Migraine and psychiatric comorbidity: a review of clinical findings. J Headache Pain. 2011;12:115–25.
30. Choong CK, Ford JH, Nyhuis AW, Joshi SG, Robinson RL, Aurora SK, Martinez JM. Clinical characteristics and treatment patterns among patients diagnosed with cluster headache in U.S. healthcare claims data. Headache. 2017;57:1359–74.
31. Jürgens TP, Gaul C, Lindwurm A, Dresler T, Paelecke-Habermann Y, Schmidt-Wilcke T, Lürding R, Henkel K, Leinisch E. Impairment in episodic and chronic cluster headache. Cephalalgia. 2011;31:671–82.
32. Liang JF, Chen YT, Fuh JL, Li SY, Liu CJ, Chen TJ, Tang CH, Wang SJ. Cluster headache is associated with an increased risk of depression: a nationwide population-based cohort study. Cephalalgia. 2012;33:182–9.
33. Govare A, Leroux E. Licit and illicit drug use in cluster headache. Curr Pain Headache Rep. 2014;18:413. https://doi.org/10.1007/s11916-014-0413-8.
34. US Department of Health and Human Services. Patterns of tobacco use among U.S. youth, young adults, and adults. In: The health consequences of smoking: 50 years of progress: a report of the surgeon general. Atlanta: Centers for Disease Control and Prevention (US); 2014. p. 701–70.
35. Giskes K, Kunst AE, Benach J, Borrell C, Costa G, Dahl E, Dalstra JAA, Federico B, Helmert U, Judge K, Lahelma E, Moussa K, Ostergren PO, Platt S, Prattala R, Rasmussen NK, Mackenbach JP. Trends in smoking behaviour between 1985 and 2000 in nine European countries by education. J Epidemiol Community Health. 2005;59:395–401.
36. Barloese MCJ. Neurobiology and sleep disorders in cluster headache. J Headache Pain. 2015;16:78. https://doi.org/10.1186/s10194-015-0562-0.
37. Germain A, Buysse DJ, Nofzinger E. Sleep-specific mechanisms underlying posttraumatic stress disorder: integrative review and neurobiological hypotheses. Sleep Med Rev. 2008;12:185–95.
38. Seifert CL, Valet M, Pfaffenrath V, Boecker H, Rüther KV, Tölle TR, Sprenger T. Neurometabolic correlates of depression and disability in episodic cluster headache. J Neurol. 2011;258:123–31.
39. Leone M, Cecchini AP. Short-lasting unilateral neuralgiform headache attacks: where is the headache generator? Brain. 2016;139:2578–89.

40. Jensen RM, Lyngberg A, Jensen RH. Burden of cluster headache. Cephalalgia. 2007;27:535–41.
41. Miller S, Watkins L, Matharu M. Treatment of intractable chronic cluster headache by occipital nerve stimulation: a cohort of 51 patients. Eur J Neurol. 2017;24:381–90.
42. Akram H, Miller S, Lagrata S, Hyam J, Jahanshahi M, Hariz M, Matharu M, Zrinzo L. Ventral tegmental area deep brain stimulation for refractory chronic cluster headache. Neurology. 2016;86:1676–82.
43. Fontaine D, Lazorthes Y, Mertens P, Blond S, Géraud G, Fabre N, Navez M, Lucas C, Dubois F, Gonfrier S, Paquis P, Lantéri-Minet M. Safety and efficacy of deep brain stimulation in refractory cluster headache: a randomized placebo-controlled double-blind trial followed by a 1-year open extension. J Headache Pain. 2010;11:23–31.
44. Ertsey C, Manhalter N, Bozsik G, Áfra J, Jelencsik I. Health-related and condition-specific quality of life in episodic cluster headache. Cephalalgia. 2004;24:188–96.
45. D'Amico D, Rigamonti A, Solari A, Leone M, Usai S, Grazzi L, Bussone G. Health-related quality of life in patients with cluster headache during active periods. Cephalalgia. 2002;22:818–21.
46. Torkamani M, Ernst L, Cheung LS, Lambru G, Matharu M, Jahanshahi M. The neuropsychology of cluster headache: cognition, mood, disability, and quality of life of patients with chronic and episodic cluster headache. Headache. 2015;55:287–300.
47. Ware JE, Sherbourne CD. The MOS 36-item short-form health survey (SF-36). I. Conceptual framework and item selection. Med Care. 1992;30:473–83.
48. EuroQol Group. EuroQol-a new facility for the measurement of health-related quality of life. Health Policy. 1990;16:199–208.
49. Pathak D, Martin B, Kwong J, Batenhorst A. Evaluation of the migraine specific quality of life questionnaire (MSQ version 2.0) using confirmatory factor analysis. Qual Life Res. 1998;13:707–17.
50. Bagley CL, Rendas-Baum R, Maglinte GA, Yang M, Varon SF, Lee J, Kosinski M. Validating migraine-specific quality of life questionnaire v2.1 in episodic and chronic migraine. Headache. 2012;52:409–21.
51. Rendas-Baum R, Bloudek LM, Maglinte GA, Varon SF. The psychometric properties of the migraine-specific quality of life questionnaire version 2.1 (MSQ) in chronic migraine patients. Qual Life Res. 2013;22:1123–33.
52. Raggi A, Giovannetti AM, Schiavolin S, Leonardi M, Bussone G, Grazzi L, Usai S, Curone M, Di Fiore P, D'Amico D. Validating the migraine-specific quality of life questionnaire v2.1 (MSQ) in Italian inpatients with chronic migraine with a history of medication overuse. Qual Life Res. 2014;23(4):1273–7.
53. Jürgens TP, Barloese M, May A, Láinez JM, Schoenen J, Gaul C, Goodman AM, Caparso A, Jensen RH. Long-term effectiveness of sphenopalatine ganglion stimulation for cluster headache. Cephalalgia. 2017;37:423–34.
54. Hakim SM. Warfarin for refractory chronic cluster headache: a randomized pilot study. Headache. 2011;51:713–25.
55. Gaul C, Finken J, Biermann J, Mostardt S, Diener HC, Müller O, Wasem J, Neumann A. Treatment costs and indirect costs of cluster headache: a health economics analysis. Cephalalgia. 2011;31:1664–72.
56. Narouze S, Kapural L, Casanova J, Mekhail N. Sphenopalatine ganglion radiofrequency ablation for the management of chronic cluster headache. Headache. 2009;49:571–7.
57. Kosinski M, Bayliss MS, Bjorner JB, Ware JE Jr, Garber WH, Batenhorst A, Cady R, Dahlöf CG, Dowson A, Tepper S. A six-item short-form survey for measuring headache impact: the HIT-6. Qual Life Res. 2003;12:963–74.
58. Stewart WF, Lipton RB, Kolodner K, Liberman J, Sawyer J. Reliability of the migraine disability assessment score in a population-based sample of headache sufferers. Cephalalgia. 1999;19:107–14.
59. Jacobson GP, Ramadan NM, Aggarwal SK, Newman CW. The Henry Ford hospital headache disability inventory (HDI). Neurology. 1994;44:837–42.

60. Chibnall JT, Tait RC. The pain disability index: factor structure and normative data. Arch Phys Med Rehabil. 1994;75:1082–6.
61. Minen MT, Seng EK, Holroyd KA. Influence of family psychiatric and headache history on migraine-related health care utilization. Headache. 2014;54:485–92.
62. Fernández-de-las-Peñas C, Benito-González E, Palacios-Ceña M, Wang K, Castaldo M, Arendt-Nielsen L. Identification of subgroups of patients with tension type headache with higher widespread pressure pain hyperalgesia. J Headache Pain. 2017;18:43.
63. Rozen TD, Fishman RS. Cluster headache in the United States of America: demographics, clinical characteristics, triggers, Suicidality, and personal burden. Headache. 2012;52:99–113.
64. Speight J, Barendse SM. FDA guidance on patient reported outcomes. BMJ. 2010;341:c2921.
65. Washington AE, Lipstein SH. The Patient-Centered Outcomes Research Institute--promoting better information, decisions, and health. N Engl J Med. 2011;365(15):e31.
66. Fleurence RL, Forsythe LP, Lauer M, Rotter J, Ioannidis JPA, Beal A, Frank L, Selby JV. Engaging patients and stakeholders in research proposal review: the Patient-Centered Outcomes Research Institute. Ann Intern Med. 2014;161:122–30.
67. Sarchielli P, Granella F, Prudenzano MP, Pini LA, Guidetti V, Bono G, Pinessi L, Alessandri M, Antonaci F, Fanciullacci M, Ferrari A, Guazzelli M, Nappi G, Sances G, Sandrini G, Savi L, Tassorelli C, Zanchin G. Italian guidelines for primary headaches: 2012 revised version. J Headache Pain. 2012;13(Suppl 2):S31–70.
68. May A, Leone M, Afra J, Linde M, Sándor PS, Evers S, Goadsby PJ, EFNS Task Force. EFNS guidelines on the treatment of cluster headache and other trigeminal-autonomic cephalalgias. Eur J Neurol. 2006;13:1066–77.
69. Martelletti P, Jensen RH, Antal A, Arcioni R, Brighina F, de Tommaso M, Franzini A, Fontaine D, Heiland M, Jürgens TP, Leone M, Magis D, Paemeleire K, Palmisani S, Paulus W, May A, European Headache Federation. Neuromodulation of chronic headaches: position statement from the European Headache Federation. J Headache Pain. 2013;14:86.
70. Halker R, Vargas B, Dodick DW. Cluster headache: diagnosis and treatment. Semin Neurol. 2010;30:175–85.
71. Goadsby PJ, Cittadini E, Burns B, Cohen AS. Trigeminal autonomic cephalalgias: diagnostic and therapeutic developments. Curr Opin Neurol. 2008;21:323–30.
72. May A. Update on the diagnosis and management of trigemino-autonomic headaches. J Neurol. 2006;253:1525–32.
73. Francis GJ, Becker WJ, Pringsheim TM. Acute and preventive pharmacologic treatment of cluster headache. Neurology. 2010;75:463–73.
74. Abu Bakar N, Torkamani M, Tanprawate S, Lambru G, Matharu M, Jahanshahi M. The development and validation of the cluster headache quality of life scale (CHQ). J Headache Pain. 2016;17:79.
75. Gooriah R, Buture A, Ahmed F. Evidence-based treatments for cluster headache. Ther Clin Risk Manag. 2015;11:1687–96.
76. Robbins MS, Starling AJ, Pringsheim TM, Becker WJ, Schwedt TJ. Treatment of cluster headache: the American headache society evidence-based guidelines. Headache. 2016;56:1093–106.
77. Leone M, Giustiniani A, Cecchini AP. Cluster headache: present and future therapy. Neurol Sci. 2017;38(Suppl 1):45–50.
78. Kingston WS, Dodick DW. Treatment of cluster headache. Ann Indian Acad Neurol. 2018;21(Suppl 1):S9–S15.
79. Sargent JD, Walters ED, Green EE. Psychosomatic self-regulation of migraine headaches. Semin Psychiatry. 1973;5:415–28.
80. Benson H, Klemchuk HP, Graham JR. The usefulness of the relaxation response in the therapy of headache. Headache. 1974;13:49–52.
81. Adler CS, Adler SM. The pragmatic application of biofeedback to headaches: a five-year clinical follow-up. Paper presented at the Seventh Annual Meeting of the Biofeedback Research Society; Colorado Springs; 1976.

82. Blanchard EB, Andrasik F, Jurish SE, Teders SJ. The treatment of cluster headache with relaxation and thermal biofeedback. Biofeedback Self Regul. 1982;7:185–91.
83. Dahlke LAM, Sable JJ, Andrasik F. Behavioral therapy: emotion and pain, a common anatomical background. Neurol Sci. 2017;38(Suppl 1):S157–61.
84. Jensen R, Zeeberg P, Dehlendorff C, Olesen J. Predictors of outcome of the treatment programme in a multidisciplinary headache Centre. Cephalalgia. 2010;30:1214–24.

Chapter 15
Neurophysiology of Cluster Headache and Other Trigeminal Autonomic Cephalalgias

Gianluca Coppola, Armando Perrotta, Francesco Pierelli, and Giorgio Sandrini

Abbreviations

BR	Blink reflex
CH	Cluster headache
CPT	Cold pressor test
DBS	Deep brain stimulation
EEG	Electroencephalography
ERPs	Event-related potentials
HCs	Healthy controls
IDAP	Intensity dependence of cortical auditory evoked potentials
LEPs	Laser evoked potentials
LFPs	Local field potentials
nBR	Nociceptive blink reflex
non-REM	Non-rapid eye movement

G. Coppola (✉)
Department of Medico-Surgical Sciences and Biotechnologies, Sapienza University of Rome
Polo Pontino, Latina, Italy

A. Perrotta
INM-Neuromed, Headache Clinic, Pozzilli (IS), Italy
e-mail: armando.perrotta@neuromed.it

F. Pierelli
Department of Medico-Surgical Sciences and Biotechnologies, Sapienza University of Rome
Polo Pontino, Latina, Italy

INM-Neuromed, Headache Clinic, Pozzilli (IS), Italy
e-mail: francesco.pierelli@uniroma1.it

G. Sandrini
Headache Science Center and Headache Unit, National Neurological Institute C. Mondino
Foundation, Pavia, Italy

Department of Brain and Behavioral Sciences, University of Pavia, Pavia, Italy
e-mail: giorgio.sandrini@unipv.it

© Springer Nature Switzerland AG 2020
M. Leone, A. May (eds.), *Cluster Headache and other Trigeminal Autonomic Cephalgias*, Headache, https://doi.org/10.1007/978-3-030-12438-0_15

NWR	Nociceptive withdrawal reflex
REM	Rapid eye movement
SSEPs	Somatosensory evoked potentials
SUNA	Short-lasting unilateral neuralgiform headache attacks with cranial autonomic symptoms
SUNCT	Short-lasting unilateral neuralgiform headache attacks with conjunctival injection and tearing
TACs	Trigeminal autonomic cephalalgias
TMS	Transcranial magnetic stimulation
TST	Temporal summation threshold
VEP	Visual evoked potential

15.1 Introduction

The conditions collectively termed trigeminal autonomic cephalalgias (TACs) include cluster headache (CH), paroxysmal hemicrania, short-lasting unilateral neuralgiform headache attacks with conjunctival injection and tearing (SUNCT), short-lasting unilateral neuralgiform headache attacks with cranial autonomic symptoms (SUNA), and hemicrania continua. These syndromes differ in attack duration and frequency and present different responses to therapy [1].

Neurophysiological methods, despite having no role in the routine activity of headache clinics [2], are commonly employed as atraumatic and noninvasive means of assessing neural functional integrity of the various subcortical-cortical structures claimed to be involved in the pathophysiology as well as in the peculiar phenotypical presentation of TACs.

Cluster headache is the most extensively studied TAC. Researchers, using cortical evoked potentials, brainstem reflexes, and spinal withdrawal reflexes, have described several interesting brain response abnormalities in this disorder. The results suggest that neurophysiological patterns may fluctuate between active and remission periods and differ according to certain clinical features of the headache.

This chapter aims to provide a complete and systematic outline of the results provided by different neurophysiological techniques that have been used to study the pathophysiology of TACs.

15.2 Electroencephalography and Microelectrode Recording During Deep Brain Stimulation in Cluster Headache

Electroencephalography, being of no use in the diagnosis of primary headaches [2], , is not recommended in the routine clinical evaluation of patients affected by TACs.

In the research setting, Silvestri and colleagues [3] performed a polysomnographic study in a group of 13 untreated episodic CH patients, 3 of whom experienced attacks during the recording. However, these three patients did not show abnormalities *on electroencephalography* (EEG), which, on the contrary, revealed abnormalities in two female patients with a family or personal history of epilepsy or head injury, and in one patient, also female, without personal or family antecedents. In the latter patient, non-rapid eye movement (non-REM) sleep EEG examination showed diffuse generalized rapid (4–5 c/s) polyspike and wave complexes bilaterally, mainly over the anterior derivations [3]. Another study failed to detect specific EEG findings in children with CH [4].

A few studies have evaluated patients implanted with devices for deep brain stimulation (DBS) of the ipsilateral hypothalamus (this is a treatment option for chronic CH patients refractory to other treatments) [5]. Recording of local field potentials (LFPs) from microelectrodes revealed tonic firing patterns with discharge rates ranging from 13 to 35 Hz; LFPs were unresponsive to sensory, motor, autonomic and emotional stimuli [6, 7], except in one case, reported to be sensitive to tactile stimulation of the ophthalmic branch of the trigeminal nerve, contralateral to the recording side [8]. Other authors observed, in a single patient during a CH attack, a prominent peak of hypothalamic LFP spectra recorded from the DBS electrode, with the LFPs showing a power increase of around 20 Hz. This activity lasted only a few minutes and was not detected at cortical level. These results were felt to argue for a role of hypothalamic activation in the generation of CH [9, 10].

15.3   Polysomnography and Sleep Dysfunction in Cluster Headache

Cluster headache and sleep are interrelated. Up to 80% of CH patients are woken during the night because of an attack [11], especially within the first 2 h of sleep onset, mostly between 1 and 3 a.m. [11–13].

Few polysomnographic studies have been carried out in CH.

Using a controlled study design in a population of 40 CH patients (21 episodic studied during an active cluster period, and 19 chronic), Barloese [11] investigated the macrostructure of sleep as well as arousals, and the relationship between spontaneous CH attacks and sleep (considering both sleep in general and specific sleep phenomena). They found a longer time to onset of rapid eye movement (REM) sleep (REM latency) and a lower percentage of REM sleep in patients versus controls; comparison of patients who did not suffer attacks during recording with those who did report attacks (during both sleep and wakefulness) revealed that both groups had reduced REM sleep. Moreover, the authors reported decreased cortical activation, as reflected in a decreased number of EEG arousals per hour of sleep, in the patients versus the controls [11]. In one case, these alterations remitted after the cluster phase [14]. Vetrugno et al. [15] found reduced sleep efficiency, fragmented sleep, and increased periodic limb movements during sleep in three male chronic

CH patients. All these sleep abnormalities improved 4 months after implantation of DBS of the posterior hypothalamus [15].

Although some authors have reported an association between nocturnal CH attacks and REM sleep periods [16–18], others have not confirmed this [11]. This aspect is thus still debated. In a study involving a large sample of patients, no difference in the macrostructural composition of sleep was found between patients and controls, apart from a lower REM density in the former [11]. A relationship between REM-related attacks and sleep apneic events has been observed in both episodic and chronic CH by some authors [19–22], but not others [23, 24].

15.4 Evoked Potentials

Evoked potential studies have been used to investigate the central pathogenesis of CH. Different sensory modalities have been used (Table 15.1).

Table 15.1 Innocuous cortical evoked potential studies performed in cluster headache

Authors	Sensory modality	Stimulation parameters	Diagnosis	Results
Polich et al. [25]	VEPs	Full-field checkerboard, 1.9 Hz reversal rate, 0.25 and 1 degrees of visual angle	10 male CH, 10 HCs	No differences between groups
Boiardi et al. [26]	VEPs	Full-field checkerboard, 1.6 Hz reversal rate, 55 min of arc	20 (18 males) CH, 20 HCs	P100 amplitudes were significantly lower than in controls, on the pain side only
Boiardi et al. [27]	VEPs and BAEPs	VEP: full-field checkerboard, 1.6 Hz reversal rate, 55 min of arc; BAEPs: 11 Hz, 70 dB	14 male CH, 14 HCs	VEPs: P100 amplitudes were significantly lower than in controls, on the pain side only; BAEPs: I–V latencies were increased on the pain side
Bussone et al. [29]	BAEPs	Repetition rate of 11 Hz, 70 dB	16 (12 episodic and 4 chronic) CH, 16 HCs	I–V latencies were increased in CH patients both during and outside an attack, and normalized during lithium therapy
Afra et al. [30]	IDAP	Repetition rate of 0.55 Hz at four intensities (40, 50, 60 and 70 dB)	15 (11 males) CH [during the bout, outside an attack], 13 HCs	ASF slopes of auditory evoked potentials were steep in CH patients compared with HCs, both during and outside a bout

Table 15.1 (continued)

Authors	Sensory modality	Stimulation parameters	Diagnosis	Results
Firenze et al. [31]	SSEPs	Median nerve stimulation contralateral to the headache side, 0.2 stimulus duration, twitching threshold, repetition rate of 2 Hz	10 male CH [during the bout, outside an attack, and again during an attack induced by intravenous administration of histamine], 20 HCs	During a bout, outside an attack, SSEP amplitudes were found to be like those of HCs, while they were reduced during an attacks induced by intravenous administration of histamine
Cosentino et al. [32]	TMS	Paired-pulse focal TMS over the hand motor cortex (120% of RMT) of both hemispheres. Measurements: ICF and SICI, CSP, input-output curves (I-O curves)	25 episodic CH patients (21 males) [13 outside bout, 12 during a bout], 13 HCs	RMT and CSP values did not differ between groups. Both inside and outside bouts, ICF was more pronounced in the hemisphere ipsilateral to the headache side with respect to the contralateral one, and also with respect to values recorded from both hemispheres in HCs. Only in patients evaluated during a bout were significantly higher SICI values were found in the motor cortex ipsilateral to the headache side compared to the contralateral one. Compared with what was found in HCs, a steeper slope was recorded from both hemispheres of CH patients evaluated outside a bout, and from the motor cortex contralateral to the headache side in patients during a bout

BAEPs brainstem auditory evoked potentials, *CH* cluster headache, *HCs* healthy controls, *IDAP* intensity dependence of cortical auditory evoked potentials, *SSEPs* somatosensory evoked potentials, *TMS* transcranial magnetic stimulation, *VEPs* visual evoked potentials, *RMT* resting motor threshold ICF: intracortical facilitation, *SICI* short intracortical inhibition, *CSP* cortical silent period

15.4.1 Visual Evoked Potentials

An early study by Polich et al. [25] failed to find any significant differences in visual evoked potential (VEP) latencies and amplitudes between a group of ten male CH patients and matched controls. However, when VEP responses were assessed over both occipital regions (O1 and O2, 10–20 EEG system), P100 amplitudes were found to be significantly lower in patients than in controls, on the pain side only, during a pain-free period, not due to pupillary asymmetry [26, 27]. This finding was interpreted as reflecting cerebral neurotransmitter dysfunction in CH. Further investigations are needed to elucidate whether it is related to a possible abnormal asymmetrical activation of the posterior hypothalamus to thalamus pathway [28].

15.4.2   Auditory Evoked Potentials

Measurement of brainstem auditory evoked potentials is a useful electrophysiological method for studying brainstem functional integrity.

A larger asymmetry of the I–V interpeak latency, increased on the symptomatic side [27], was detected in both episodic and chronic CH with respect to healthy controls (HCs), irrespective of whether patients were recorded during or outside an attack [29]. Interestingly, this neurophysiological pattern normalized during prophylactic intervention with lithium [29].

Afra and co-workers [30] recorded intensity dependence of cortical auditory evoked potentials (IDAP) in 15 episodic CH patients during both the active and the remission phase. They found steeper amplitude-stimulus intensity function slopes in CH patients than in controls, in both phases, and this difference was not related to patients' clinical features. Since IDAP is a surrogate marker of central nervous system serotonin transmission, the authors argued that their results reflect diminished serotonergic activity in raphe-hypothalamic serotonergic pathways in CH patients.

15.4.3   Somatosensory Evoked Potentials

Only one study involving the use of somatosensory evoked potentials (SSEPs) has been performed in CH (a group of ten patients). SSEPs were recorded, after median nerve stimulation at the wrist, during an active period but outside an attack, and then during an attack induced by intravenous administration of histamine (40 µg) [31]. In the first condition (during a bout but outside an attack), the patients showed normal SSEP patterns; however, during a severe histamine-induced attack, the amplitudes of the N20-P25 complex were significantly decreased in comparison with outside the attack, and in comparison with values recorded in HCs. This histamine-related effect on SSEPs seems to be specific to CH, since it was not found in other primary headache disorders, such as migraine and tension-type headache [31].

15.4.4   Motor Evoked Potentials

Transcranial magnetic stimulation (TMS) is a noninvasive method used to study the excitability of the underlying cortical area.

To date, only one TMS study has been performed in CH [32]: in this study, episodic CH patients, recorded in active and remission periods, showed normal thresholds for the elicitation of motor evoked potentials and normal duration of the cortical silent period. Using paired-pulse TMS, intracortical facilitation, recorded both in active and remission phases, was found to be increased in the hemisphere ipsilateral to the headache side versus the contralateral one, and compared with values recorded from both hemispheres in healthy volunteers. Only patients evaluated during the active phase showed significantly lower short intracortical inhibition in the motor cortex ipsilateral to the headache side compared with the contralateral one.

15.4.5   Event-Related Potentials and P300

Few studies have investigated cognitive event-related potentials (ERPs) in CH. Evers et al. [33, 34], using a visual oddball paradigm, evaluated the P300 component in CH patients and found, in active (but not remission) periods, a delayed latency as compared with HCs, but normal amplitude, reaction time, and cognitive habituation. Furthermore, P300 latency, amplitude, and reaction time were found to be significantly increased in chronic CH during the cluster period as compared with remission and with all other conditions [34]. The same authors also studied a group of chronic paroxysmal hemicrania patients during indomethacin treatment and detected normal ERP parameters [33, 34]. Prophylactic drugs normalized the ERP latencies in episodic, but not in chronic, CH. No significant correlations were found between ERP data and disease duration, attack duration and daily frequency of attacks in the different groups of patients [33, 34]. In one visual ERP study, P300 amplitude was decreased in CH patients in comparison with HCs, irrespective of the headache side [35].

Event-related potentials have also been investigated using an auditory paradigm in CH [36]. The authors found significantly diminished middle-latency P200 amplitudes in CH patients compared with HCs, but no significant differences in P300 or N100 amplitudes, and no increased latencies for any of the ERP components considered [36] (Table 15.2).

15.4.6   Pain-Related Evoked Potentials

Electrical or laser pulse stimulation of the superficial skin layers is a reliable and objective way of studying pain-evoked brain responses in the trigeminal or extracranial systems.

Trigeminal somatosensory evoked potentials were recorded in 28 CH patients in an active period and repeated in 22 during remission. Recordings were made after electrically stimulating the corner of the mouth (third trigeminal nerve division) on both sides. Data recorded in cluster periods showed the N2 latency to be delayed on the affected side versus the non-affected side, and compared with latency data

Table 15.2 Cognitive event-related potentials and noxious-related pain-related cortical evoked potential studies performed in cluster headache

Authors	Sensory modality	Stimulation parameters	Diagnosis	Results
Evers et al. [33]	ERPs (P300 component)	Visual oddball paradigm	37 (32 males) CH [11 during remission, 26 during active phase], 8 CPH, 30 HCs	Delayed P300 latency with normal habituation in CH patients during active phase. CPH patients showed normal ERP parameters
Evers et al. [34]	ERPs (P300 component)	Visual oddball paradigm	61 (32 males) CH [50 episodic during active phase, 11 chronic], 12 CPH, 20 HCs	Delayed P300 latency with normal habituation more marked in chronic CH patients than in episodic CH patients during active phase. CPH patients showed normal ERP parameters
Casale et al. [36]	ERPs (P300 component)	Auditory paradigm	27 (21 males) CH, 25 HCs	Significantly smaller P200 amplitude in CH patients than in controls. No significant differences in P300 or N100 amplitudes were detected, or increased latencies for any of the ERP components considered
Wang et al. 2014 [35]	ERPs (P300 component)	Visual oddball paradigm	17 (15 males) CH, 15 HCs	P300 amplitude was decreased in CH patients compared with HCs, without side-to-side differences. No differences in P300 latency or in reaction times were detected
van Vliet et al. [37]	TSEPs	Electrical stimuli were delivered to both sides on the corner of the mouth in all subjects at three times the sensory threshold	28 male episodic CH patients during active phase [repeated in 22 also during remission], 22 HCs	TSEP N2 component latency was more delayed during the active phase on the affected side versus the non-affected side, compared with HCs and recordings outside the active phase. N1 latency was significantly delayed on the affected (during the active phase) and unaffected side (in remission phase only) compared with HCs
Ellrich et al. [39]	LEPs	YAG laser stimulation of the cutaneous innervation territory of the supraorbital nerve	25 (21 males) CH patients (16 episodic [7 during and 10 outside the active phase], 9 chronic), 10 HCs	In chronic CH patients on the headache side, the LEP N1c component occurred later, while the P2 amplitude was smaller than on the non-headache side. In episodic CH patients during the active phase, P2 latency was shorter on the headache side. In episodic CH outside the active phase the N2-P2 ratio was lower on the headache side

Table 15.2 (continued)

Authors	Sensory modality	Stimulation parameters	Diagnosis	Results
Holle et al. [38]	PREPs	The PREP was recorded using two planar concentric surface electrodes placed above the entry zone of the supraorbital nerve	66 (49 males) CH patients (46 episodic [7 during and 28 outside the active phase], 20 chronic), 30 HCs	In chronic CH patients, the authors found a decreased N2 latency ratio ([latency headache side/latency non-headache side] × 100) compared with HCs, which was not detected in episodic CH either during or outside the active phase

CH cluster headache, *CPH* chronic paroxysmal hemicrania, *ERPs* event-related potentials, *HCs* healthy controls, *TSEPs* trigeminal somatosensory evoked potentials, *LEPs* laser evoked potentials, *PREP* pain-related evoked potentials

recorded in HCs and in patients during remission. N1 latencies were found to be significantly delayed in CH patients on both sides (affected, only in active periods, and non-affected, only during remission) compared with HCs [37].

In another study, use of a concentric electrode placed over the supraorbital division of the trigeminal nerve to elicit pain-related evoked potentials revealed a decreased N2 latency ratio (headache side/non-headache side) in chronic CH patients compared with HCs, but not in episodic CH during either active or remission periods [38]. Perception and pain thresholds as well as P2 amplitude and latency ratios showed no significant between-groups differences [38].

Ellrich and colleagues [39] measured YAG laser evoked potentials (LEPs) and found similar LEP component values and pain thresholds between CH patients and HCs. In chronic CH patients, N1c was delayed on the headache side, while the P2 amplitude was larger on the non-affected side. In episodic CH patients during a cluster period, P2 latency was found to be reduced on the headache side compared with the contralateral one. In episodic CH during remission, the N2-P2 ratio was lower on the affected than on the non-affected side [39]. Unfortunately, the authors did not compare mean LEP parameters between CH patients and HCs but limited their analysis to an assessment of whether each single patient's LEP values exceeded the normal limits. They found that 19 out of 26 patients showed pathological deviation on some LEP parameter, although no typical pattern emerged [39].

15.5 Electromyographic Reflex Responses

15.5.1 Brainstem Reflexes

Side-to-side asymmetry in CH patients was also observed using the blink reflex (BR), a surrogate marker of brainstem trigeminal system integrity. Episodic CH patients, investigated during the active phase, showed higher R2 threshold [40] and amplitude [41] values on the headache side than contralaterally. The threshold of the corneal reflex, another brainstem reflex, was reduced on the affected side in a mixed group of episodic CH (investigated during the active phase) and chronic CH patients, but normal when recorded during the remission phase [42].

In ten episodic CH patients, also recorded during an active period, Lozza et al. [43] found a significantly faster R2 BR recovery curve on the headache side after a paired supraorbital stimulus, possibly secondary to a sensitization process within the trigeminal nucleus caudalis. Additionally, the same patients showed a faster R2 recovery curve on both the headache and the non-headache side when the supraorbital stimulus was preconditioned by an index finger stimulation. Since injection of the opioid antagonist naloxone transiently reversed this bilateral R2 sensitizing response, the authors hypothesized, in line with more recent neuroimaging findings [44, 45], that the faster R2 recovery they observed reflects hypoactivity of reticular nuclei, due to reduced descending opiatergic inhibition [43].

These lateralized BR abnormalities were further confirmed by the use of a nociception-specific concentric electrode to evoke reflex blinking. Both in episodic and in chronic CH patients, the authors found a decreased R2 latency ratio ([latency headache side/latency non-headache side] × 100) compared with controls, while the R2 area-under-the-curve ratio was increased only in active episodic CH patients compared with HCs. However, when considering the raw R2 latencies, only those of the non-headache side in episodic CH patients investigated during a bout were delayed compared with those of HCs [38] (Table 15.3).

After the initial observation, by Formisano et al. [46], of abnormal habituation of the R2 BR component in a small number of CH patients during attacks, the habituation process was further explored outside attacks and in comparison with controls. Habituation of both the conventional R2 and the R3 BR components was found to be impaired in CH patients compared with HCs, although only the usual headache side was investigated [47]. It is worth noting that the lack of habituation in the CH patients was even more pronounced than that found in episodic migraine [47]. These abnormalities in the processing of painful trigeminal stimuli were further investigated in a study involving the use of a nociception-specific concentric stimulating electrode, which showed that the R2 reflex area and habituation were reduced on the headache side in comparison with the non-headache side in episodic CH [48]. More recently, the habituation to trigeminal nociceptive stimulation has been investigated using different stimulation frequencies (SF, 0.05, 0.1, 0.2, 0.3, 0.5, 1 Hz). The authors demonstrated a frequency-dependent habituation deficit of the R2 component of the nociceptive BR (nBR) in episodic CH at higher stimulation frequency, and both during the active and remission period. This abnormal temporal pattern of pain processing may suggest a trait-dependent dysfunction of some underlying pain-related subcortical structures, rather than a state-dependent functional abnormality due to the recurrence of the headache attacks during the active period [49]. Conversely, Holle et al. [50] did not detect habituation deficit of the nBR R2 component in episodic and chronic CH, either during or outside active periods, but the inclusion of patients under multiple prophylactic medications may have biased the results.

Table 15.3 Blink reflex studies performed in cluster headache

Authors	Sensory modality	Stimulation parameters	Diagnosis	Results
Pavesi et al. [40]	Blink reflex	Electrical stimulation of the supraorbital nerve	18 (13 males) CH (5 chronic and 13 episodic [8 during and 5 outside active phase]), 15 HCs	Almost all patients were under prophylactic pharmacological treatment. Episodic CH patients during active phase showed R2 threshold values on the headache side exceeding those of the non-affected one
Formisano et al. [46]	Blink reflex	Blink reflex habituation	8 CH patients during attack vs. between attacks	Abnormal habituation of the blink reflex in CH patients during the attack
Raudino [41]	Blink reflex	Electrical stimulation of the supraorbital nerve	12 episodic CH during active phase, 15 HCs	At the same stimulus intensity, the amplitude of the R2 response on the symptomatic side was significantly lower than on the asymptomatic side
Sandrini et al. [42]	Corneal reflex	Electrical stimulation	21 (17 males) CH (episodic [during and outside active phase] and chronic), 9 HCs	The pain threshold of the corneal reflex was reduced on the headache side in a mixed group of episodic (active phase) and chronic CH patients, and normal outside the active phase
Lozza et al. [43]	Blink reflex	Blink reflex recovery curve after paired supraorbital electrical stimulations and after paired supraorbital and index finger stimulations	10 (9 males) episodic CH during active phase, 10 HCs	Faster R2 blink reflex recovery curve on the symptomatic side after paired supraorbital stimuli. Faster R2 blink reflex recovery curve both on the symptomatic and on the asymptomatic side after index finger conditioning stimulation
Magis et al. [45]	Brink reflex	Concentric electrode stimulation of the supraorbital nerve in the forehead before and after ONS device implantation	8 drug-resistant chronic CH	ONS did not significantly modify pain thresholds. The amplitude of the nociceptive blink reflex increased with longer durations of ONS
Perrotta et al. [57]	Blink reflex	Blink reflex habituation	27 (22 males) episodic CH patients during active phase, 20 HCs	A significant habituation deficit in the R2 and R3 BR components was found in CH patients compared with both HCs and migraineurs

(continued)

Table 15.3 (continued)

Authors	Sensory modality	Stimulation parameters	Diagnosis	Results
Holle et al. [50]	Nociception-specific blink reflex	The blink reflex was recorded using 2 planar concentric surface electrodes placed above the entry zone of the supraorbital nerve	66 (49 males) CH patients (46 episodic [7 during and 28 outside active phase], 20 chronic), 30 HCs	Almost all patients were under prophylactic pharmacological treatment. In all CH patients, authors found a decreased R2 latency ratio ([latency headache side/latency non-headache side]*100) compared with HCs. AUC ratio was increased only in episodic CH patients during the active phase compared with HCs. With regard to the latency of R2 component of the blink reflex, only those of the non-headache side in episodic CH patients investigated during an active period were delayed compared with those of HCs
Di Lorenzo et al. [51]	Nociception-specific blink reflex	Nociceptive blink reflex habituation before and after treatment with dopamine agonist rotigotine	1 male drug-resistant chronic CH patient	Normalization of the baseline reduced habituation of the R2 component of the nociceptive blink reflex was observed during rotigotine treatment
Haane et al. [54]	Nociception-specific blink reflex	Electrical stimulation using nociception-specific concentric electrode on both the affected and non-affected side	8 male CH patients (5 episodic and 3 chronic)	Transcutaneous supraorbital nerve stimulation could have a prophylactic effect in episodic and chronic cluster headache
Coppola et al. [48]	Nociception-specific blink reflex	Nociceptive blink reflex habituation	18 (16 males) episodic CH patients during active phase, 18 HCs	Reduced pain threshold, R2 reflex area, and habituation were found on the affected side compared with the non-affected side
Haane et al. [53]	Nociception-specific blink reflex	Supraorbital nociceptive blink reflex recording before, during, and every 2 h thereafter up until 6 h after O_2 inhalation	10 male CH patients (3 episodic, 5 chronic, and 2 on their first cluster)	Oxygen showed no significant effect, immediately or over time, on the nociception-specific blink reflex parameters

CH cluster headache, *HCs* healthy controls, *ONS* occipital nerve stimulation, *AUC* area under the curve

In one patient with drug-resistant chronic CH whose clinical condition improved following administration of the transdermal dopamine agonist rotigotine, concurrent normalization of the baseline reduced habituation of the R2 nBR component was observed [51]. This observation led the authors to suggest that a malfunction in descending aminergic (especially dopaminergic) control may play a role in CH pathogenesis.

In a group of drug-resistant chronic CH patients submitted to invasive occipital nerve stimulator implantation, Magis et al. [52] observed that the amplitude of the nBR response increased with more protracted occipital nerve stimulation, although this did not significantly modify pain thresholds.

Oxygen did not modify both immediately and over time the nociception-specific BR parameters, in ten CH patients (mixed population of both episodic and chronic males) both during the active phase, between attacks [53]. As a chance observation, the same authors noticed that the transcutaneous supraorbital nerve stimulation used to elicit reflex blinking may have a prophylactic effect in episodic and chronic CH, warranting its testing in a specific study [54].

15.5.2 Spinal Reflexes

The nociceptive withdrawal (or flexor) reflex (NWR) of the lower limb is a reflex response induced by nociceptive stimulation and intended to protect the body from potentially damaging stimuli. The NWR is a reliable and objective measure of experimental pain in humans and animals [55]. Furthermore, as the NWR parameters are under the influence of supraspinal pain control systems, the NWR also serves as a tool for studying the endogenous pain system (Table 15.4).

In TACs (predominantly CH), the NWR has been employed to study extracephalic sensitization of the pain pathways and the functional activity of the endogenous pain system. A lowered threshold for the NWR and for subjective electrically induced pain has been reported in episodic CH during the active compared with the remission phase [56, 57]. Furthermore, both episodic CH patients during the active phase and chronic CH patients had lower electrically induced pain and NWR thresholds on the affected versus the unaffected side [56]. Surprisingly, two different studies [56, 58] failed to document significant reductions in NWR and pain sensation thresholds in chronic CH, probably due to the small sample sizes. Due to the circadian rhythmicity of the NWR threshold, this response has also been used to verify potential abnormalities in the circadian activity of the nociceptive system in CH, considered a counterpart of the cyclic occurrence of CH attacks [58]. The authors found significantly preserved circadian rhythmicity of the NWR threshold in episodic CH during both active and remission periods, but the sensitization within the nociceptive system was coupled with a phase shift of the normal circadian rhythmic variations in the NWR threshold during the active period when compared with the remission period. On the contrary, no circadian rhythmicity of the NWR threshold was observed in chronic CH patients [58].

Table 15.4 Nociceptive spinal reflexes and experimental subjective pain sensation studies in cluster headache and other trigeminal autonomic cephalalgias

Authors	Sensory modality	Stimulation parameters	Diagnosis	Results
Sandrini et al. [56]	NWR and electrically induced pain threshold	Electrical stimulation of the sural nerve	23 (19 males) CH during and 28 (25 males) outside active phase, 18 CCH (16 males)	No patient was under prophylactic pharmacological treatment. Episodic CH patients during the active phase showed lower NWR and electrically induced pain threshold values on the headache side. No differences were detected in chronic CH
Perrotta et al. [57]	NWR threshold and TST of the NWR, cold pressor test	Electrical stimulation of the sural nerve, cold pressor test	10 (8 males) CH during and outside active phase	No patient was under prophylactic pharmacological treatment. Episodic CH patients during the active phase showed lower NWR threshold and TST values on the headache side coupled with a defective activity of the CPT on NWR threshold and TST
Nappi et al. [58]	NWR threshold	Electrical stimulation of the sural nerve	14 (14 males) CH during and 11 (11 males) outside active phase, 6 chronic CH (6 males)	No patient was under prophylactic pharmacological treatment. Episodic CH showed a significant circadian rhythmicity of the NWR threshold. A clear shift of the phase was observed in the active period, while a loss of circadian rhythmicity was seen in chronic CH
Fernandez de La Penas et al. [59]	Quantitative sensory testing	Mechanical pain threshold at trigeminal and ulnar, radial and median nerve level	16 (16 males) CH outside active phase	No patient was under prophylactic pharmacological treatment. Episodic patients showed bilateral trigeminal and extratrigeminal mechanical hyperalgesia during the remission period
Bono et al. [60]	Quantitative sensory testing	Mechanical pain threshold at trigeminal and deltoid level	41 (35 males) CH during and 14 (14 males) outside active phase, 17 CCH (17 males)	No patient was under prophylactic pharmacological treatment. Episodic CH patients during the active phase and chronic CH patients showed lower pressure pain threshold values on the headache side

Table 15.4 (continued)

Authors	Sensory modality	Stimulation parameters	Diagnosis	Results
Ellrich et al. [61]	Quantitative sensory testing	Thermal threshold on the periorbital area	10 (6 males) CH during and 7 (7 males) outside active phase, 9 CCH (9 males)	Episodic and chronic CH showed reduced warmth, cold, and pressure pain on the symptomatic side
Antonaci et al. [63]	Quantitative sensory testing, NWR, blink reflex, and corneal reflex	Mechanical pain threshold, blink reflex threshold, sural nerve stimulation	12 (6 males) chronic paroxysmal hemicrania, 12 (7 males) hemicrania continua	Both paroxysmal hemicrania and hemicrania continua patients showed lower NWR, electrically induced pain, and pressure pain threshold values on the headache side Corneal reflex thresholds were significantly reduced bilaterally in paroxysmal hemicrania

CH cluster headache, *NWR* nociceptive withdrawal reflex, *TST* temporal summation threshold, *CPT* cold pressor test

An interesting property of the NWR response is that it can be evoked through the temporal summation of non-nociceptive stimuli. Temporal summation of sensory neuronal responses to non-nociceptive or nociceptive stimuli is a form of neural plasticity that shifts the sensory inflow from tactile to nociceptive or amplifies the nociceptive responses. In humans, the temporal summation of pain can be tested using the temporal summation threshold (TST) of the NWR. Like the NWR threshold, the TST can be modulated by supraspinal descending pain control systems.

Perrotta et al. [57] studied the functional activity of the descending diffuse noxious inhibitory control (or conditioned pain modulation system) elicited by a cold pressor test (CPT) in a group of episodic CH patients during active and remission phases. CH patients during active periods showed a significant reduction of the TST when compared both with controls and with CH patients during the remission phase. Only during this phase, was the CPT found to have no effect on the TST or on the NWR threshold and area. The authors concluded that CH patients have a dysfunction of the supraspinal pain control system that depends on the clinical activity of the disease and leads to facilitation of pain processing, predisposing to CH attacks [57].

15.5.3 Experimental Subjective Pain Sensation

Subjective pain sensation, both cephalic and extracephalic, is usually investigated through mechanical or thermal stimulation of the skin and recording of the subjective pain sensation reported by the subject. This method can reveal sensitization of the pain pathways as a consequence of local or widespread abnormal pain processing, clinically expressed as hyperalgesia.

In TACs, mechanical pressure-induced pain has been explored in subjects with episodic and chronic CH. The authors found diffuse bilateral cephalic and extracephalic mechanical hyperalgesia in episodic CH patients during the remission phase when compared with controls [59]. However, the findings of this study are limited by the lack of data from CH patients during the active phase. In a previous study, a lower mechanical pressure pain threshold was detected on the symptomatic side in episodic CH during the active phase and in chronic CH [60]. Thermal stimulation has been used in episodic CH to investigate thresholds for the sensory perception of warmth and cold in the periorbital area. The patients showed reduced perception of warmth and cold on the symptomatic side [61]. In a prospective and controlled study, the thermal thresholds for warm and cold sensations as well as the thermal thresholds for heat and cold pain were examined bilaterally at the cephalic (forehead), extracephalic (ventral forearm, lateral lower leg) levels in chronic CH patients who received or not DBS implantation and in a group of HCs. Authors found that DBS induces an increase of cold pain solely at the cephalic level (forehead) and ipsilateral to the stimulation side both when compared with HCs and with non-implanted CH patients [62]. Interestingly, these results were obtained only after long-term DBS (for months), not after short-term interruption of DBS (stimulator on/off) [62].

15.5.4   Other TACs

To the best of our knowledge, very few neurophysiological studies explored trigeminal and extratrigeminal sensory pathways in TACs other than CH. To date, only one study explored the habituation to painful trigeminal stimulation in episodic PH. By studying the habituation of the nBR R2 component, the authors revealed a clear deficit in habituation to trigeminal pain that resembles what has been observed in episodic CH. These results demonstrated that the clinical similarities in the different subtypes of TACs are in parallel with a trait-dependent dysfunction in pain processing. We are aware of only one study on sensitization of the pain pathways in patients with chronic paroxysmal hemicrania and hemicrania continua. In both groups, pressure pain threshold, subjective pain perception after sural nerve stimulation, and the NWR threshold were reduced, most markedly on the affected side, compared with the values recorded in healthy subjects [63]. Moreover, corneal reflex thresholds were significantly reduced on both sides only in chronic paroxysmal hemicrania patients.

15.6   Conclusions

Despite the considerable advances in modern neuroimaging techniques seen in recent years, the mechanisms of CH attack initiation, recurrence, and resolution remain to be clearly identified. A major role of posterior hypothalamic activation in initiating and maintaining attacks has been suggested [64]. Pathophysiological involvement of the pain neuromatrix, now termed the salient network, and of the central descending opiatergic pain control system, has also been observed [65]. Neurophysiology techniques have provided some insights, which can be summarized as follows:

- The very few studies of spontaneous EEG cortical activity have not revealed peculiar electrocortical features in CH patients, but a systematic study of a larger sample of patients would be useful to confirm these observations. Conversely, LFP recordings in patients implanted with DBS devices consistently disclosed a tonic firing pattern in the posterior hypothalamus with a frequency of around 20 Hz coinciding with the onset of an attack.
- In polysomnographic studies, CH patients have been found to show a longer REM latency, a lower percentage of REM sleep, and a decreased number of EEG arousals compared with HCs. Some authors have reported an association between REM sleep and nocturnal CH attacks and thus suggested that REM sleep may be either one of several triggering events and/or a perpetuating factor of cluster attacks. It has been proposed that a hypothalamic dysregulation may somehow be responsible both for sleep-related complaints and for CH recurrence with its strong chronobiological features [11, 66].
- Innocuous or noxious evoked potential and TMS studies of CH have revealed signs of abnormal levels of cortical excitability, more prominent on the headache side, interpreted as due to asymmetrical cerebral neurotransmitter dysfunction. It remains to be established whether these findings pointing to abnormal cortical excitability in CH patients are primary dysfunctions determining the recurrence of strictly lateralized pain or rather secondary signs of this recurrence.
- Cognitive ERP studies, in conjunction with the findings provided by non-cognitive evoked potential studies, support the hypothesis that CH cannot be a disorder of exclusively peripheral origin. The extent to which the findings observed in studies using cognitive ERPs might be ascribed to real cognitive, mood, and affective changes in CH patients remains to be determined.
- In CH, lateralized abnormalities have also been observed at the trigeminal and spinal levels, using blink and lower limb flexion reflexes, respectively. These findings may be explained as due mainly to side-specific sensitization of anatomical structures involved in cephalic and extracephalic pain processing (e.g., wide dynamic range neurons in the ipsilateral trigeminal nucleus caudalis) on the headache side. The facilitating response at spinal level may be due to a process of widespread central sensitization triggered by the recurrence of CH attacks, further reinforced by a malfunctioning descending brainstem pain control system. In some cases, acute or prophylactic treatments can reverse these dysfunctions.
- Most of the authors did not found peculiar dysfunctions in chronic CH patients as compared with episodic CH patients.
- The few ERP and reflex data available support the hypothesis that CH and paroxysmal hemicrania have both common and specific basic neurophysiological mechanisms and thus that the central structures involved in the pathophysiology of both conditions could be at least in part different.

To reduce discrepancies between studies, greater attention should be paid to ensure more accurate patient selection and inclusion. Moreover, although the posterior hypothalamus is generally recognized as playing a pivotal role in the pathophysiology of CH, its specific role in determining the functional abnormalities of the cluster brain must be questioned. More investigation of this particular area is needed in order to solve the puzzling pathophysiology of this brain disorder.

References

1. Headache Classification Committee of the International Headache Society (IHS). The International Classification of Headache Disorders, 3rd edition (beta version). Cephalalgia. 2013;33:629–808.
2. Sandrini G, Friberg L, Coppola G, et al. Neurophysiological tests and neuroimaging procedures in non-acute headache (2nd edition). Eur J Neurol. 2011;18:373–81.
3. Silvestri R, Narbone MC, De Domenico P, et al. Generalized EEG abnormalities in cluster headache. Ital J Neurol Sci. 1996;17:179.
4. Martens D, Oster I, Gottschlling S, et al. Cerebral MRI and EEG studies in the initial management of pediatric headaches. Swiss Med Wkly. 2012;142:w13625.
5. Leone M, Franzini A, Bussone G. Stereotactic stimulation of posterior hypothalamic gray matter in a patient with intractable cluster headache. N Engl J Med. 2001;345:1428–9.
6. Broggi G, Franzini A, Leone M, et al. Update on neurosurgical treatment of chronic trigeminal autonomic cephalalgias and atypical facial pain with deep brain stimulation of posterior hypothalamus: results and comments. Neurol Sci. 2007;28(Suppl 2):S138–45.
7. Bartsch T, Pinsker MO, Rasche D, et al. Hypothalamic deep brain stimulation for cluster headache: experience from a new multicase series. Cephalalgia. 2008;28:285–95.
8. Cordella R, Carella F, Leone M, et al. Spontaneous neuronal activity of the posterior hypothalamus in trigeminal autonomic cephalalgias. Neurol Sci. 2007;28:93–5.
9. Brittain J-S, Green AL, Jenkinson N, et al. Local field potentials reveal a distinctive neural signature of cluster headache in the hypothalamus. Cephalalgia. 2009;29:1165–73.
10. Nager W, Münte TF, Marco-Pallares J, et al. Beta-oscillations in the posterior hypothalamus are associated with spontaneous cluster headache attack. J Neurol. 2010;257:1743–4.
11. Barloese MCJ. Neurobiology and sleep disorders in cluster headache. J Headache Pain. 2015;16:78.
12. Manzoni GC, Terzano MG, Bono G, et al. Cluster headache—clinical findings in 180 patients. Cephalalgia. 1983;3:21–30.
13. Chervin RD, Zallek SN, Lin X, et al. Timing patterns of cluster headaches and association with symptoms of obstructive sleep apnea. Sleep Res Online. 2000;3:107–12.
14. Della Marca G, Vollono C, Rubino M, et al. A sleep study in cluster headache. Cephalalgia. 2006;26:290–4.
15. Vetrugno R, Pierangeli G, Leone M, et al. Effect on sleep of posterior hypothalamus stimulation in cluster headache. Headache. 2007;47:1085–90.
16. Dexter JD, Riley TL. Studies in nocturnal migraine. Headache. 1975;15:51–62.
17. Pfaffenrath V, Pöllmann W, Rüther E, et al. Onset of nocturnal attacks of chronic cluster headache in relation to sleep stages. Acta Neurol Scand. 1986;73:403–7.
18. Kayed K, Sjaastad O. Nocturnal and early morning headaches. Ann Clin Res. 1985;17:243–6.
19. Kudrow L, McGinty DJ, Phillips ER, et al. Sleep apnea in cluster headache. Cephalalgia. 1984;4:33–8.
20. Chervin RD, Zallek SN, Lin X, et al. Sleep disordered breathing in patients with cluster headache. Neurology. 2000;54:2302–6.

21. Graff-Radford SB, Newman A. Obstructive sleep apnea and cluster headache. Headache. 2004;44:607–10.
22. Pelin Z, Bozluolcay M. Cluster headache with obstructive sleep apnea and periodic limb movements during sleep: a case report. Headache. 2005;45:81–3.
23. Terzaghi M, Ghiotto N, Sances G, et al. Episodic cluster headache: NREM prevalence of nocturnal attacks, time to look beyond macrostructural analysis? Headache. 2010;50:1050–4.
24. Zaremba S, Holle D, Wessendorf TE, et al. Cluster headache shows no association with rapid eye movement sleep. Cephalalgia. 2012;32:289–96.
25. Polich J, Ehlers CL, Dalessio DJ. Pattern-shift visual evoked responses and EEG in migraine. Headache. 1986;26:451–6.
26. Boiardi A, Carenini L, Frediani F, et al. Visual evoked potentials in cluster headache: central structures involvement. Headache. 1986;26:70–3.
27. Boiardi A, Frediani F, Leone M, et al. Cluster headache: Lack of central modulation? Funct Neurol. 1988;3:79–87.
28. Kagan R, Kainz V, Burstein R, et al. Hypothalamic and basal ganglia projections to the posterior thalamus: possible role in modulation of migraine headache and photophobia. Neuroscience. 2013;248:359–68.
29. Bussone G, Sinatra MG, Boiardi A, et al. Brainstem auditory evoked potential (BAEPs) in cluster headache (CH): new aspects for a central theory. Headache. 1986;26:67–9.
30. Afra J, Ertsey C, Bozsik G, et al. Cluster headache patients show marked intensity dependence of cortical auditory evoked potentials during and outside the bout. Cephalalgia. 2005;25:36–40.
31. Firenze C, Del Gatto F, Mazzotta G, et al. Somatosensory-evoked potential study in headache patients. Cephalalgia. 1988;8:157–62.
32. Cosentino G, Brighina F, Brancato S, et al. Transcranial magnetic stimulation reveals cortical hyperexcitability in episodic cluster headache. J Pain. 2015;16:53–9.
33. Evers S, Bauer B, Suhr B, et al. Cognitive processing in primary headache: a study on event-related potentials. Neurology. 1997;48:108–13.
34. Evers S, Bauer B, Suhr B, et al. Cognitive processing is involved in cluster headache but not in chronic paroxysmal hemicrania. Neurology. 1999;53:357–63.
35. Wang R, Dong Z, Chen X, et al. Cognitive processing of cluster headache patients: evidence from event-related potentials. J Headache Pain. 2014;15:66.
36. Casale MS, Baratto M, Cervera C, et al. Auditory evoked potential abnormalities in cluster headache. Neuroreport. 2008;19:1633–6.
37. van Vliet J, Vein A, Le Cessie S, et al. Impairment of trigeminal sensory pathways in cluster headache. Cephalalgia. 2003;23:414–9.
38. Holle D, Gaul C, Zillessen S, et al. Lateralized central facilitation of trigeminal nociception in cluster headache. Neurology. 2012;78:985–92.
39. Ellrich J, Jung K, Ristic D, et al. Laser-evoked cortical potentials in cluster headache. Cephalalgia. 2007;27:510–8.
40. Pavesi G, Granella F, Brambilla S, et al. Blink reflex in cluster headache: evidence of a trigeminal system dysfunction. Cephalalgia. 1987;6:100–2.
41. Raudino F. The blink reflex in cluster headache. Headache. 1990;30:584–5.
42. Sandrini G, Alfonsi E, Ruiz L, et al. Impairment of corneal pain perception in cluster headache. Pain. 1991;47:299–304.
43. Lozza A, Schoenen J, Delwaide PJ. Inhibition of the blink reflex R2 component after supraorbital and index finger stimulations is reduced in cluster headache: an indication for both segmental and suprasegmental dysfunction? Pain. 1997;71:81–8.
44. Sprenger T, Willoch F, Miederer M, et al. Opioidergic changes in the pineal gland and hypothalamus in cluster headache: a ligand PET study. Neurology. 2006;66:1108–10.
45. Magis D, Bruno MA, Fumal A, et al. Central modulation in cluster headache patients treated with occipital nerve stimulation: an FDG-PET study. BMC Neurol. 2011;11:25.
46. Formisano R, Cerbo R, Ricci M, et al. Blink reflex in cluster headache. Cephalalgia. 1987;7:353–4.

47. Perrotta A, Serrao M, Sandrini G, et al. Reduced habituation of trigeminal reflexes in patients with episodic cluster headache during cluster period. Cephalalgia. 2008;28:950–9.

48. Coppola G, Di Lorenzo C, Bracaglia M, et al. Lateralized nociceptive blink reflex habituation deficit in episodic cluster headache: correlations with clinical features. Cephalalgia. 2015;35:600–7.

49. Perrotta A, Coppola G, Anastasio MG, et al. Trait- and frequency-dependent dysfunctional habituation to trigeminal nociceptive stimulation in trigeminal autonomic cephalalgias. J Pain. 2018;19:1040–8. https://doi.org/10.1016/j.jpain.2018.03.015.

50. Holle D, Zillessen S, Gaul C, et al. Habituation of the nociceptive blink reflex in episodic and chronic cluster headache. Cephalalgia. 2012;32:998–1004.

51. Di Lorenzo C, Coppola G, Pierelli F. A case of cluster headache treated with rotigotine: clinical and neurophysiological correlates. Cephalalgia. 2013;33:1272–6.

52. Magis D, Allena M, Bolla M, et al. Occipital nerve stimulation for drug-resistant chronic cluster headache: a prospective pilot study. Lancet Neurol. 2007;6:314–21.

53. Haane DYP, Plaum A, Koehler PJ, et al. High-flow oxygen therapy in cluster headache patients has no significant effect on nociception specific blink reflex parameters: a pilot study. J Headache Pain. 2016;17:7.

54. Haane DY, Koehler PJ. Nociception specific supraorbital nerve stimulation may prevent cluster headache attacks: serendipity in a blink reflex study. Cephalalgia. 2014;34:920–6.

55. Sandrini G, Serrao M, Rossi P, et al. The lower limb flexion reflex in humans. Prog Neurobiol. 2005;77:353–95.

56. Sandrini G, Antonaci F, Lanfranchi S, et al. Asymmetrical reduction of the nociceptive flexion reflex threshold in cluster headache. Cephalalgia. 2000;20:647–52.

57. Perrotta A, Serrao M, Ambrosini A, et al. Facilitated temporal processing of pain and defective supraspinal control of pain in cluster headache. Pain. 2013;154:1325–32.

58. Nappi G, Sandrini G, Alfonsi E, et al. Impaired circadian rhythmicity of nociceptive reflex threshold in cluster headache. Headache. 2002;42:125–31.

59. Fernández-de-las-Peñas C, Ortega-Santiago R, Cuadrado ML, et al. Bilateral widespread mechanical pain hypersensitivity as sign of central sensitization in patients with cluster headache. Headache. 2011;51:384–91.

60. Bono G, Antonaci F, Sandrini G, et al. Pain pressure threshold in cluster headache patients. Cephalalgia. 1996;16:62–6.

61. Ellrich J, Ristic D, Yekta SS. Impaired thermal perception in cluster headache. J Neurol. 2006;253:1292–9.

62. Jürgens TP, Leone M, Proietti-Cecchini A, et al. Hypothalamic deep-brain stimulation modulates thermal sensitivity and pain thresholds in cluster headache. Pain. 2009;146:84–90.

63. Antonaci F, Sandrini G, Danilov A, et al. Neurophysiological studies in chronic paroxysmal hemicrania and hemicrania continua. Headache. 1994;34:479–83.

64. Leone M, Bussone G. Pathophysiology of trigeminal autonomic cephalalgias. Lancet Neurol. 2009;8:755–64.

65. Iacovelli E, Coppola G, Tinelli E, et al. Neuroimaging in cluster headache and other trigeminal autonomic cephalalgias. J Headache Pain. 2012;13:11–20.

66. Graff-Radford SB, Teruel A. Cluster headache and obstructive sleep apnea: are they related disorders? Curr Pain Headache Rep. 2009;13:160–3.

Chapter 16
Trigeminal Neuralgia: Channels, Pathophysiology, and Therapeutic Challenges

Daniele Cazzato, Stine Maarbjerg, Lars Bendtsen, and Giuseppe Lauria

16.1 Introduction

Trigeminal neuralgia (TN) is defined by the International Classification of Headache Disorders-3 (ICHD-3) as a condition characterized by recurrent unilateral brief electric shock-like, shooting, stabbing, or sharp pain, abrupt in onset and termination, limited to the distribution of one or more divisions of the trigeminal nerve, and triggered by innocuous stimuli. In ICHD-3 a new subclassification of TN into three subtypes was proposed: *idiopathic* TN with no neurovascular contact or neurovascular contact without morphological changes of the trigeminal nerve and without significant electrophysiological findings; *classical* TN with neurovascular compression with morphological changes of the trigeminal nerve; and *symptomatic* TN when there is another underlying neurological disease such as multiple sclerosis or a space-occupying lesion affecting the ipsilateral trigeminal nerve in the root entry zone [1].

D. Cazzato
Neurophysiology and Neuroalgology Units, Department of Clinical Neuroscience,
IRCCS Foundation "Carlo Besta" Neurological Institute, Milan, Italy
e-mail: daniele.cazzato@istituto-besta.it

S. Maarbjerg · L. Bendtsen
Department of Neurology, Danish Headache Center, Rigshospitalet—Glostrup, University of Copenhagen, Copenhagen, Denmark
e-mail: stine.maarbjerg@regionh.dk; lars.bendtsen@regionh.dk

G. Lauria (✉)
Department of Biomedical and Clinical Sciences "Luigi Sacco", University of Milan, Milan, Italy

Neuroalgology Unit, Department of Clinical Neuroscience, IRCCS Foundation "Carlo Besta" Neurological Institute, Milan, Italy
e-mail: giuseppe.lauriapinter@istituto-besta.it; giuseppe.lauria@unimi.it

© Springer Nature Switzerland AG 2020   209
M. Leone, A. May (eds.), *Cluster Headache and other Trigeminal Autonomic Cephalgias*, Headache, https://doi.org/10.1007/978-3-030-12438-0_16

The clinical picture is characterized by painful paroxysms lasting from seconds to minutes, with highly variable frequency ranging from a few to hundreds of attacks per day. Long remission periods that can last years are seen in most patients. The pain is sharp and severe, and it can be triggered by trivial non-painful sensory stimuli in the area of trigeminal nerve distribution, such as light touch and cold wind, or by simple actions including chewing, talking, washing the face, or brushing the teeth. During the refractory period typically following a pain attack, patients can remain completely asymptomatic or experience background dull pain of variable intensity.

16.2 Pathophysiology

The finding of a neurovascular conflict at brain magnetic resonance imaging (MRI) in a high percentage of patients and the prolonged pain relief achieved by the microvascular decompression have suggested that nerve compression could have a primary role in the pathogenesis of TN [2, 3]. However, the presence of a neurovascular conflict does not necessarily induce TN, and not all the patients diagnosed with TN have a neurovascular conflict. Therefore, it is possible that individual susceptibility and/or specific conditions are needed to determine the development of TN. Moreover, how vascular compression can cause the clinical picture and explain its course remains speculative. Repetitive pulsatile microvascular compression has been proposed to cause nerve demyelination, as supported by neuropathology studies and the increased incidence of TN in multiple sclerosis patients with brainstem demyelinating lesions in the trigeminal root entry zone [4]. In TN patients with multiple sclerosis, one study found that both brainstem plaque and neurovascular compression were associated with the painful side thus suggesting a dual crush mechanism in this patient category [5].

The analysis of the pathophysiological mechanisms should consider the following crucial issues: (1) How do abnormal sensory impulses occur either spontaneously or triggered by non-painful stimuli and spread beyond the trigger area? (2) How do attacks abruptly stop and the triggering mechanism become temporary refractory?

Pathological findings confirming demyelination of trigeminal fibers and electrophysiological evidence of spontaneous discharge generation in focally demyelinated axons suggest that pulsatile compression of demyelinated axons may be responsible for initiating aberrant discharges in some patients. Nerve injury triggers the release of inflammatory mediators inducing alteration of primary afferent neurons. Changes in the expression of Na^+, K^+, and Ca^{2+} channels can increase nerve excitability, enhance ectopic and spontaneous activity, and reduce nociceptors threshold making them more responsive to low-intensity stimuli [6, 7]. Demyelinated nerve fibers can acquire the ability of producing after discharges, namely, bursts of spontaneous firing triggered by brief low-intensity stimulation lasting for tens of seconds after the stimulus removal. At the site of vascular compression, the close apposition of myelin-devoid axons is thought to facilitate the ephaptic transmission of the impulses. The ephaptic cross-talk between nerve fibers conveying light touch and those conveying pain has been proposed as a possible explanation for the generation of excruciating attack in response to light mechanical triggering stimuli. The spreading of nerve impulses can cause the recruitment of nerve fibers conveying pain in a synchronous fashion, amplifying the neural response and inducing the spread of the lightening sensation.

The abrupt termination of the pain attack and the ensuing refractory period are thought to occur because of a prolonged hyperpolarization shift triggered by the repetitive firing of primary sensory neurons in the dorsal root ganglia (DRG). Ca^{2+} ions that enter the neuron during the burst activate calcium-activated potassium channels and increase the outflow of potassium ions which produce the neuronal hyperpolarization, firing termination, and refractoriness of the nerve fibers to further excitation. However, in experimental setting, the duration of the refractory period is much shorter than that experienced by the patients, suggesting that other unknown factors likely intervene.

16.3   Ion Channels and Trigeminal Neuralgia

The clinical evidence that carbamazepine and oxcarbazepine, which are sodium channel blockers, can provide fast and prolonged control in the majority of TN patients is used as an indirect clue in support of the role of sodium channel altered functioning in the pathophysiology of TN.

Most of the experimental studies suggesting that sodium channels could play key roles in the pathophysiology of TN have been performed applying the chronic constriction injury method to the infraorbital branch of the trigeminal nerve, providing a model to recapitulate human TN [8]. However, such model probably better mimics the nerve damage seen in painful posttraumatic trigeminal neuropathy.

Genetic mutations of sodium channel genes have been described in rare Mendelian disorders affecting pain perception, ranging from extremely painful conditions to complete insensitivity to pain. In particular, homozygous or compound heterozygous mutations inactivating $SCN9A$ gene, which encode for $Na_v1.7$ α-subunit, and mutations of $SCN11A$ encoding for $Na_v1.9$ α-subunit result in congenital insensitivity to pain [9–11]. Conversely, missense heterozygous gain-of-function mutations in $SCN9A$ produce dominantly inherited pain syndromes such as inherited erythromelalgia and paroxysmal extreme pain disorder [12]. Further clinical studies have demonstrated the association between heterozygous gain-of-function mutations of $SCN9A$, $SCN10A$, and $SCN11A$ genes, encoding for $Na_v1.7$, $Na_v1.8$, and $Na_v1.9$ α-subunits, respectively, and painful idiopathic small fiber neuropathy, a condition characterized by burning and paroxysmal pain, neuropathic pain, hyperalgesia, allodynia, and autonomic dysfunctions usually presenting with a length-dependent "gloves and stockings" distribution [13–15]. Gene mutations identified in the context of SFN are best described as variants, since some of them can have a minor allele frequency up to 3–7% and their penetrance is not yet known.

At electrophysiological testing, these mutations produce a range of dysfunctions including enhanced excitability of nociceptor membrane, hypoexcitability of sympathetic neurons, and altered channel functioning such as impaired slow inactivation or impaired fast and slow inactivation [16]. Overall, these sodium channel gene variants might be part of a complex genetic and molecular mosaic predisposing individuals to develop neuropathic pain.

Recently, sodium and calcium channel genes have been sequenced in a small series of patients with TN. A de novo missense mutation of *SCN8A* encoding for the $Na_v1.6$ α-subunit has been described in one patient with TN and neurovascular compression. The $Na_v1.6$ subunit is widely expressed in the central and peripheral nervous system and is crucial for the initial membrane depolarization that occurs during the generation of the action potential in excitable cells. Gain-of-function mutations in $Na_v1.6$ have previously been linked to epilepsy and cognitive impairment with or without ataxia. The electrophysiological characterization of the mutated $Na_v1.6$ revealed that the p.Met136Val substitution potentiates transient and resurgent sodium currents and leads to increased excitability of trigeminal ganglion neurons expressing the mutant channel, therefore suggesting a pathophysiological role of $Na_v1.6$ [17].

Other studies investigated the expression of three different sodium channels in TN patients. The quantification of mRNA extracted from homogenized gingival biopsies from patients and controls demonstrated the upregulation of $Na_v1.3$ and the downregulation of $Na_v1.7$, whereas no differences emerged in the expression of $Na_v1.8$ [18]. Interestingly, other works showed the upregulation of $Na_v1.3$ and the downregulation of $Na_v1.7$, $Na_v1.8$, and $Na_v1.9$ in the CION model [15]. Conversely, no changes in $Na_v1.3$, $Na_v1.8$, and $Na_v1.9$ expression have been found in DRG neurons after transection of the centrally projecting axons by dorsal rhizotomy.

Silencing of the $Na_v1.9$ subunit was found to prevent mice from developing CION-induced mechanical and thermal allodynia [19]. Intriguingly, mutations in this α-subunit can result in enhanced pain or complete loss of pain perception in man [11, 15]. However, this finding appears to be in contrast with other reports revealing only a minor role for this sodium channel subunit in other somatic neuropathic pain models, thus prompting possible distinct mechanisms of neuropathic pain [20, 21].

The emerging concept of "channelopathy" in several painful conditions prompted investigating further families of ion channels involved in the pathway of pain sensation. In particular, transient receptor potential (TRP), calcium, and potassium channels have been studied in a TN model.

TRP channels are a wide group of nonselective ion channels among which specific subtypes are involved in pain and thermal stimuli transduction. The capsaicin receptor transient receptor potential vanilloid 1 (TRPV1) activated by capsaicin, heat, and other painful stimuli has been the first identified [22]. In the CION model, TRPV1 was found to be overexpressed in trigeminal neurons and involved in heat hyperalgesia but not in mechanical allodynia. The antagonist capsazepine could abolish the heat hyperalgesia without changing the behavior related to mechanical stimuli. Cold allodynia is known to be associated with TRPM8 activation, which is enhanced by the receptor agonist menthol and abolished by its antagonist capsazepine [23, 24]. TRPA1, also involved in painful cold sensation, has been studied in trigeminal neuropathic pain models. TRPA1 knockout mice do not develop non-evoked nociceptive, mechanical allodynia and cold hypersensitivity behaviors. Consistently, TRPA1 selective antagonists showed the rescue of the painful phenotype in CION mice. Conversely, loss of TRPA1 channel in knockout mice does not prevent heat hyperalgesia that therefore appears not to be related to this TRP channel subtype [25].

The painful phenotype of CION model has been also associated with a significant downregulation in trigeminal neurons of large-conductance, calcium-activated potassium channels (BKCa) both at mRNA and protein level. On the electrophysiological ground, it reflected into a decreased BKCa current and lower threshold intensity of action potential in neurons [26].

Second-line pharmacological treatments of TN include gabapentinoids. These compounds block the $\alpha_2\delta_1$calcium channels ($Ca_v\alpha_2\delta_1$) of nociceptors at presynaptic level, reducing the release of neurotransmitters at the dorsal horn where they exert the pharmacological action. $Ca_v\alpha_2\delta_1$ channels have been demonstrated to be upregulated in the trigeminal neurons of the CION model. The increased expression in the dorsal horns was associated with increased excitatory synaptogenesis and increased frequency of miniature excitatory postsynaptic currents in dorsal horn neurons that can be blocked by gabapentinoids [27]. This evidence provided further experimental support for their clinical use in TN.

The role of calcium channels has also been investigated in central processing of pain. Electroencephalogram and magnetoencephalogram studies revealed an increase of low-frequency thalamocortical oscillations in patients with neuropathic pain compared to healthy controls. This activity is thought to be mediated by T-type Ca^{2+} channels inducing thalamic burst firing which is a well-defined underlying mechanism for low-frequency oscillations. The CION model of $Ca_v3.1$ knockout mice has been used to investigate the role of T-type calcium channel in trigeminal neuropathic pain. Results revealed a decrease of trigeminal neuropathic pain associated with reduced low-frequency rhythms in mice lacking of $Ca_v3.1$ channel compared to wild type, therefore suggesting a possible role of $Ca_v3.1$ channels in pathophysiology of trigeminal neuropathic pain [28].

While disentangling the role of ion channels in TN can provide a better understanding of its pathophysiology, the identification of new molecular mechanisms represents the opportunity to identify new druggable target.

16.4 Treatment

Recommendations for medical treatment are generally the same in classical, idiopathic, and symptomatic TN [29]. Figure 16.1 outlines a proposed work-up and treatment algorithm. An MRI of the brain and brainstem, ECG, and laboratory testing should be part of early work-up.

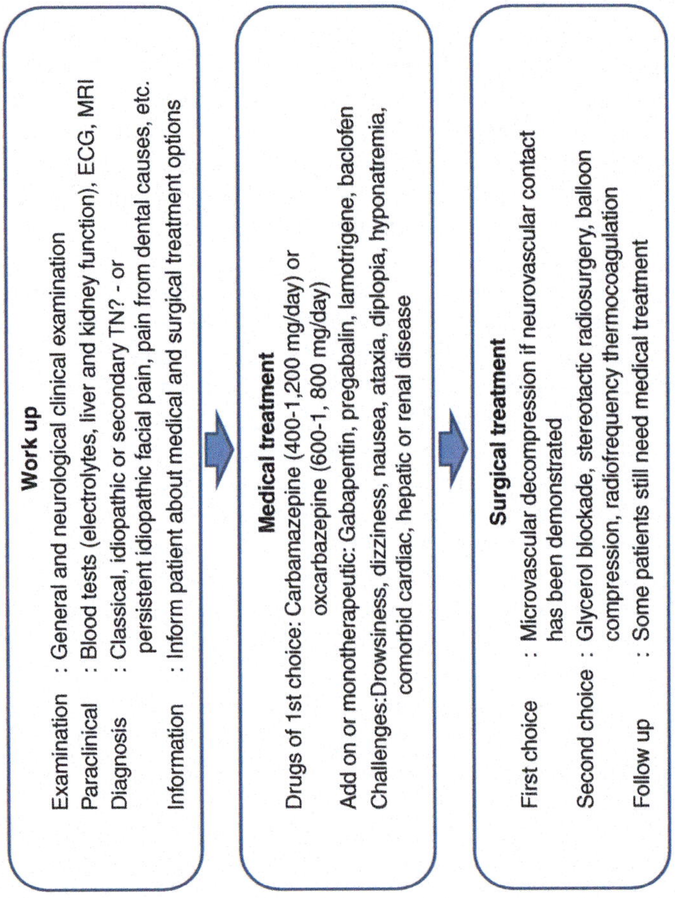

Work up

Examination : General and neurological clinical examination

Paraclinical : Blood tests (electrolytes, liver and kidney function), ECG, MRI

Diagnosis : Classical, idiopathic or secondary TN? - or persistent idiopathic facial pain, pain from dental causes, etc.

Information : Inform patient about medical and surgical treatment options

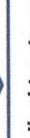

Medical treatment

Drugs of 1st choice: Carbamazepine (400-1,200 mg/day) or oxcarbazepine (600-1, 800 mg/day)

Add on or monotherapeutic: Gabapentin, pregabalin, lamotrigene, baclofen

Challenges:Drowsiness, dizziness, nausea, ataxia, diplopia, hyponatremia, comorbid cardiac, hepatic or renal disease

Surgical treatment

First choice : Microvascular decompression if neurovascular contact has been demonstrated

Second choice : Glycerol blockade, stereotactic radiosurgery, balloon compression, radiofrequency thermocoagulation

Follow up : Some patients still need medical treatment

Fig. 16.1 Work-up and management of trigeminal neuralgia

First-line treatment is sodium channel blockers, either carbamazepine or oxcarbazepine [29]. Laboratory testing should be performed to ensure normal renal and liver function and normal sodium level prior to prescription of medication. ECG is warranted because carbamazepine and oxcarbazepine are contraindicated in patients with atrial ventricular block. They have the same mechanism of action, namely, the blockade of voltage-gated sodium channels in a frequency-dependent manner. It is thought that this stabilizes the hyperexcited neural membranes and inhibits repetitive firing. Sodium channel blockers are effective in most TN patients, and the numbers needed to treat for carbamazepine is 1.7 [30]. However, side effects including somnolence, drowsiness, dizziness, rash, and tremor are frequent [31], and the numbers needed to harm for carbamazepine are 3.4 for minor and 24 for severe side effects [30]. Furthermore, carbamazepine-induced Stevens-Johnson syndrome and toxic epidermal necrolysis have been described to be more frequent in Asiatic population carrying HLA-B*1502 allele [32]. Oxcarbazepine may be preferred because of a minor risk of drug interactions and better tolerability in comparison with carbamazepine [33]. Typical doses are 400–1200 mg/day for carbamazepine and 600–1800 for oxcarbazepine, but higher doses up to 2000 mg/day may be needed. They have a good effectiveness, and carbamazepine can provide up to 100% of pain relief in about 70% of patients, although over time response tends to wane, ensuring a sustained pain relief in fewer patients. Carbamazepine was reported to have a higher percentage of discontinuation due to all kinds of side effects, except for sodium depletion, for which discontinuation only occurred with oxcarbazepine [31]. It is possible that the efficacy of sodium channel blockers is lower in the subgroup of patients [34] with concomitant continuous pain [35]. It can be hypothesized that add-on therapy with gabapentin, pregabalin, or amitriptyline is particularly useful in this group of patients, but this has not been investigated.

Very often high dosages are necessary to achieve a satisfactory pain relief; thus patients can complain of disabling side effects, which are a major reason of drug withdrawal. In one study, worsening of pain with time and development of late resistance only occurred in a very small minority of patients [31]. A recent small open-label retrospective study indicated efficacy of eslicarbazepine, a third-generation antiepileptic drug [36].

According to the international guidelines, it is advised that "if any of these sodium-channel blockers is ineffective, referral for a surgical consultation would be a reasonable next step" [29]. Surgery should also be considered when drugs, although effective, cannot reach the therapeutic dosage due to adverse events. From a clinical perspective, it may be reasonable to try out both carbamazepine and oxcarbazepine sequentially. Furthermore, many TN patients benefit from add-on treatment combining carbamazepine or oxcarbazepine with gabapentin, pregabalin, lamotrigine, or baclofen. Combination treatment should be considered when carbamazepine or oxcarbazepine cannot reach full dosage because of side effects. Each of the before-mentioned drugs may also have efficacy as mono-therapeutic agents, although the available evidence is very weak.

Some recent studies have indicated that onabotulinumtoxinA (Botox) could be efficacious in TN [37]. However, injection paradigms and doses varied among the studies making it difficult to draw conclusions. A phase 2 trial recently published has shown promising efficacy and safety profile of a selective sodium channel blocker in TN [38].

At severe exacerbations in-hospital treatment may be necessary for titration of antiepileptic drugs and rehydration. Exacerbation can be treated with intravenous loading of fosphenytoin, even though there is no evidence-based data in support.

Since medical treatment is generally recommended because of severe pain, there is only little information about the natural course of the disease. However, a retrospective study conducted over 40 years of observation reported that about 29% of patient experienced only one episode of facial pain, 19% two episodes, 24% three episodes, and 28% four to eleven episodes. Most of relapses occurred within 5 years from the first episodes, whereas in a quarter of patients, recurrence was reported after a pain-free period of more than 10 years [39].

In medically refractory patients with MRI evidence of neurovascular conflict, microvascular decompression (MVD) is first-choice treatment [29]. This procedure implies craniotomy and posterior fossa exploration for identification of the affected trigeminal nerve and the conflicting blood vessel. A recent study has demonstrated that the presence of neurovascular compression with morphological changes and male gender are both positive predictors of excellent outcome [40]. Microvascular decompression provides immediate pain relief in up to 90% and the longest duration of pain freedom in comparison with other surgical techniques as it provides significant pain relief in 73% of TN patients at a 5-year follow-up. Minor complications such as new aching or burning pain, sensory loss, and other mild or transient cranial nerve dysfunctions occur in 2–7%. Major complications such as major cranial nerve dysfunction (2%), stroke (0.3%), and death (0.2%) are rare, yet it is important to inform patients on the potential risks [41]. However, most studies did not provide the rate of surgical complications or efficacy as assessed by an independent examiner; therefore frequency of complications might be higher, and the rate of efficacy might be lower. The conventional opinion that multiple sclerosis is a contraindication to microvascular decompression has recently been confuted by a study showing that in multiple sclerosis patients with TN, a neurovascular conflict may act as a concurring mechanism in producing focal demyelination of the primary afferents at the root entry zone [5].

Second-choice neurosurgical treatments are lesioning peripheral procedures targeting the trigeminal ganglion by chemical glycerol blockade, balloon mechanic compression, or radiofrequency thermocoagulation. Stereotactic radiosurgery (Gamma Knife) targets the trigeminal root by convergent beams of radiation. Overall, these second-line procedures are efficacious in approximately 50% of the patients after 5 years. Complications such as sensory loss (12–50%), masticatory problems after balloon compression (up to 50%), and new burning or aching pain (12%) can occur [29].

The abovementioned treatment recommendations are mainly based on expert opinion. There is a lack of robust scientific evidence for effect and side effects of both medical and surgical treatment of TN.

References

1. Zakrzewska JM, Linskey ME. Trigeminal neuralgia. BMJ. 2014;348:g474. http://www.ncbi. nlm.nih.gov/pubmed/24534115
2. Jannetta PJ. Arterial compression of the trigeminal nerve at the pons in patients with trigeminal neuralgia. J Neurosurg. 1967;26(1part2):159–62. http://www.ncbi.nlm.nih.gov/ pubmed/6018932
3. Jannetta PJ. Microsurgical approach to the trigeminal nerve for tic douloureux. Basel: Karger Publishers; 1976. p. 180–200. https://www.karger.com/Article/FullText/428328
4. Love S, Coakham HB. Trigeminal neuralgia: pathology and pathogenesis. Brain. 2001;124(Pt 12):2347–60. https://www.ncbi.nlm.nih.gov/pubmed/11701590.
5. Truini A, Prosperini L, Calistri V, Fiorelli M, Pozzilli C, Millefiorini E, et al. A dual concurrent mechanism explains trigeminal neuralgia in patients with multiple sclerosis. Neurology. 2016;86(22):2094–9.
6. Woolf CJ, Ma Q. Nociceptors-noxious stimulus detectors. Neuron. 2007;55(3):353–64.
7. Waxman SG, Zamponi GW. Regulating excitability of peripheral afferents: emerging ion channel targets. Nat Neurosci. 2014;17(2):153–63.
8. Bennett GJ, Xie YK. A peripheral mononeuropathy in rat that produces. Pain. 1988;33:87–107. https://doi.org/10.1016/0304-3959(88)90209-6.
9. Ahmad S, Dahllund L, Eriksson AB, Hellgren D, Karlsson U, Lund PE, et al. A stop codon mutation in SCN9A causes lack of pain sensation. Hum Mol Genet. 2007;16(17):2114–21.
10. Yuan J, Matsuura E, Higuchi Y, Hashiguchi A, Nakamura T, Nozuma S, et al. Hereditary sensory and autonomic neuropathy type IID caused by an SCN9A mutation. Neurology. 2013;80(18):1641–9.
11. Leipold E, Liebmann L, Korenke GC, Heinrich T, Giesselmann S, Baets J, et al. A de novo gain-of-function mutation in SCN11A causes loss of pain perception. Nat Genet. 2013;45(11):1399–404. http://www.ncbi.nlm.nih.gov/pubmed/24036948
12. Bennett DLH, Woods CG. Painful and painless channelopathies. Lancet Neurol. 2014;13(6):587–99.
13. Faber CG, Hoeijmakers JGJ, Ahn HS, Cheng X, Han C, Choi JS, et al. Gain of function Na V1.7 mutations in idiopathic small fiber neuropathy. Ann Neurol. 2012;71(1):26–39.
14. Faber CG, Lauria G, Merkies ISJ, Cheng X, Han C, Ahn H-S, et al. Gain-of-function Nav1.8 mutations in painful neuropathy. Proc Natl Acad Sci U S A. 2012;109(47):19444–9. http:// www.pnas.org/content/109/47/19444.long
15. Huang J, Han C, Estacion M, Vasylyev D, Hoeijmakers JGJ, Gerrits MM, et al. Gain-of-function mutations in sodium channel NaV1.9 in painful neuropathy. Brain. 2014;137(6):1627–42.
16. Waxman SG. Painful Na-channelopathies: an expanding universe. Trends Mol Med. 2013;19(7):406–9. https://doi.org/10.1016/j.molmed.2013.04.003.
17. Tanaka BS, Zhao P. A gain-of-function mutation in Nav1.6 in a case of trigeminal neuralgia. Mol Med. 2016;22(1):1. http://www.molmed.org/content/pdfstore/16_131_Tanaka.pdf
18. Siqueira SRDT, Alves B, Malpartida HMG, Teixeira MJ, Siqueira JTT. Abnormal expression of voltage-gated sodium channels Nav1.7, Nav1.3 and Nav1.8 in trigeminal neuralgia. Neuroscience. 2009;164(2):573–7. https://doi.org/10.1016/j.neuroscience.2009.08.037.
19. Lulz AP, Kopach O, Santana-Varela S, Wood JN. The role of Nav1.9 channel in the development of neuropathic orofacial pain associated with trigeminal neuralgia. Mol Pain. 2015;11:1–7.
20. Leo S, D'Hooge R, Meert T. Exploring the role of nociceptor-specific sodium channels in pain transmission using Nav1.8 and Nav1.9 knockout mice. Behav Brain Res. 2010;208(1):149–57. https://doi.org/10.1016/j.bbr.2009.11.023.
21. Minett MS, Falk S, Santana-Varela S, Bogdanov YD, Nassar MA, Heegaard AM, et al. Pain without nociceptors? Nav1.7-independent pain mechanisms. Cell Rep. 2014;6(2):301–12. https://doi.org/10.1016/j.celrep.2013.12.033.

22. Caterina MJ, Schumacher MA, Tominaga M, Rosen TA, Levine JD, Julius D. The capsaicin receptor: a heat-activated ion channel in the pain pathway. Nature. 1997;389(6653):816–24. http://www.ncbi.nlm.nih.gov/pubmed/9349813

23. Urano H, Ara T, Fujinami Y, Yukihiro Hiraoka B. Aberrant TRPV1 expression in heat hyperalgesia associated with trigeminal neuropathic pain. Int J Med Sci. 2012;9(8):690–7.

24. Zuo X, Ling JX, Xu GY, Gu JG. Operant behavioral responses to orofacial cold stimuli in rats with chronic constrictive trigeminal nerve injury: effects of menthol and capsazepine. Mol Pain. 2013;9(1):28.

25. Trevisan G, Benemei S, Materazzi S, De Logu F, De Siena G, Fusi C, et al. TRPA1 mediates trigeminal neuropathic pain in mice downstream of monocytes/macrophages and oxidative stress. Brain. 2016;139(5):1361–77.

26. Liu C-Y, Lu Z-Y, Li N, Yu L-H, Zhao Y-F, Ma B. The role of large-conductance, calcium-activated potassium channels in a rat model of trigeminal neuropathic pain. Cephalalgia. 2015;35(1):16–35. http://journals.sagepub.com/doi/10.1177/0333102414534083

27. Li KW, Yu YP, Zhou C, Kim DS, Lin B, Sharp K, et al. Calcium channel $\alpha 2\delta 1$ proteins mediate trigeminal neuropathic pain states associated with aberrant excitatory synaptogenesis. J Biol Chem. 2014;289(10):7025–37.

28. Choi S, Yu E, Hwang E, Llinás RR. Pathophysiological implication of Ca $_v$ 3.1 T-type Ca $^{2+}$ channels in trigeminal neuropathic pain. Proc Natl Acad Sci U S A. 2016;113(8):2270–5. http://www.pnas.org/lookup/doi/10.1073/pnas.1600418113

29. Cruccu G, Gronseth G, Alksne J, Argoff C, Brainin M, Burchiel K, et al. AAN-EFNS guidelines on trigeminal neuralgia management. Eur J Neurol. 2008;15(10):1013–28.

30. Wiffen PJ, Derry S, Moore RA, McQuay HJ. Carbamazepine for acute and chronic pain in adults. Cochrane Database Syst Rev. 2011;(1):CD005451.

31. Di Stefano G, La Cesa S, Truini A, Cruccu G. Natural history and outcome of 200 outpatients with classical trigeminal neuralgia treated with carbamazepine or oxcarbazepine in a tertiary centre for neuropathic pain. J Headache Pain. 2014;15(1):1–5.

32. Tangamornsuksan W, Chaiyakunapruk N, Somkrua R, Lohitnavy M, Tassaneeyakul W. Relationship between the HLA-B*1502 allele and carbamazepine-induced Stevens-Johnson syndrome and toxic epidermal necrolysis: a systematic review and meta-analysis. JAMA Dermatol. 2013;149(9):1025–32. http://www.ncbi.nlm.nih.gov/pubmed/23884208

33. Beydoun A. Safety and efficacy of oxcarbazepine: results of randomized, double-blind trials. Pharmacotherapy. 2000;20(8):152S–8S. http://www.ncbi.nlm.nih.gov/pubmed/10937814

34. Vincent M, Wang S. Headache classification committee of the International Headache Society (IHS) the international classification of headache disorders, 3rd edition. Cephalalgia. 2018;38(1):1–211. http://journals.sagepub.com/doi/10.1177/0333102417738202

35. Maarbjerg S, Wolfram F, Gozalov A, Olesen J, Bendtsen L. Significance of neurovascular contact in classical trigeminal neuralgia. Brain. 2015;138(2):311–9.

36. Sanchez-Larsen A, Sopelana D, Diaz-Maroto I, Perona-Moratalla AB, Gracia-Gil J, García-Muñozguren S, et al. Assessment of efficacy and safety of eslicarbazepine acetate for the treatment of trigeminal neuralgia. Eur J Pain. 2018;22(6):1080–7. http://www.ncbi.nlm.nih.gov/pubmed/29369456

37. Morra ME, Elgebaly A, Elmaraezy A, Khalil AM, Altibi AMA, TL-H V, et al. Therapeutic efficacy and safety of Botulinum Toxin A Therapy in Trigeminal Neuralgia: a systematic review and meta-analysis of randomized controlled trials. J Headache Pain. 2016;17(1):63. http://thejournalofheadacheandpain.springeropen.com/articles/10.1186/s10194-016-0651-8

38. Zakrzewska JM, Palmer J, Morisset V, Giblin GM, Obermann M, Ettlin DA, et al. Safety and efficacy of a Nav1.7 selective sodium channel blocker in patients with trigeminal neuralgia: a double-blind, placebo-controlled, randomised withdrawal phase 2a trial. Lancet Neurol. 2017;16(4):291–300. https://doi.org/10.1016/S1474-4422(17)30005-4.

39. Katusic S, Beard CM, Bergstralth E, Kurland LT. Incidence and clinical features of trigeminal neuralgia, Rochester, Minnesota, 1945-1984. Ann Neurol. 1990;27(1):89–95. http://www.ncbi.nlm.nih.gov/pubmed/2301931
40. Heinskou TB, Rochat P, Maarbjerg S, et al. Prognostic factors for outcome of microvascular decompression in trigeminal neuralgia. Cephalalgia. 2018;. in press
41. Barker FG, Jannetta PJ, Bissonette DJ, Larkins MV, Jho HD. The long-term outcome of microvascular decompression for trigeminal neuralgia. N Engl J Med. 1996;334(17):1077–83. http://www.nejm.org/doi/abs/10.1056/NEJM199604253341701

Chapter 17
Migraine and Cluster Headache: Differences and Similarities

Fu-Chi Yang, Todd J. Schwedt, and Shuu-Jiun Wang

Abbreviations

CH	Cluster headache
ICHD-III	International Classification of Headache Disorders 3rd edition
TAC	Trigeminal autonomic cephalalgia
CAS	Cranial autonomic symptoms
CSD	Cortical spreading depression
DBS	Deep brain stimulation
IHS	International Headache Society
GON	Greater occipital nerve
TCC	Trigeminocervical complex
CGRP	Calcitonin gene-related peptide
NO	Nitric oxide
NKA	Neurokinin A
MRS	Magnetic resonance spectroscopy
fMRI	Functional magnetic resonance imaging
FC	Functional connectivity
VBM	Voxel-based morphometry

F.-C. Yang
Department of Neurology, Tri-Service General Hospital, National Defense Medical Center,
Taipei, Taiwan

T. J. Schwedt
Department of Neurology, Mayo Clinic, Phoenix, AZ, USA

S.-J. Wang (✉)
Brain Research Center, National Yang-Ming University, Taipei, Taiwan

Faculty of Medicine, School of Medicine, National Yang-Ming University, Taipei, Taiwan

Neurological Institute, Taipei Veterans General Hospital, Taipei, Taiwan
e-mail: sjwang@vghtpe.gov.tw

© Springer Nature Switzerland AG 2020
M. Leone, A. May (eds.), *Cluster Headache and other Trigeminal Autonomic
Cephalgias*, Headache, https://doi.org/10.1007/978-3-030-12438-0_17

GMV   Gray matter volume
DTI   Diffusion tensor imaging
WM   White matter

17.1 Introduction

Migraine and cluster headache (CH) are widely regarded as two of the most disabling primary headache disorders. According to the International Classification of Headache Disorders (ICHD-III) criteria, there is a clear diagnostic distinction between migraine and CH [1]. Migraine—which affects approximately 10% of the global adult population with female predominance [2]—is characterized by recurrent attacks of 4–72 h moderate-to-severe headache of pulsating quality, aggravation during routine activities, and the presence of nausea, vomiting, photophobia, and phonophobia [2]. Patients with migraine can also experience autonomic, affective, and cognitive symptoms before (premonitory phase), during, or after (postdrome) each headache episode [3]. Furthermore, approximately one-third of patients with migraine experience transient focal neurological deficits or "auras" (e.g., visual, speech and/or language, sensory, motor, brainstem, or retinal deficits) [4]. CH is much less prevalent than migraine (0.1% of the population) and occurs more frequently in men than in women [5]. CH is the most common form of trigeminal autonomic cephalalgias (TACs) and has been regarded as one of the most painful conditions people can experience, with a pain intensity estimated to be 100–1000 times worse than migraine [6, 7]. CH attacks are characterized primarily by severe, unilateral, and relatively short-lasting (15–180 min) headache episodes. These episodes occur in association with ipsilateral cranial autonomic symptoms (CAS) such as conjunctival injection and/or lacrimation, nasal congestion and/or rhinorrhea, eyelid edema, forehead and facial sweating, and miosis and/or ptosis [7] (ICHD-3 criteria). CH is also characterized by circadian and circannual rhythmicity: CH attacks may occur at the same time(s) each day during episodes that last for weeks or months (in-bout period), separated by pain-free remission periods (out-of-bout period) [7]. Although the characteristic features of migraine and CH are very different, in practice there can be substantial overlap in the clinical presentations of the two disorders [8].

Furthermore, research indicates that migraine and CH share some pathophysiologic mechanisms, such as head pain being mediated by activation of neuronal pathways within the trigeminovascular system [9, 10]. Previous research suggests that the pathophysiology of migraine may involve the diencephalon and brainstem, regions that might also be involved in cluster headache [11]. Additional studies have indicated that cortical spreading depression (CSD)—a wave of neuronal hyperactivity followed by cortical depression—is the most likely pathophysiological mechanism underlying the generation of migraine auras [12]. Neuroimaging studies and the reported efficacy of deep brain stimulation (DBS) have suggested that CH attacks involve the ipsilateral hypothalamus, particularly during the active headache period [13].

In this chapter, we review the similarities and differences in the clinical and pathophysiological characteristics of these two headache disorders.

17.2 Differences and Similarities in the Clinical Features of CH and Migraine

17.2.1 Pain Location and Duration

In both migraine and CH, the location of the pain is primarily in the first division of the trigeminal nerve, with more than three-quarters of patients with CH reporting periorbital pain localization [7, 14]. Although approximately two-thirds of patients with migraine report unilateral pain, pain can be bilateral or begin unilaterally before developing into generalized pain. The headache side may also change within the same attack [15].

The pain of a CH attack is almost exclusively side-locked, and the patient usually experiences attacks consistently on the same side of the head. However, studies have reported that approximately 17% of patients with migraine also experience side-locked headaches [16]. Moreover, some patients with CH experience pain that shifts sides during attacks, and very rarely pain can occur on both sides during a single attack [14, 15]. This shift may occur following invasive treatment such as unilateral occipital nerve stimulation [17]. Most CH attacks last between 30 and 120 minutes, seldom persisting for more than 3 h (when untreated) [15]; however, most migraine attacks last for at least 4 h and may last for 2–3 days if untreated [18].

17.2.2 Circannual and Circadian Periodicity

Many patients with CH experience extended periods of time in which headache attacks recur from one every other day to up to eight per day. These in-bout periods last for weeks or months, during which time most patients experience one to two attacks per day. These periods are followed by headache-free periods of weeks to years (out-of-bout periods) [7]. Furthermore, patients with CH tend to experience attacks at the same time(s) each day. This pattern may persist for days or weeks, and a nocturnal preponderance is commonly observed [15]. CH may also exhibit seasonal periodicity, with the onset of in-bout periods occurring once or twice yearly, especially in the spring and autumn (following solstices) [7, 19].

This consistent circannual and circadian periodicity is rarely observed in patients with migraine. The median migraine attack frequency is 1.5 attacks per month, although approximately 10% of patients experience migraine attacks at least weekly [18]. However, some reports have indicated that migraine attacks with aura peak once per year in May [20], and some patients with migraine may similarly experience frequent headaches during a limited period (several weeks to months), which may even recur during the same season. This condition has often been described as cyclical migraine [21]. Studies have also demonstrated that patients with cyclical migraine respond well to lithium carbonate, which is generally accepted as a standard prophylactic therapy for CH [19, 21].

17.2.3   Cranial Autonomic Symptoms (CAS)

CH attacks are usually accompanied by ipsilateral CAS, including conjunctival injection, lacrimation, nasal congestion, eyelid edema, forehead/facial sweating, miosis, and ptosis [7]. These distinct CAS are suggestive of a parasympathetic discharge with a sympathetic deficit, although the precise reason for unilateral CAS in patients with CH remains unknown. Researchers have hypothesized that ipsilateral activation of the hypothalamus during headache attacks may stimulate ipsilateral while simultaneously suppressing contralateral, trigeminal autonomic reflexes [22]. However, patients with CH may also experience bilateral CAS such as conjunctival injection or facial/forehead sweating [23, 24]. This may be because the trigeminal autonomic reflex includes an often minor contralateral component, likely due to crossover within the brainstem [25].

These CAS are also observed in 67–95% of patients with migraine. Therefore, migraines accompanied by autonomic symptoms may clinically mimic CH [23, 26]. However, patients with migraine mainly experience a single CAS, which tends to be less consistent, bilateral, less severe, and unrelated to the headache side [27]. In contrast, patients with CH are more likely to report multiple and more severe CAS [14, 23]. Collectively, these differences in the clinical characteristics of CAS may aid physicians in differentiating CH from migraine with CAS.

17.2.4   Aura Symptoms

Although aura symptoms usually involve visual sensations (flashing lights, scintillating scotomas), they may occasionally include facial and limb paresthesias, speech disturbances, weakness, vertigo, and mild ataxia. Previously, such symptoms were regarded as being solely characteristic of migraine with aura [4]; however, aura symptoms have been reported in up to 20% of patients with CH [28, 29]. Furthermore, Asian patients with CH tend to present less frequent aura symptoms (approximately 1%) than Western patients [30]. Studies have also indicated that only 1.8% of patients with CH have comorbid migraine with aura [31].

17.2.5 Restlessness

While headaches during migraine attacks are usually aggravated by movement or routine physical activity [18], between 51% and 99.2% of patients with CH experience restlessness and/or agitation during attacks [7, 14]. Thus, individuals with migraine typically remain quite still during attacks (e.g., lying in bed), while those with CH often pace or rock during CH attacks. Despite the agitated behavior that is common during CH attacks, physical activity can worsen headache intensity in a minority of patients with CH. Although it was previously believed that the pain of CH attacks is not exacerbated by activity or movement, more recent studies have reported that approximately 7–45.8% of patients with CH also experience aggravation of headache pain during physical activity or movement [30, 32]. While restlessness and avoidance of movement are hallmarks of CH and migraine, respectively, Asian patients with CH tend to exhibit less frequent pacing/restlessness than Western patients [30].

17.2.6 Other Features

Nausea and vomiting are commonly observed during acute migraine attacks [18, 33]. Sensory hypersensitivity is also observed in most patients with migraine, with photophobia and phonophobia occurring in up to 90% of patients [18, 33]. Interestingly, a high proportion of patients with CH also report at least one accompanying symptom (photophobia, phonophobia, nausea, or vomiting) typically associated with migraine [7, 14]. Studies have reported that 27–53% of patients with CH experience nausea, 12–32% experience vomiting, 54–78% experience photophobia, and 15–49% experience phonophobia [7, 14]. Individuals with CH more commonly report unilateral photophobia and phonophobia, while those with migraine nearly always report that these symptoms are bilateral [34]. Some patients with CH have also reported a variety of triggers for their attacks (e.g., certain foods, odors, or chocolate), many of which are supposed triggers of migraine attacks as well [19].

Although premonitory symptoms such as fatigue, apathy, irritability, yawning, and neck pain/stiffness are not included in the International Headache Society (IHS) classification criteria for migraine, such symptoms are known to precede migraine attacks in the majority of patients with migraine [15, 35]. However, these symptoms are also observed in approximately 8–11% of patients with CH [15, 36].

Once regarded as a characteristic feature of migraine, allodynia—which can be a clinical feature of peripheral or central sensitization—has also been observed in 40–49% of patients with CH [37, 38]. In summary, although features such as nausea, vomiting, sensory hypersensitivities, and premonitory symptoms occur more frequently with migraine attacks, they can also be observed in patients with CH, potentially delaying diagnosis of CH (Table 17.1).

Table 17.1 Comparisons of the clinical features between CH and migraine

	CH	Migraine
Prevalence	Approximately 0.1%	Approximately 10%
Sex predominance	Majority male	Majority female
Location of pain	Primarily in the first division of the trigeminal nerve, one-sided, around the eyes	Primarily in the first division of the trigeminal nerve, one-sided or both sides
Duration of each headache attack (when untreated)	15–180 min	4–72 h
Intensity of pain	Severe or very severe	Moderate or severe
Occurrence of attacks	Multiple attacks daily for weeks during the in-bout period (0.5–8/day)	Usually 1–7 per month
Circannual and circadian periodicity	Common	Rare
Cranial autonomic symptoms	Most accompanied by ipsilateral cranial autonomic symptoms Consistent, severe, ipsilateral to headache side	Approximately 67–95% of patients Inconsistent, less severe, bilateral
Aura	Rare	Approximately 1/3 of patients
Restlessness and/or agitation during attacks	Approximately 51% and 99.2% of patients	Rare
Headache exacerbated by activity or movement	Approximately 7–45.8% of patients	Approximately up to 90% of patients
Nausea and vomiting during attacks	Nausea, approximately 27–53% of patients; vomiting, 12–32% of patients	Approximately 50–90% of patients
Photophobia and/or phonophobia	Photophobia, approximately 54–78% of patients; phonophobia, 15–49% of patients	Approximately up to 90% of patients
Premonitory symptoms	Approximately 8–11% of patients	Approximately up to 88% of patients
Allodynia	Approximately 40–49% of patients	Approximately up to 62% of patients

CH cluster headache

Prophylactic treatment is important for both CH and migraine. Some prophylactic treatments are similarly effective for patients with CH and for those with migraine, such as calcium channel blockers (i.e., verapamil) and anticonvulsants (i.e., sodium valproate, topiramate). However, others such as beta-blockers and tricyclic antidepressants are more effective in patients with migraine than in those with CH [39, 40]. In contrast, oxygen and lithium are more often used in patients with CH.

While many women with migraine notice that their headaches greatly improve during the second and third trimesters of pregnancy, few large-scale prospective studies have investigated the effect of pregnancy on patients with CH, as the condition is observed in less than 0.3% of pregnancies [41]. In one previous study, approximately 25% of pregnant women with CH reported that an expected cluster period did not develop during gestation, although many reported that clusters began soon after delivery. Additionally, the majority of these women reported that CH attacks did not change in frequency or intensity during pregnancy [42]. Menstruation, the use of oral contraceptives, and menopause also exert a much smaller influence on CH attacks than on migraine attacks. However, CH may have an impact on women with the condition, who may refrain from having children due to their symptoms [42].

17.3 Pathophysiological Similarities and Differences Between CH and Migraine

17.3.1 The Trigeminovascular System

In CH and migraine, headache pain originates from activation of the trigeminovascular system. The trigeminovascular system consists of the neurons innervating the cerebral vessels whose cell bodies are located in the trigeminal ganglion [43]. This ganglion contains bipolar cells: the peripheral fiber making a synaptic connection with the vessels in the meninges, the extracranial arteries, and those in the circle of Willis; and the centrally projecting fiber synapsing in the caudal brainstem or high cervical cord [43]. Furthermore, the peripheral fibers—which are mainly found in the ophthalmic division of the trigeminal nerve—exhibit synaptic connections with the dura mater, vessels, and other widespread brain structures involved in pain processing [44, 45]. In CH, activation of the trigeminovascular system may trigger CAS through the trigeminal autonomic reflex [46]. The trigeminal nucleus caudalis exhibits a connection with the superior salivatory nucleus, from which the parasympathetic efferent fibers of the facial nerve arise. Activation of these parasympathetic fibers may result in symptoms such as rhinorrhea, lacrimation, nasal congestion, ptosis, and miosis [47]. Furthermore, fibers originating from the superior salivatory nucleus synapse in the pterygopalatine ganglia, with postganglionic fibers innervating the cerebral vessels as well as the lacrimal and nasal glands [47]. This explains why blockade of the sphenopalatine ganglion may relieve the symptoms of CH attacks in some patients [48]. It is widely accepted that high-flow oxygen is an efficient abortive therapy for acute CH attacks [49]. Indeed, previous animal studies have suggested that oxygen may produce these effects by acting on parasympathetic outflow to the cranial vasculature and trigeminovascular system [50].

Although most migraine pain is localized to the ophthalmic division of the trigeminal nerve, some patients report headache sites outside this region, such as in the occipital area, the area of innervation for the greater occipital nerve (GON) [51]. This may be due to the convergence of trigeminal and cervical afferent neurons in the trigeminocervical complex (TCC)—the region of the brainstem in contact with the caudal portion of the trigeminal nucleus caudalis and the dorsal horn of the C1–C2 segments of the spinal cord [51]. Additionally, the pathophysiology of migraine attacks involves both central and peripheral sensitization. Peripheral sensitization is associated with the activation of primary afferent nociceptive neurons [52]: A first-order neuron in the trigeminal ganglion receives input from dura-level blood vessels. This signal is then transmitted to a second-order neuron in the trigeminal brainstem nuclear complex, followed by a third-order neuron in the thalamus to the sensory cortex [53]. The major clinical symptom associated with first-order-neuron sensitization is throbbing pain that is aggravated by physical activity or certain postures that increase intracranial pressure (e.g., coughing) [53]. Moreover, sensitization of the nociceptors innervating the meninges may also result in intracranial hypersensitivity [54].

The central sensitization hypothesis suggests that, when peripheral sensitization later spreads to second-order neurons in the trigeminovascular system, cutaneous allodynia (pain evoked by applying non-noxious stimuli to normal skin) will occur [55]. Furthermore, the sensitization of third-order neurons in the thalamus is clinically expressed as extracranial hypersensitivity [54]. Thus, altered sensory processing in the brainstem may lead to hyperexcitability of TCC neurons [56]. Central sensitization may contribute to reducing the pain threshold, aggravating the pain response, and resulting in typically non-painful stimuli being perceived as painful (i.e., allodynia) [57]. Interestingly, central sensitization is also believed to be a risk factor for increasing headache frequency, such as transforming from episodic migraine to chronic migraine [55, 58].

17.3.2 Neuropeptide Release

Release of vasoactive neuropeptides from trigeminovascular sensory afferents results in vasodilatation, leakage of plasma protein from blood vessels, and mast cell degranulation [59, 60]. Following activation of the trigeminal fibers or trigeminal ganglion, neuropeptides such as calcitonin gene-related peptide (CGRP), substance P, vasoactive intestinal peptide (VIP), and pituitary adenylate cyclase-activating polypeptide (PACAP) [61] are released. These neuropeptides have been associated with the pathophysiology of both CH and migraine [60].

CGRP is also a powerful vasodilator that may contribute to dilation of the dura vessels [62]. Previous studies have also reported that substance P-immunoreactive fibers are more highly concentrated around the cerebral arteries, while CGRP-immunoreactive fibers are more highly concentrated around the middle meningeal artery [62]. Animal studies have demonstrated that small nerve fibers containing CGRP and substance P arise from the trigeminal ganglion and innervate the dura mater [62], thereby allowing for the transmission of nociceptive information from nerves innervating meningeal blood vessels to the trigeminal nucleus caudalis [63]. Accumulating evidence also suggests that migraine can be successfully treated using antibodies against CGRP, CGRP receptor antagonists, and CGRP-regulating triptans [64, 65]. Such findings support an important role for CGRP in migraine and other primary headache disorders [66–69].

Previous studies have demonstrated that elevated plasma concentrations of CGRP, substance P, and VIP occur during migraine attacks and during CH attacks (for a review see [70]). Furthermore, since VIP is derived from parasympathetic afferents, elevated plasma VIP may be associated with parasympathetic activation, which has been linked to CH pathophysiology [71]. Nitric oxide (NO), which may interact with CGRP, is also a potent vasodilator in the meningeal circulation [71]. The interaction between NO and CGRP may contribute to vasodilation and peripheral sensitization of perivascular afferent fibers [72]. Furthermore, infusion of nitro-vasodilators can trigger CH attacks, supporting a key role for NO in CH pathophysiology and nociceptive processing, as well as migraine [73].

Research has further revealed that substance P and neurokinin A (NKA) may increase vascular permeability in response to trigeminal nerve activation [74]. Moreover, it has been hypothesized that activation of substance P neurons in the ophthalmic and maxillary divisions can cause all the symptoms of an acute CH attack, and this could explain the observed improvement in symptoms following blockade of the Gasserian or sphenopalatine ganglia [75]. Although there is a potentially prominent link between the release of several important neuropeptides in migraine and CH pathophysiology, further research is required to fully elucidate this relationship and its role in triggering and maintaining individual attacks.

17.3.3 Structural and Functional Brain Changes

17.3.3.1 Cluster Headache

Clinically, the circadian rhythmicity and ipsilateral cranial autonomic features of CH underlie the hypothesis that the disorder may involve the hypothalamus [76, 77]. Indeed, functional imaging studies have documented increased ipsilateral posterior hypothalamic activation in patients with CH during acute attacks [78–80]. Proton magnetic resonance spectroscopy (MRS) studies have provided additional evidence in support of the hypothesis that CH is caused by hypothalamic neuronal dysfunction [81, 82]. In addition to the hypothalamus, several regions of the pain matrix have been strongly implicated in CH, including the anterior cingulate cortex, posterior thalamus, basal ganglia, insula, and the cerebellar hemispheres [79, 80, 83]. Furthermore, dynamic functional differences in the central descending pain-modulatory system have been observed between in-bout (without acute attacks) and out-of-bout periods [84].

Several functional magnetic resonance imaging (fMRI) studies have reported abnormal functional connectivity (FC) between the hypothalamus and other brain areas (i.e., areas of the pain network) in patients with CH experiencing acute attacks [85, 86]. Additionally, FC disruptions in nontraditional pain-processing areas (e.g., occipital and salience networks) may also be involved in CH pathophysiology [87, 88]. These FC differences in nontraditional pain-processing areas have also been associated with the patient's in- or out-of-bout status [88, 89], advancing our understanding of network functionality in episodic CH.

Using T1 voxel-based morphometry (VBM), structural imaging studies have demonstrated changes in the gray matter volume (GMV) of the hypothalamus and several pain-processing regions in patients with CH [83, 90–93]. GMV differences have also been observed between in-bout and out-of-bout periods. These changes in GMV may reflect an insufficient capacity to modulate pain in frontal areas, which may contribute to the pathophysiology of shifts in bout status among patients with CH [92].

Several diffusion tensor imaging (DTI) studies have documented controversial microstructural white matter (WM) changes in patients with CH, while others have reported no differences between patients with CH and healthy controls [91]. Still other studies have reported changes primarily in regions related to the pain matrix [94, 95]. Such discrepancies may be attributable to differences in bout status among the study populations. An additional study documented dynamic microstructural differences in the frontal and limbic WM between patients with CH and healthy controls (with the exception of the cerebellum), noting that these changes persisted during the out-of-bout period [96]. Consistent anatomical connections have also been observed between these altered areas and the hypothalamus [96]. These findings may also partially explain the shifts between in-bout and out-of-bout periods in patients with CH.

17.3.3.2 Migraine

Functional neuroimaging studies have demonstrated differences in brain activation patterns during migraine attacks compared to the interictal phase, highlighting the potential importance of brainstem regions such as the dorsal midbrain, dorsolateral pons, and trigeminal nucleus caudalis and of the hypothalamus for generating acute migraine attacks [97, 98]. Increased activation has also been observed in the red nucleus, substantia nigra, posterior thalamus, cerebellum, insula, cingulate, prefrontal cortices, hippocampus, and anterior temporal pole during migraine attacks [10, 97–99]. However, these areas do not appear to be specific to migraine and are collectively referred to as the "pain matrix," which exhibits increased activation in other pain disorders that are thought to occur secondary to central hypersensitivity (e.g., low back pain, irritable bowel syndrome, fibromyalgia, and cardiac pain) [100].

Evidence obtained from fMRI studies indicates that activation of the thalamic pulvinar occurs during migraine attacks accompanied by extracephalic allodynia, suggesting that sensitization of posterior thalamic neurons may mediate the spread of multimodal allodynia and hyperalgesia beyond the locus of the migraine headache [101]. Patients with episodic migraine also experience greater pain-induced activation in regions primarily associated with the cognitive aspects of pain perception, including attending to pain and pain memory [102]. Therefore, enhanced cognitive pain processing by migraineurs may reflect cerebral hyper-sensitivity, which may in turn be associated with high expectations and hyper-vigilance for pain [102]. Migraine may also be associated with altered FC in the insular region during the interictal state, especially with the dorsal pons [103]. Moreover, the FC of various brain regions and networks may be altered during the pain stage of migraine attacks [104]. More recently, Schulte and May inves-tigated the different stages of the native migraine cycle in a single patient with episodic migraine. The authors observed heightened hypothalamic, pontine, tri-geminal nucleus caudalis and visual cortex activity shortly before the onset of migraine pain. Furthermore, the FC between the hypothalamus and trigeminal nucleus caudalis/dorsal rostral pons differed between the pre-ictal and ictal phases, providing evidence that changes in hypothalamic FC occur during differ-ent stages of the migraine cycle [105].

In addition to functional alterations, VBM and DTI studies have also demon-strated GMV reductions in the insula, motor/premotor cortex, prefrontal cortex, cingulate cortex, posterior parietal cortex, and orbitofrontal cortex in patients with migraine, along with thickening of the somatosensory cortex and increased gray matter density in the caudate [106–108]. Furthermore, several reports have indicated that such changes in areas mostly related to pain processing may be associated with the frequency and duration of migraine attacks [106–108]. Similarly, these structural changes have also been observed in patients with other chronic pain disorders, including osteoarthritis, chronic low back pain, and pel-vic pain [109].

The accumulated evidence from structural and functional neuroimaging stud-ies draws a complex picture of the central mechanisms underlying CH and migraine, with some key similarities and differences. First, the hypothalamus and the dorsal rostral pons likely play key roles during the acute stages of migraine, similar to the key role of the hypothalamus in acute CH attacks. Furthermore, the trigeminal nuclei are essential for headache generation in both migraine and CH [110]. Recent evidence suggests that the hypothalamus is not only a potential generator of CH attacks but also a generator of migraine-like accompanying symptoms [105]. Furthermore, the descending projections of the hypothalamus may activate or disinhibit the trigeminal nucleus caudalis and the dorsal rostral pons, both of which are thought to be specifically associated with the activation of migraine attacks [105]. Additionally, the activation of the tri-geminal system via trigeminal autonomic reflexes may explain the variation in CAS observed in patients with CH who exhibit migraine-like accompanying fea-tures [111]. Finally, although these structural and functional changes in pain-related areas can be observed in patients with CH and in those with migraine, some overlap is also observed with other chronic pain disorders, suggesting that CH and migraine may also be related to these pain disorders. However, unique to CH are the dynamic changes in the structure and functional linkage of pain-modulatory networks—as well as regions outside of the traditional pain-process-ing networks—that occur between in-bout and out-of-bout periods. Such changes may indeed be more specific to the pathophysiology of CH.

17.4   Conclusions

Both migraine and CH are disorders of the trigeminovascular system with complex pathophysiological origins. Although the two conditions can be differentiated based on differences in clinical symptoms, neurochemical mechanisms, and neuroimaging patterns, some overlap (e.g., some clinical features and similar responses to triptans) can be observed between the two. Identifying the similarities and differences between CH and migraine may advance the current understanding of the shared pathophysiology of these two conditions and aid in the development of novel therapeutic strategies.

References

1. Headache Classification Committee of the International Headache Society (IHS). The international classification of headache disorders, 3rd edition. Cephalalgia. 2018;38:1–211.
2. Lipton RB, et al. Migraine prevalence, disease burden, and the need for preventive therapy. Neurology. 2007;68:343–9.
3. Giffin NJ, Lipton RB, Silberstein SD, Olesen J, Goadsby PJ. The migraine postdrome: an electronic diary study. Neurology. 2016;87:309–13.
4. Rasmussen BK, Olesen J. Migraine with aura and migraine without aura: an epidemiological study. Cephalalgia. 1992;12:221–8.. discussion 186
5. Broner SW, Cohen JM. Epidemiology of cluster headache. Curr Pain Headache Rep. 2009;13:141–6.
6. Rozen TD. Cluster headache as the result of secondhand cigarette smoke exposure during childhood. Headache. 2010;50:130–2.
7. Bahra A, May A, Goadsby PJ. Cluster headache: a prospective clinical study with diagnostic implications. Neurology. 2002;58:354–61.
8. Bahra A, Goadsby PJ. Diagnostic delays and mis-management in cluster headache. Acta Neurol Scand. 2004;109:175–9.
9. Bahra A, Matharu MS, Buchet C, Frackowiak RSJ, Goadsby PJ. Brainstem activation specific to migraine headache. Lancet. 2001;357:1016–7.
10. Denuelle M, Fabre N, Payoux P, Chollet F, Geraud G. Hypothalamic activation in spontaneous migraine attacks. Headache. 2007;47:1418–26.
11. Akerman S, Holland PR, Goadsby PJ. Diencephalic and brainstem mechanisms in migraine. Nat Rev Neurosci. 2011;12:570–84.
12. Ayata C. Cortical spreading depression triggers migraine attack: pro. Headache. 2010;50:725–30.
13. Leone M, et al. Lessons from 8 years' experience of hypothalamic stimulation in cluster headache. Cephalalgia. 2008;28:789–97.
14. Gaul C, et al. Differences in clinical characteristics and frequency of accompanying migraine features in episodic and chronic cluster headache. Cephalalgia. 2012;32:571–7.
15. Peatfield R. Migrainous features in cluster headache. Curr Pain Headache Rep. 2001;5:67–70.
16. Leone M, et al. Clinical considerations on side-locked unilaterality in long-lasting primary headaches. Headache. 1993;33:381–4.
17. Burns B, Watkins L, Goadsby PJ. Treatment of medically intractable cluster headache by occipital nerve stimulation: long-term follow-up of eight patients. Lancet. 2007;369:1099–106.
18. Stewart WF, Shechter A, Lipton RB. Migraine heterogeneity. Disability, pain intensity, and attack frequency and duration. Neurology. 1994;44:S24–39.

19. Applebee AM, Shapiro RE. Cluster-migraine: does it exist? Curr Pain Headache Rep. 2007;11:154–7.
20. Alstadhaug KB, Bekkelund S, Salvesen R. Circannual periodicity of migraine? Eur J Neurol. 2007;14:983–8.
21. Medina JL, Diamond S. Cyclical migraine. Arch Neurol. 1981;38:343–4.
22. Young WB, Rozen TD. Bilateral cluster headache: case report and a theory of (failed) contralateral suppression. Cephalalgia. 1999;19:188–90.
23. Kaniecki RG. Cranial autonomic symptoms in migraine: headache characteristics and comparison with cluster. Headache. 2010;50:680.
24. Bigal ME. Objective assessment of bilateral conjunctival injection during cluster headache attacks—commentary. Headache. 2007;47:943.
25. Lambert GA, Bogduk N, Goadsby PJ, Duckworth JW, Lance JW. Decreased carotid arterial resistance in cats in response to trigeminal stimulation. J Neurosurg. 1984;61:307–15.
26. Obermann M, et al. Prevalence of trigeminal autonomic symptoms in migraine: a population-based study. Cephalalgia. 2007;27:504–9.
27. Lai T, Fuh J, Wang S. Cranial autonomic symptoms in migraine: characteristics and comparison with cluster headache. J Neurol Neurosurg Psychiatry. 2008;80:1116–9.
28. Rozen TD. Cluster headache with aura. Curr Pain Headache Rep. 2011;15:98–100.
29. Silberstein SD, Niknam R, Rozen TD, Young WB. Cluster headache with aura. Neurology. 2000;54:219–21.
30. Lin KH, et al. Cluster headache in the Taiwanese—a clinic-based study. Cephalalgia. 2004;24:631–8.
31. Taga A, Russo M, Manzoni GC, Torelli P. Cluster headache with accompanying migraine-like features: a possible clinical phenotype. Headache. 2017;57:290–7.
32. Rozen TD, Fishman RS. Cluster headache in the United States of America: demographics, clinical characteristics, triggers, suicidality, and personal burden. Headache. 2012;52:99–113.
33. Silberstein SD. Migraine symptoms: results of a survey of self-reported migraineurs. Headache. 1995;35:387–96.
34. Irimia P, Cittadini E, Paemeleire K, Cohen AS, Goadsby PJ. Unilateral photophobia or phonophobia in migraine compared with trigeminal autonomic cephalalgias. Cephalalgia. 2008;28:626–30.
35. Rossi P, Ambrosini A, Buzzi MG. Prodromes and predictors of migraine attack. Funct Neurol. 2005;20:185–91.
36. Blau JN, Engel HO. Premonitory and prodromal symptoms in cluster headache. Cephalalgia. 1998;18:91–3.
37. Ashkenazi A, Young WB. Dynamic mechanical (brush) allodynia in cluster headache. Headache. 2004;44:1010–2.
38. Marmura MJ, Abbas M, Ashkenazi A. Dynamic mechanical (brush) allodynia in cluster headache: a prevalence study in a tertiary headache clinic. J Headache Pain. 2009;10:255–8.
39. Ashkenazi A, Schwedt T. Cluster headache-acute and prophylactic therapy. Headache. 2011;51:272–86.
40. Silberstein SD, et al. Evidence-based guideline update: pharmacologic treatment for episodic migraine prevention in adults. Neurology. 2012;78:1337–45.
41. Pearce CF, Hansen WF. Headache and neurological disease in pregnancy. Clin Obstet Gynecol. 2012;55:810–28.
42. vanVliet J, Favier I, Helmerhorst FM, Haan J, Ferrari MD. Cluster headache in women: relation with menstruation, use of oral contraceptives, pregnancy, and menopause. J Neurol Neurosurg Psychiatry. 2006;77:690–2.
43. May A, Goadsby PJ. The trigeminovascular system in humans: pathophysiologic implications for primary headache syndromes of the neural influences on the cerebral circulation. J Cereb Blood Flow Metab. 1999;19:115–27. https://doi.org/10.1097/00004647-199902000-00001.
44. Olesen J, Burstein R, Ashina M, Tfelt-Hansen P. Origin of pain in migraine: evidence for peripheral sensitisation. Lancet Neurol. 2009;8:679–90.

45. Liu-Chen LY, Mayberg MR, Moskowitz MA. Immunohistochemical evidence for a substance P-containing trigeminovascular pathway to pial arteries in cats. Brain Res. 1983;268:162–6.
46. Goadsby PJ, Lipton RB. A review of paroxysmal hemicranias, SUNCT syndrome and other short-lasting headaches with autonomic feature, including new cases. Brain. 1997;120:193–209.
47. Goadsby PJ, Edvinsson L. Human in vivo evidence for trigeminovascular activation in cluster headache neuropeptide changes and effects of acute attacks therapies. Brain. 1994;117:427–34.
48. Narouze SN. Role of sphenopalatine ganglion neuroablation in the management of cluster headache. Curr Pain Headache Rep. 2010;14:160–3.
49. Cohen AS, Burns B, Goadsby PJ. High-flow oxygen for treatment of cluster headache. JAMA. 2009;302:2451.
50. Akerman S, Holland PR, Summ O, Lasalandra MP, Goadsby PJ. A translational in vivo model of trigeminal autonomic cephalalgias: therapeutic characterization. Brain. 2012;135:3664–75.
51. Cutrer FM. Pathophysiology of migraine. Semin Neurol. 2010;30:120–30.
52. Burstein R, Zhang X, Levy D, Aoki KR, Brin MF. Selective inhibition of meningeal nociceptors by botulinum neurotoxin type A: therapeutic implications for migraine and other pains. Cephalalgia. 2014;34:853–69.
53. Mathew NT. Pathophysiology of chronic migraine and mode of action of preventive medications. Headache. 2011;51:84–92.
54. Bartsch T, Goadsby PJ. Increased responses in trigeminocervical nociceptive neurons to cervical input after stimulation of the dura mater. Brain. 2003;126:1801–13.
55. Burstein R, Yarnitsky D, Goor-Aryeh I, Ransil BJ, Bajwa ZH. An association between migraine and cutaneous allodynia. Ann Neurol. 2000;47:614–24.
56. Dodick D, Silberstein S. Central sensitization theory of migraine: clinical implications. Headache. 2006;46:S182–91.
57. McMahon SB, Lewin GR, Wall PD. Central hyperexcitability triggered by noxious inputs. Curr Opin Neurobiol. 1993;3:602–10.
58. Noseda R, Burstein R. Migraine pathophysiology: anatomy of the trigeminovascular pathway and associated neurological symptoms, CSD, sensitization and modulation of pain. Pain. 2013;154(Suppl):S44–53.
59. Geppetti P, Nassini R, Materazzi S, Benemei S. The concept of neurogenic inflammation. BJU Int. 2008;101:2–6.
60. Williamson DJ, Hargreaves RJ. Neurogenic inflammation in the context of migraine. Microsc Res Tech. 2001;53:167–78.
61. Vécsei L, Tuka B, Tajti J. Role of PACAP in migraine headaches. Brain. 2014;137:650–1.
62. Meßlinger K, Hanesch U, Baumgärtel M, Trost B, Schmidt RF. Innervation of the dura mater encephali of cat and rat: ultrastructure and calcitonin gene-related peptide-like and substance P-like immunoreactivity. Anat Embryol. 1993;188:219–37.
63. Mayberg MR, Zervas NT, Moskowitz MA. Trigeminal projections to supratentorial pial and dural blood vessels in cats demonstrated by horseradish peroxidase histochemistry. J Comp Neurol. 1984;223:46–56.
64. Goadsby PJ, et al. A controlled trial of Erenumab for episodic migraine. N Engl J Med. 2017;377:2123–32.
65. Silberstein SD, et al. Fremanezumab for the preventive treatment of chronic migraine. N Engl J Med. 2017;377:2113–22.
66. Goadsby PJ, Akerman S, James Storer R. Evidence for postjunctional serotonin (5-HT1) receptors in the trigeminocervical complex. Ann Neurol. 2001;50:804–7.
67. Olesen J, et al. Calcitonin gene-related peptide receptor antagonist BIBN 4096 BS for the acute treatment of migraine. N Engl J Med. 2004;350:1104–10.
68. Ho TW, Edvinsson L, Goadsby PJ. CGRP and its receptors provide new insights into migraine pathophysiology. Nat Rev Neurol. 2010;6:573–82.

69. Dodick DW, et al. Safety and efficacy of ALD403, an antibody to calcitonin gene-related peptide, for the prevention of frequent episodic migraine: a randomised, double-blind, placebo-controlled, exploratory phase 2 trial. Lancet Neurol. 2014;13:1100–7.
70. Riesco N, Cernuda-Morollón E, Pascual J. Neuropeptides as a marker for chronic headache. Curr Pain Headache Rep. 2017;21:18.
71. Goadsby PJ, Edvinsson L, Ekman R. Vasoactive peptide release in the extracerebral circulation of humans during migraine headache. Ann Neurol. 1990;28:183–7.
72. Strecker T, Dux M, Messlinger K. Nitric oxide releases calcitonin-gene-related peptide from rat dura mater encephali promoting increases in meningeal blood flow. J Vasc Res. 2002;39:489–96.
73. Thomsen LL, Olesen J. Nitric oxide in primary headaches. Curr Opin Neurol. 2001;14:315–21.
74. DiMarzo V, Blumberg PM, Szallasi A. Endovanilloid signaling in pain. Curr Opin Neurobiol. 2002;12:372–9.
75. Hardebo JE. The involvement of trigeminal substance P neurons in cluster headache. An hypothesis. Headache. 1984;24:294–304.
76. Pringsheim T. Cluster headache: evidence for a disorder of circadian rhythm and hypothalamic function. Can J Neurol Sci. 2002;29:33–40.
77. Leone M, Bussone GA. Review of hormonal findings in cluster headache. Evidence for hypothalamic involvement. Cephalalgia. 1993;13:309–17.
78. May A, Bahra A, Büchel C, Frackowiak RSJ, Goadsby PJ. Hypothalamic activation in cluster headache attacks. Lancet. 1998;352:275–8.
79. May A, Bahra A, Büchel C, Frackowiak RSJ, Goadsby PJ. PET and MRA findings in cluster headache and MRA in experimental pain. Neurology. 2000;55:1328–35.
80. Sprenger T, et al. Specific hypothalamic activation during a spontaneous cluster headache attack. Neurology. 2004;62:516–7.
81. Lodi R, et al. Study of hypothalamic metabolism in cluster headache by proton MR spectroscopy. Neurology. 2006;66:1264–6.
82. Wang S-J, Lirng J-F, Fuh J-L, Chen J-J. Reduction in hypothalamic H-MRS metabolite ratios in patients with cluster headache. J Neurol Neurosurg Psychiatry. 2006;77:622–5.
83. May A, et al. Correlation between structural and functional changes in brain in an idiopathic headache syndrome. Nat Med. 1999;5:836–8.
84. Sprenger T, et al. Altered metabolism in frontal brain circuits in cluster headache. Cephalalgia. 2007;27:1033–42.
85. Rocca MA, et al. Central nervous system dysregulation extends beyond the pain-matrix network in cluster headache. Cephalalgia. 2010;30:1383–91.
86. Qiu E, et al. Abnormal brain functional connectivity of the hypothalamus in cluster headaches. PLoS One. 2013;8:e57896.
87. Qiu E, Tian L, Wang Y, Ma L, Yu S. Abnormal coactivation of the hypothalamus and salience network in patients with cluster headache. Neurology. 2015;84:1402–8.
88. Yang F-C, et al. Altered hypothalamic functional connectivity in cluster headache: a longitudinal resting-state functional MRI study. J Neurol Neurosurg Psychiatry. 2015;86(4):437–45. https://doi.org/10.1136/jnnp-2014-308122.
89. Chou K-H, et al. Bout-associated intrinsic functional network changes in cluster headache: a longitudinal resting-state functional MRI study. Cephalalgia. 2017;37(12):1152–63. https://doi.org/10.1177/0333102416668657.
90. Matharu MS. Functional and structural neuroimaging in primary headache syndromes. London: University of London; 2006.
91. Absinta M, et al. Selective decreased grey matter volume of the pain-matrix network in cluster headache. Cephalalgia. 2012;32:109–15.
92. Yang FC, et al. Altered gray matter volume in the frontal pain modulation network in patients with cluster headache. Pain. 2013;154:801–7.
93. Naegel S, et al. Cortical plasticity in episodic and chronic cluster headache. NeuroImage Clin. 2014;6:415–23.

94. Szabó N, et al. White matter disintegration in cluster headache. J Headache Pain. 2013;14:1–6.
95. Teepker M, et al. Diffusion tensor imaging in episodic cluster headache. Headache. 2012;52:274–82.
96. Chou K-H, et al. Altered white matter microstructural connectivity in cluster headaches: a longitudinal diffusion tensor imaging study. Cephalalgia. 2014;34:1040–52.
97. Afridi SK, et al. A positron emission tomographic study in spontaneous migraine. Arch Neurol. 2005;62:1270–5.
98. Weiller C, et al. Brain stem activation in spontaneous human migraine attacks. Nat Med. 1995;1:658–60.
99. Cao Y, Aurora SK, Nagesh V, Patel SC, Welch KM. Functional MRI-BOLD of brainstem structures during visually triggered migraine. Neurology. 2002;59:72–8.
100. Baliki MN, Geha PY, Apkarian AV, Chialvo DR. Beyond feeling: chronic pain hurts the brain, disrupting the default-mode network dynamics. J Neurosci. 2008;28:1398–403.
101. Burstein R, et al. Thalamic sensitization transforms localized pain into widespread allodynia. Ann Neurol. 2010;68:81–91.
102. Schwedt TJ, et al. Enhanced pain-induced activity of pain-processing regions in a case-control study of episodic migraine. Cephalalgia. 2014;34:947–58.
103. Tso AR, Trujillo A, Guo CC, Goadsby PJ, Seeley WW. The anterior insula shows heightened interictal intrinsic connectivity in migraine without aura. Neurology. 2015;84:1043–50.
104. Amin FM, et al. Change in brain network connectivity during PACAP38-induced migraine attacks: a resting-state functional MRI study. Neurology. 2016;86:180–7.
105. Schulte LH, May A. The migraine generator revisited: continuous scanning of the migraine cycle over 30 days and three spontaneous attacks. Brain. 2016;139:1987–93.
106. Maleki N, et al. Migraine attacks the basal ganglia. Mol Pain. 2011;7:71.
107. DaSilva AFM, Granziera C, Snyder J, Hadjikhani N, Alexandre FM. Thickening in the somatosensory cortex of patients with migraine. Neurology. 2007;69:1990–5.
108. Kim JH, et al. Regional grey matter changes in patients with migraine: a voxel-based morphometry study. Cephalalgia. 2008;28:598–604.
109. Baliki MN, Schnitzer TJ, Bauer WR, Apkarian AV. Brain morphological signatures for chronic pain. PLoS One. 2011;6:e26010.
110. Hoffmann J, et al. Evidence for orexinergic mechanisms in migraine. Neurobiol Dis. 2015;74:137–43.
111. Barbanti P, et al. The phenotype of migraine with unilateral cranial autonomic symptoms documents increased peripheral and central trigeminal sensitization. A case series of 757 patients. Cephalalgia. 2016;36:1334–40.

Chapter 18
The Short-Lasting Headaches Including Hypnic Headache

Anna Cohen and Giorgio Lambru

18.1 The Short-Lasting Unilateral Neuralgiform Headache Attacks (SUN)

18.1.1 Introduction

The SUN constellation incorporates SUNCT (short-lasting unilateral neuralgiform headache attacks with conjunctival injection and tearing) and SUNA (short-lasting unilateral neuralgiform headache attacks with cranial autonomic symptoms). As with the other TACs, these are attacks of severe unilateral head and facial pain, with associated ipsilateral autonomic features such as conjunctival injection, lacrimation, nasal blockage, rhinorrhoea, eyelid oedema, facial sweating, feeling of ear fullness, miosis and/or ptosis [1]. Attacks can be either spontaneous or triggered by cutaneous triggers such as touching the face or scalp, washing or brushing hair, chewing, brushing teeth, cold wind on the face, and also light (including sunlight and fluorescent lights). Table 18.1 lists the Classification Criteria for SUN.

When SUNCT was first described in the 1980s, the cranial autonomic symptoms including conjunctival injection and tearing ('C' and 'T' in the nomenclature) were noted to be prominent [2]. However subsequent patients were identified with an almost identical syndrome, with cranial autonomic symptoms, but lacking either conjunctival injection or tearing or both. This syndrome was labelled SUNA (cranial 'a'utonomic symptoms) [3]. Although the SUNCT syndrome has been validated, very limited data are available for SUNA, despite the diagnostic criteria were set to suggest that SUNCT forms a subset of a the broader SUNA entity [4]. For this

A. Cohen (✉)
Royal Free Hospital London, Luton and Dunstable University Hospital, London, UK
e-mail: anna.cohen@nhs.net

G. Lambru
Guy's and St Thomas' Hospital, London, UK

© Springer Nature Switzerland AG 2020
M. Leone, A. May (eds.), *Cluster Headache and other Trigeminal Autonomic Cephalgias*, Headache, https://doi.org/10.1007/978-3-030-12438-0_18

Table 18.1 International Headache Classification for SUN [4]

3.3 Short-lasting unilateral neuralgiform headache attacks
Description:
Attacks of moderate or severe, strictly unilateral head pain lasting seconds to minutes, occurring at least once a day and usually associated with prominent lacrimation and redness of the ipsilateral eye
Diagnostic criteria
A. At least 20 attacks fulfilling criteria B–D
B. Moderate or severe unilateral head pain, with orbital, supraorbital, temporal and/or other trigeminal distribution, lasting for 1–600 s and occurring as single stabs, series of stabs or in a sawtooth pattern
C. At least one of the following cranial autonomic symptoms or signs, ipsilateral to the pain
1. Conjunctival injection and/or lacrimation
2. Nasal congestion and/or rhinorrhoea
3. Eyelid oedema
4. Forehead and facial sweating
5. Miosis and/or ptosis
D. Attacks have a frequency of at least once a day for more than half of the time when the disorder is active
E. Not better accounted for by another ICHD-3 diagnosis

reason the two conditions are currently classified as a separate subtype, although studies on this are ongoing.

18.1.2 Epidemiology

SUNCT is relatively rare, with a recent study showing a prevalence of 6.6/100,000 and an incidence of 1.2/100,000 [5]. The disorder seems to have a male preponderance, with a gender ratio of 2:1. In a small case series of nine SUNA patients, the disorder seemed to display a female preponderance with a gender ratio of 2:1. The typical age of onset is between 40 and 70 years, with a mean age of onset at 48 years [6].

18.1.3 Clinical Phenotype

Headache attacks in SUN are strictly unilateral with a slight preponderance of right-sided attacks. However patients with unilateral, side-alternating attacks and seldom patients with bilateral attacks have been reported [6]. The pain in SUN is predominantly centred over the periorbital, retro-orbital and temporal regions, though 1/3 of patients experience pain radiation in the second branch of the trigeminal territory and 1/3 of SUNA patients can experience pain in the third branch of the trigeminal territory.

Pain (Verbal Rating Scale from 0 to 10)

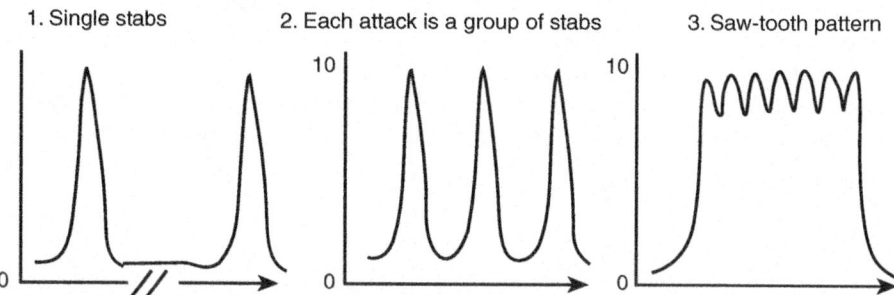

Fig. 18.1 The three types of clinical picture of attacks of SUNCT/SUNA. From: Short-lasting unilateral neuralgiform headache attacks with conjunctival injection and tearing (SUNCT) or cranial autonomic features (SUNA)—a prospective clinical study of SUNCT and SUNA. Brain. 2006;129(10):2746–2760. doi:10.1093/brain/awl202. Brain I © The Author (2006). Published by Oxford University Press on behalf of the Guarantors of Brain. All rights reserved. For Permissions, please email: journals.permissions@oxfordjournals.org

Classically the attacks last a few seconds or minutes at a time, in a 'stab'-like pattern. However these stabs can group together to give the impression of a longer-lasting attack, or if multiple stabs occur without resolution of the pain to baseline between the stabs, then a 'sawtooth' pattern is experienced, and this may last up to an hour [6]. This may lead to diagnostic confusion, and the syndrome may be mistaken for cluster headache or paroxysmal hemicrania. Figure 18.1 depicts the three types of attacks in SUN.

By definition, all of the SUNCT patients have both ipsilateral conjunctival injection and lacrimation accompanying the attacks. Almost half of the patients also report ipsilateral eyelid oedema, ptosis, nasal blockage and rhinorrhoea associated with their attacks. A small percent of the SUNCT patients reports facial flushing and facial sweating.

The other TACs also have agitation in their list of features; typically during an attack, patients cannot sit still and feel the need to rock or pace the floor. This is thought to be due to activation in the region of the posterior hypothalamus, which has been reported in all the TACs [7–10]. Agitation is thought to be also a feature of SUN [6], though this is not included in the current diagnostic criteria.

The vast majority of SUNCT patients could trigger their attacks by various cutaneous stimulations. Touching the face ipsilaterally to the side of the pain, chewing, eating, wind blowing on the face, washing the face and brushing teeth were the most prevalent types of triggers. Alcohol seems not to be a trigger unlike cluster headache. The majority of SUN patients denies the presence of a refractory period, which is the ability of triggering an attack immediately after the cessation of the previous one. This seems to constitute a meaningful distinguishing clinical feature to trigeminal neuralgia, which traditionally manifests refractory periods after triggered attacks [6].

The SUN headache syndromes can be episodic or chronic, just as in cluster headache or paroxysmal hemicrania. Unlike cluster headache, SUN presents more frequently with the chronic form ab initio or evolved from an episodic form. In the episodic form, bouts of SUNCT last between 7 days and 1 year and can remit for usually a year, up to 7 years [6]. In the chronic form, as in the other TACs, attacks are present for at least a year with no more than 7 days' break [1].

18.1.4   Differential Diagnosis of SUN

The differential diagnosis of the SUN headaches includes any short-lasting unilateral headache attack with ipsilateral autonomic features, that is, cluster headache and paroxysmal hemicrania. However the attacks in PH are longer lasting and less frequent than in SUN (2–30 min, several or many attacks per day), and those in CH are longer and less frequent still (up to 180 min, from one every other day up to eight attacks per day) [1, 4]. Another clinical feature that may help differentiating SUN from the other TACs is the presence of attacks triggered by cutaneous/intraoral stimulation. These triggers do not occur in the other TACs. In complex cases or poor patient history, diagnostic trials of certain medications such as sumatriptan 6 mg subcutaneous injection, high flow oxygen (100%, 12–15 litres/minute) and indometacin can help in ruling out cluster headache and the indometacin-sensitive headaches.

SUN may also be confused with trigeminal neuralgia (TN), in view of the multiple neuralgiform short-lasting attacks of unilateral facial pain. However, although autonomic symptoms may be present in TN due to the trigeminal autonomic reflex, the autonomic symptoms are generally much more prominent in SUN [11]. Also the agitation seen in SUN is presumed to be of hypothalamic origin [12] and is a defining feature of the TACs. Furthermore the lack of refractory period between attacks of SUN [6], such that an attack of SUN can be triggered immediately on top of a previous attack, can generally distinguish SUN in its purest form from TN. SUN can coexist with TN as two separate entities [13].

18.1.5   Secondary/Symptomatic SUN

SUN is a primary headache syndrome, but as with the other TACs, there may be a structural cause or lesion which results in the SUN headache syndrome. To date there are many causes of secondary or symptomatic SUN, which are detailed in Table 18.2. These mainly involve pituitary lesions such as adenomata; posterior fossa lesions such as infarcts or neuro-inflammatory disease; or direct local effects onto the trigeminal nerve such as vascular loops, which are also found in up to 80% of cases of TN.

Pituitary lesions are well recognised to cause any type of headache syndrome, most commonly migraine. However studies have shown that SUNCT

Table 18.2 Causes of secondary/symptomatic SUNCT and SUNA

Location of lesion	Pituitary lesions	Posterior fossa	Local lesions
Presumed mechanism of action	Via pituitary-hypothalamic axis	Local action on trigeminal nerve root or trigemino-cervical complex or ascending pathways	Local action on trigeminal nerve
Examples	Macrodenomata Microadenomata	Arteriovenous malformations Brainstem cavernous haemangioma Associated with HIV/AIDS Osteogenesis imperfecta Craniostosis Ischaemic brainstem and medullary infarctions[a] Pilocytic astrocytomas in V root entry zone Devic's syndrome (neuromyelitis optica) Plaque of multiple sclerosis in the pons, cerebral peduncle and medulla Vertebral artery dissection Pathological white matter changes in multiple sclerosis Epidermoid cyst in cerebellopontine angle	Vascular loops compressing trigeminal nerve Pontine capillary telangiectasia and developmental venous anomaly Meningoencephalitis Metastatic intraorbital carcinoid Associated with chronic sinusitis After herpes zoster infection of V1 trigeminal nerve

[a]There is one case report also of medullary infarction causing coexistent SUNCT and trigeminal neuralgia [13]

and SUNA are present in higher proportions in cohorts of patients with pituitary adenomata (5% in one series of 88 patients) [14] than in the general population (usually quoted as 6.6 per 100,000 population) [5]. Both micro- and macro-adenomata are able to cause a secondary SUN syndrome; therefore it is not purely due to the size of the lesion and its local mass effect; rather it is thought to be due to neurohormonal mechanisms. Table 18.2 lists some of the recognised causes of secondary SUN.

18.1.6   Diagnostic Workup

It is recommended that patients with SUNCT or SUNA, especially those with atypical features or with abnormal findings on neurological examination, should have MRI imaging of the brain, particularly to rule out any pituitary or posterior fossa lesions. Dedicated fine cut or high-resolution scanning through the trigeminal nerves should also be performed to look for neurovascular conflict to the ipsilateral trigeminal nerve [15].

18.1.7 Medical and Surgical Treatments

The management of SUN have historically been considered challenging. Due to the rarity of these disorders, no randomised placebo-controlled trials have ever been conducted. The series published so far have included very small numbers of patients and have produced data on a very limited number of medications. As far as SUNA is concerned, it is still unclear whether medications effective in SUNCT are also effective in SUNA.

18.1.8 Abortive Treatments

Since the attacks are very short lasting, abortive therapy strategies are not a useful concept in SUNCT/SUNA.

18.1.9 Preventive Treatments

Several case reports and small case series have shown the efficacy of lamotrigine in SUNCT, with a response rate of almost 70% [8]. The dose reported to be effective in SUN ranges between 50 and 600 mg/day. On the basis of the current evidence and although no randomised-controlled trials have been published, lamotrigine is at present considered the drug of choice for the preventive treatment of SUNCT [16].

Other anticonvulsants have been reported to have some effect in SUN.

Topiramate was reported to be effective in five SUNCT patients at doses up to 300 mg daily [17, 18]. Subsequently, 11 of 21 SUNCT patients (52%) benefited from topiramate given up to a dose of 400 mg/day in an open-label study, whereas the only SUNA patient treated with topiramate did not notice any benefit [8]. A placebo-controlled trial of Topiramate in SUNCT showed that three out of five patients received some benefit in reduction of attack frequency or attack load [19].

Zonisamide, which has got similar mechanisms of action to topiramate, has been tried in a SUNCT patient who did not tolerate carbamazepine with excellent results on long-term follow-up [20].

SUNCT has been shown to respond to gabapentin, with complete suppression of attacks in three of nine patients treated with 800 to 2700 mg daily [21–23]. When tried in an open-label fashion in 22 SUNCT and 5 SUNA patients at up to 3600 mg daily, it was reported to be effective in 60% of SUNA but only 45% of SUNCT patients [8].

Carbamazepine was beneficial in 11 of 33 (33%) of SUNCT patients. Among these, 8 of the 33 patients had a partial response, and 3 had a complete or almost complete response [24]. In a recent open-label series of 36 SUNCT and 5 SUNA patients treated with carbamazepine, 40% of SUNCT and 20% of SUNA patients reported a favourable response [8]. Two case reports only support the effectiveness of oxcarbazepine in the prevention of SUNCT [25, 26].

OnabotulinumtoxinA infiltrated at four points around the orbit, 10 U at each site, was reported to be consistently effective in a SUNCT patient refractory to oral treatments after 2.5 years of follow-up [27].

18.1.10   Transitional Treatments

There can be a lag of several days to a few weeks before the efficacy of preventive treatments becomes apparent. Transitional treatments, which produce a rapid suppression of the attacks for a limited period of time, can be used when waiting for the beneficial effect of a preventive treatment to become evident.

The administration of intravenous (IV) lidocaine at a rate of 1.3 to 3.3 mg/kg/h suppressed the headaches in four patients with SUNCT syndrome [28]. Subsequently 11 SUNCT and 4 SUNA patients reported a favourable outcome during administration of IV lidocaine at the dose of 1.5–3.5 mg/kg/h. Seven SUNCT patients were pain free for times varying between the duration of the infusion to 6 months. Three SUNCT patients had reduced attack frequency or severity, and one was lost to follow-up. All SUNA patients were pain free for 2 days to 12 weeks [8]. It is advisable to use IV lidocaine as a short-term treatment in patients who present in a so-called SUNCT status [29] and also in order to avoid breakthrough attacks while switching from one preventive drug to another in patients with high load of attacks. Twenty-four-hour ECG monitoring is mandatory during the infusion.

A suboccipital injection of a combination of lidocaine and a steroid was beneficial in five out of eight SUNCT patients [8]. Greater occipital nerve injections may render the patient pain free for weeks or months, allowing the introduction and dose escalation of preventive medications. Oral or intravenous corticosteroids have been reported to be effective in some cases of SUNCT. Partial or complete responses have been described. However in most of the initial cases, corticosteroids were used in combination with other oral medicines, which may have potentially biased their overall effect. Similarly to cluster headache, there can be a recrudescence of pain on either lowering the dose or discontinuing the corticosteroids. Intravenous methylprednisolone was reported to suppress SUNCT attacks completely [30, 31]. More evidence is needed before recommending oral or intravenous corticosteroids for the management of SUN.

18.1.11   Surgical Management

Some patients with the chronic form of SUNCT and SUNA are refractory to the available medical treatments. The extent of this problem is unknown. This group of patients are left with severe disability. For these patients surgical approaches may be justified. The approaches can be subdivided into three main groups:

ablative procedures of the trigeminal nerve, microvascular decompression of the trigeminal nerve and neurostimulation techniques.

18.1.12 Ablative Procedures of the Trigeminal Nerve

Data on ablative procedures on the trigeminal nerve are limited to isolated cases reports, and there is considerable potential for bias due to under-reporting of unsuccessful cases or those with adverse outcomes. Additionally, these procedures may have irreversible complications, such as residual hypoesthesia, anaesthesia dolorosa and keratitis. Procedures that have been tried in SUNCT syndrome include retrogasserian glycerol rhizolysis, percutaneous trigeminal ganglion compression, trigeminal ganglion thermocoagulation and gamma knife surgery. In view of the poor quality of data and the destructive nature, these procedures are not indicated in SUN.

18.1.13 Microvascular Decompression of the Trigeminal Nerve

Trigeminal microvascular decompression is considered the surgical treatment of choice for refractory trigeminal neuralgia with evidence of trigeminal neurovascular conflict [32]. In view of the clinical overlap between TN, SUNCT and SUNA, Williams and Broadley systematically looked for trigeminal neurovascular conflict with dedicated trigeminal MRI scans and found a high proportion of ipsilateral vascular loops in contact with the trigeminal nerve in SUNCT and SUNA (88%, $n = 15/17$) [5]. Ninety percent of the aberrant vessels were pressing on the symptomatic trigeminal nerve, compared to only 7% abutting on the asymptomatic nerve. This supported the notion of microvascular decompression (MVD) being a potential treatment for these conditions. To date, ten case reports and a case series of nine SUNCT and SUNA patients, who underwent MVD of the trigeminal nerve, have been reported [33–39]. After a median follow-up of 14 months (range: 0.5–32 months), 12 of 19 (63%) of cases were pain free, whereas in the remaining patients, the procedure had little or no effect. Two patients suffered from persistent complications, such as ataxia and hearing loss, whereas in five cases transient complications were only reported. Although series with longer follow-ups would be ideal to assess the long-term efficacy of MVD for chronic medically intractable SUNCT/SUNA, at present this approach may be considered a valuable option in refractory patients with ipsilateral trigeminal nerve compression due to a vascular loop, though possible benefit should be weighed against operation-related risks of permanent neurological deficits.

18.1.14   Peripheral and Central Neurostimulation

18.1.14.1   Occipital Nerve Stimulation

Similarly to cluster headache and hemicrania continua, occipital nerve stimulation has been trialled also in SUN. Preliminary positive outcomes were observed in a prospective series with a long follow-up of nine medically refractory chronic SUN. Eight out of nine patients reported a meaningful headache improvement [40]. A large uncontrolled study in 31 SUN patients showed at a mean follow-up of 44.9 months that 77% of the patients were considered responders, obtaining an improvement of at least 50% of the attacks. The surgery had favourable adverse rates with no electrode migration or erosion reported [41].

18.1.14.2   Deep Brain Stimulation of the Ventral Tegmental Area

In view of the functional imaging evidence of activation of the posterior hypothalamus region being linked to attacks of SUNCT [8] and the broad experience in the use of posterior hypothalamic region deep brain stimulation in patients with medically intractable CCH, three patients with intractable SUNCT have been treated with DBS of the posterior hypothalamus, which is now established to be the ventral tegmental area. The outcome of the three patients was promising, with a significant and sustained decrease in attack frequency, respectively, at 18-month [42], 12-month [43] and 15-month follow-up [44]. In a recent uncontrolled, open-label prospective observational study, 11 medically refractory SUN patients were treated with ipsilateral ventral tegmental area deep brain stimulation. At the final follow-up of a median of 29 months, 82% of the patients were considered responders, obtaining at least a 50% reduction in headache attacks compared to baseline [45].

The available evidence equally support the efficacy and safety of occipital nerve stimulation, trigeminal MVD and ventral tegmental area deep brain stimulation in refractory SUN. In view of the different degree of invasiveness, occipital nerve stimulation should be offered as first neuromodulation option, before more invasive procedures are considered. Refractory SUN patients should be managed in specialist centred with extensive level of expertise in surgical procedures for headache and facial pain disorders [46].

18.2   Hypnic Headache

Hypnic headache is a headache disorder which only occurs during sleep and causes awakening. It is relatively short lasting, of duration 15 min to 4 h, and does not usually cause autonomic symptoms or restlessness, although a recent review found up

Table 18.3 International
Headache Classification
Criteria for hypnic headache

4.9 Hypnic headache
A. Recurrent headache attacks fulfilling criteria B–E
B. Developing only during sleep and causing wakening
C. Occurring on ≥10 days per month for >3 months
D. Lasting ≥15 min and for up to 4 h after waking
E. No cranial autonomic symptoms or restlessness
F. Not better accounted for by another ICHD-3 diagnosis

to 15% of patients had some form of cranial autonomic symptoms [47]. Table 18.3 shows the classification criteria for hypnic headache [1].

The syndrome was originally described in 1988 [48]. Recent reviews have collated the findings of the 250 cases reported in the literature [49, 50]. The headache can be unilateral or bilateral; it usually is of a dull quality, but it can be pulsating (6%) or sharp, stabbing or burning (68%). Attacks vary in frequency from one to six attacks per night. The syndrome can be chronic or episodic with periods of headaches followed by periods of remission. The headache causes the patient to wake up, and typically patients exhibit some sort of motor behaviour: sitting up in bed, drinking, reading or watching TV. This is in contrast to migraine, where patients generally have to remain still as movement makes the pain worse, or other TACs which cause agitation and restlessness in CH [51], PH [52] and SUN [6]. Moreover, cranial autonomic symptoms are rare in hypnic headache, as opposed to that in TACs where they form part of the defining criteria.

Hypnic headache usually presents over the age of 50 years although it can present in some cases in younger patients and even children. It is commoner in women than men (F:M ratio 1.5:1) [53]. Even so, it is a rare headache, and prevalence is estimated in tertiary headache centres at 0.07–0.35% [50].

18.2.1 Pathophysiology of Hypnic Headache

The pathophysiology of hypnic headache remains elusive. A relation to obstructive sleep apnoea has been refuted [54], and hypnic headache can occur both during rapid eye movement (REM) and non-REM sleep, thus not showing a direct relationship to the stage of sleep [55]. It was also thought that melatonin was involved in the pathophysiology of hypnic headache and has been tried in treatments, but a recent study has found no correlation between melatonin levels and HH [56].

Given the strict sleep-related occurrence of these attacks, the hypothalamus has been postulated to have a role in HH with its diurnal periodicity [57]. This was borne out in a voxel-based morphometric study of 14 HH patients, whose hypothalamic grey matter volume was significantly reduced compared to healthy controls [58]. The role of the hypothalamus is well recognised in the TACs, all of which can wake patients from sleep. Migraine can also wake a patient from sleep and has some functional imaging evidence of hypothalamic activation in acute attacks [59] and in the chronic form [60]. It is unclear as to whether the hypothalamus is the main driver of the attacks, or just part of the response to pain, or involved in permission of the pain pathways reviewed [61]. Silencing of the anti-nociceptive network of periaqueductal grey (PAG), locus ceruleus and dorsal raphe nucleus doing REM sleep may also explain the preferential pattern [62].

18.2.2 Differential Diagnosis of Hypnic Headache

The differential diagnosis of hypnic headache is that of any headache that can wake a patient at night. These include nocturnal migraine, cluster headache, analgesic withdrawal syndrome, intracranial space occupying lesions causing symptoms of raised intracranial pressure, obstructive sleep apnoea syndrome, nocturnal hypoglycaemia, and nocturnal arterial hypertension.

Hypnic headache can coexist with migraine and can be associated with nausea in some cases. It can also coexist with obstructive sleep apnoea [1].

18.2.3 Diagnostic Workup

The diagnosis of hypnic headache is made on the history, but secondary causes of nocturnal headache must be ruled out. Therefore patients are required to have cranial MRI imaging, 24-h blood pressure monitoring and polysomnography or nocturnal blood glucose if required.

18.2.4 Medical Treatment

Treatment of hypnic headache, as in cluster headache and migraine, can be either abortive or preventive.

Abortive medications include caffeine, in the form of a cup of coffee or caffeine-containing analgesics [53], although care must be taken to avoid precipitating an analgesic-overuse syndrome, especially if the patient has a personal or family history of migraine. Triptans can be used in single cases [63]. Caffeine may also be used as a prophylactic treatment, with a strong cup of coffee on retiring to bed [63]. Patients may be concerned about caffeine disrupting their sleep, but if taken this way there has been no sleep disturbance found in HH [49].

As hypnic headache is so rare, the evidence for preventive treatment relies on case reports or series. Lithium has been best studied, with effectiveness in about two thirds of patients at doses of 150–600 mg daily, adjusted to plasma levels [49, 53, 63]. However adverse effects such as tremor, renal and thyroid disturbance are common with lithium, especially in the elderly population with significant comorbidities and contraindications to lithium treatment. Patients should have a course of lithium for 3–4 months, and gradual tapering of the drug thereafter, although some patients can relapse after withdrawal of the drug.

It is interesting to note that lithium is also effective in cluster headache. Lithium may preferentially affect the hypothalamus, which is important in the circadian pattern of both CH and HH [57].

Indomethacin has been tried in around 20 patients at 25–150 mg daily, with a good response in about 50%. Interestingly the responders were mostly those who had unilateral headache with subtle cranial autonomic symptoms [63], and this may relate to the beneficial effect of indomethacin on paroxysmal hemicrania.

Other medications including topiramate 25–100 mg daily in 12 patients and oxetorone 60–180 mg/day in 8 patients showed moderate benefit [53]. Verapamil and flunarizine have shown a mild effect [64], and other medications such as amitriptyline, beta-blockers and pizotifen are generally unhelpful [50, 64]. Melatonin has been tried in hypnic headache, but with limited success (only 1 of 4 cases with beneficial effect, and 4 of 33 cases in another study) [64].

Table 18.4 shows the similarities and differences between hypnic headache and the TACs.

18.3 Primary Stabbing Headache

Primary stabbing headache is characterised by short-lived episodes of stabbing pain centred over the first trigeminal division, occurring in single stabs or cluster of stabs. The attacks normally last a few seconds up to a minute and can occur on

Table 18.4 Similarities and differences between hypnic headache and the TACs

	Hypnic headache	TACs		
		Cluster headache	PH	SUN
Nocturnal occurrence	Exclusive	+	+	+
Occurrence during wakefulness	Never	+	+	+
Unilaterality	39%	100% [51]	100% [52]	98% [6]
Duration	15 min to 4 h	15–180 min	2–30 min	1–600 s
Autonomic symptoms	15% [47]	100%	100%	100%
Agitation	–	92% [51]	80% [52]	56–58% [6]
Response to medications: Lithium	++	++	–	–
Indomethacin	+	–	+++	–
Topiramate	±	+	+	+
Melatonin	±	±	–	N/A
Caffeine	++	N/A	N/A	N/A

NB. Patients with CH, PH and SUN can have attacks which remain strictly unilateral but alternate sides between attacks
N/A no data available

Table 18.5 Differentiating features of SUNCT and trigeminal neuralgia

Feature	SUNCT	Trigeminal neuralgia	Primary stabbing headache
Gender preponderance	Male	Female	Female
Site of pain	V1	V2/3	Extratrigeminal Regions in 70% of cases [4]
Severity of pain	Moderate to severe	Very severe	Severe
Duration(s)	1–600	<1–120	1–3
Autonomic features	Prominent	None	None
Refractory period	Absent	Present	Not applicable
Response to carbamazepine	Partial	Complete	None
Response to indometacin	None	None	Partial/complete

SUNCT short-lasting neuralgiform headache attacks with conjunctival injection and tearing

a daily or weekly basis. One of the cornerstone clinical features of primary stabbing headache is that the pain episodes tend to change site of occurrence within the trigeminal distribution, often occurring bilaterally or unilaterally side-alternating, normally sparing the face. This, along with the lack of accompanied cranial autonomic symptoms and the lack of cutaneous triggers, allows SUN to be distinguished from primary stabbing headache [65]. Table 18.5 shows some similarities and differences between SUN, TN and primary stabbing headache.

18.4   Cough, Exertional and Sex Headaches

18.4.1   Primary Cough Headache

Primary cough headache is that headache which is precipitated by coughing or any other Valsalva (straining) manoeuvre, in the absence of any structural neurological disorder. It is usually bilateral and posterior, with quick rise to peak pain occurring a few moments after the cough, and lasting usually only a few seconds or minutes, although some can persist in a mild to moderate form for up to an hour. The severity of the headache may be proportional to the frequency of the cough.

It is rare, affecting less than 1% of a headache clinic population, but up to 40% of patients in a respiratory clinic reported a cough.

The important differential of primary cough headache is secondary cough headache, which occurs in about 40% of patients who present with cough headache. The commonest cause is a posterior fossa lesion, mostly Arnold-Chiari type I malformations, although other lesions have been reported [1]. These include:

- CSF hypotension
- Carotid or vertebrobasilar disease

- Cranial fossa or posterior fossa tumours
- Midbrain cyst
- Basilar impression
- Platybasia
- Subdural haematoma
- Cerebral aneurysms
- Reversible cerebral vasoconstriction syndrome

Therefore diagnostic imaging is mandatory for patients with cough headache, especially as the treatment, such as indomethacin 50–200 mg daily, may be effective in reducing the symptoms of both primary and secondary cough headache and is therefore not a distinguishing feature between the two. However a recent study in 16 patients with cough headache suggested that those patients with headache induced by a positive modified Valsalva manoeuvre were more likely to have posterior fossa pathologies on MRI scan [66]. It is suggested that secondary cough headache is due to a transient increase in CSF pressure in the presence of obstruction of normal CSF dynamics. Primary cough headache appears to be caused by a different mechanism, possibly through congestion of the orbital venous plexus in the presence of jugular venous incompetence and a reduced threshold for trigeminal sensory activation [66].

Diagnostic imaging is even more important in children with cough headache, as subtentorial tumours account for over half of all space occupying lesions in the paediatric population.

18.4.2 Primary Exercise Headache

Primary exercise headache is brought on by sustained physical exertion, as opposed to a short-lasting Valsalva-type manoeuvre (primary cough headache). It can occur at high altitude or high temperatures. It is usually distinguishable by the trigger of sustained physical exertion, and the headache is longer-lasting, up to 48 h in duration, and often has a pulsating quality [1]. However some exercise headaches may be shorter in duration (less than 5 min) and have a less pulsating quality, especially in the adolescent population [67].

Primary exercise headache should also not be confused with exercise-induced migraine, where the underlying pathophysiology is migraine. Exercise headache can coexist with migraine in 46% of [68].

18.4.3 Laughter-Induced Headache

Laughter-induced headache, as the title suggests, is headache induced by laughter. The headache reaches a peak quickly after the laughter and then subsides over a few minutes. In a recent study, one patient with laughter-induced headache had cerebellar tonsillar herniation through the foramen magnum, and another patient did not [69]. It is thought that the same mechanism of transiently increasing intracerebral pressure causes symptoms in cough headache, exercise headache, and laughter-induced headache. Interestingly some patients could only induce a headache with mirthful rather than mirthless laughter, and it is possible that the areas of the brain associated in the expression of mirth may also play a role in laughter-induced headache [69].

18.4.4   Primary Headache Associated with Sexual Activity

This is described as a headache precipitated by sexual activity, either with gradual onset and increasing in intensity with increasing sexual excitement or with abrupt explosive intensity at or just before orgasm [1]. Although unilateral in 2/3 of cases and sometimes short lasting (a minute), it is generally not accompanised by autonomic activity, and can last up to 24-72 hours with severe intensity. These features plus the direct association with sexual activity makes differentiating from TACs relatively straightforward.

Importantly, primary headache associated with sexual activity is not associated with loss of consciousness, vomiting or other symptoms, whereas symptomatic sexual headache due to a subarachnoid haemorrhage, arterial dissection and reversible cerebral vasoconstriction (RCVS) may all be. At the first presentation of headache associated with sexual activity, cranial imaging including MRI and/or MRA is mandatory to exclude these secondary causes.

18.4.5   Primary Thunderclap Headache

This is a headache of high intensity and abrupt onset, reaching its peak before 1 min and lasting at least 5 min [1]. However the evidence that this is a primary headache syndrome is poor, and it is usually symptomatic of a vascular intracranial disorder, such as subarachnoid haemorrhage, venous sinus thrombosis, unruptured vascular malformation (such as aneurysm), arterial dissection, RCVS, pituitary apoplexy, meningitis, colloid cyst of third ventricle, CSF hypotension and acute sinusitis.

If accompanied by cranial autonomic symptoms due to the trigemino-autonomic reflex, then it is conceivable that it may be mistaken acutely for a TAC. However any thunderclap headache presenting de novo must be investigated fully for an underlying cause. If it were a primary TAC then there would be multiple stereotyped attacks of unilateral headache with cranial autonomic symptoms, and will be diagnosed as such.

18.4.6   Cold-Stimulus Headache

This is a short-lasting headache which is brought on by exposure of the head to very low environmental temperature, either external or by ingesting or inhaling a cold stimulus such as ice cream. It is usually bilateral and midfrontal or frontotemporal, although some patients can have unilateral, temporal, frontal or retro-orbital pain, which is usually distinguished from a TAC by the direct association with cold stimulus and lack of autonomic symptoms. Of course some SUNCT and SUNA attacks can be triggered by cold wind to the face, but SUN also occurs spontaneously. In a series of 52 patients with SUN/SUNA, only 1 had attacks which were entirely triggered [6].

18.5   Summary

This chapter has dealt with the short-lasting headaches, including SUN (short-lasting unilateral neuralgiform headache attacks) with cranial autonomic symptoms, which can be either a primary headache syndrome or symptomatic of an underlying structural disorder. The differential diagnosis, clinical characteristics and treatment options are discussed. Other short-lasting headaches are explored, including hypnic headache, primary stabbing headache and their features, and clinical characteristics are compared. Finally the other headaches are described, including cough, exertional and sex headaches, along with cold stimulus headache and primary thunderclap headache, which should be investigated appropriately in order to rule out an intracranial (usually vascular) cause.

References

1. Headache Classification Committee of the International Headache Society (IHS). The international classification of headache disorders, 3rd edition (beta version). Cephalalgia. 2013;33(9):629–808.
2. Sjaastad O, Saunte C, Salvesen R, Fredriksen T, Seim A, Roe O, et al. Shortlasting, unilateral neuralgiform headache attacks with conjunctival injection, tearing, sweating, and rhinorrhea. Cephalalgia. 1989;9(2):147–56.
3. IHS Classification. The international classification of headache disorders: 2nd edition. Cephalalgia. 2004;24(Suppl1):9–160.
4. Headache Classification Committee of the International Headache Society (IHS). The international classification of headache disorders, 3rd edition. Cephalalgia. 2018;38:1–211.. https://www.ichd-3.org/
5. Williams M, Broadley S. SUNCT and SUNA: clinical features and medical treatment. J Clin Neurosci. 2008;15(5):526–34.
6. Cohen A. Short-lasting unilateral neuralgiform headache attacks with conjunctival injection and tearing (SUNCT) or cranial autonomic features (SUNA)—a prospective clinical study of SUNCT and SUNA. Brain. 2006;129(10):2746–60.

7. May A, Bahra A, Büchel C, Frackowiak R, Goadsby P. Hypothalamic activation in cluster headache attacks. Lancet. 1998;352(9124):275–8.
8. Cohen A. Short-lasting unilateral neuralgiform headache attacks with conjunctival injection and tearing. Cephalalgia. 2007;27(7):824–32.
9. Matharu M, Cohen A, McGonigle D, Ward N, Frackowiak R, Goadsby P. Posterior hypothalamic and brainstem activation in hemicrania continua. Headache. 2004;44(8):747–61.
10. Matharu M, Cohen A, Frackowiak R, Goadsby P. Posterior hypothalamic activation in paroxysmal hemicrania. Ann Neurol. 2006;59(3):535–45.
11. Pareja J, Barón M, Gili P, Yangüela J, Caminero A, Dobato J, et al. Objective assessment of autonomic signs during triggered first division trigeminal neuralgia. Cephalalgia. 2002;22(4):251–5.
12. Sano K, Mayanagi Y, Sekino H, Ogashiwa M, Ishijima B. Results of stimulation and destruction of the posterior hypothalamus in man. J Neurosurg. 1970;33(6):689–707.
13. Lambru G, Trimboli M, Tan S, Al-Kaisy A. Medullary infarction causing coexistent SUNCT and trigeminal neuralgia. Cephalalgia. 2016;37(5):486–90.
14. Levy M, Matharu M, Meeran K, Powell M, Goadsby P. The clinical characteristics of headache in patients with pituitary tumours. Brain. 2005;128(8):1921–30.
15. Mitsikostas D, Ashina M, Craven A, Diener H, Goadsby P, Ferrari M, et al. European headache federation consensus on technical investigation for primary headache disorders. J Headache Pain. 2015;17:5.
16. May A, Leone M, Afra J, Linde M, Sándor PS, Evers S, Goadsby PJ. EFNS Task Force EFNS guidelines on the treatment of cluster headache and other trigeminal-autonomic cephalalgias. Eur J Neurol. 2006;13(10):1066–77.
17. Matharu MS, Boes CJ, Goadsby PJ. SUNCT syndrome: prolonged attacks, refractoriness and response to topiramate. Neurology. 2002;58(8):1307.
18. Rossi P, Cesarino F, Faroni J, Malpezzi MG, Sandrini G, Nappi G. Sunct syndrome successfully treated with topiramate: case reports. Cephalalgia. 2003;23(10):998–1000.
19. Weng HY, Cohen AS, Schankin C, Goadsby PJ. Phenotypic and treatment outcome data on SUNCT and SUNA, including a randomised placebo-controlled trial. Cephalalgia. 2018;38(9):1554–63.
20. Ikawa N, Imai N, Manaka S. A case of SUNCT syndrome responsive to zonisamide. Cephalalgia. 2010;31(4):501–3.
21. Graff-Radford SB. SUNCT syndrome responsive to gabapentin (neurontin). Cephalalgia. 2000;20(5):515–7.
22. Hunt C, Dodick D, Bosch E. SUNCT responsive to gabapentin. Headache. 2002;42(6):525–6.
23. Porta-Etessam J, Benito-Leon J, Martinez-Salio A, Berbel A. Gabapentin in the treatment of SUNCT syndrome. Headache. 2002;42(6):523–4.
24. Matharu M, Cohen A, Boes C, Goadsby P. Short-lasting unilateral neuralgiform headache with conjunctival injection and tearing syndrome: a review. Curr Pain Headache Rep. 2003;7(4):308–18.
25. Dora B. SUNCT syndrome with dramatic response to oxcarbazepine. Cephalalgia. 2006;26(9):1171–3.
26. Marziniak M, Breyer R, Evers S. SUNCT syndrome successfully treated with the combination of oxcarbazepine and gabapentin. Pain Med. 2009;10(8):1497–500.
27. Zabalza R. Sustained response to botulinum toxin in SUNCT syndrome. Cephalalgia. 2012;32(11):869–72.
28. Matharu M, Cohen A, Goadsby P. SUNCT syndrome responsive to intravenous lidocaine. Cephalalgia. 2004;24(11):985–92.
29. Pareja J, Caballero V, Sjaastad O. SUNCT syndrome. Status like pattern. Headache. 1996;36(10):622–4.
30. Raimondi E, Gardella L. SUNCT syndrome. Two cases in Argentina. Headache. 1998;38(5):369–71.

31. Maihöfner C, Speck V, Sperling W, Giede-Jeppe A. Complete remission of SUNCT syndrome by intravenous glucocorticoid treatment. Neurol Sci. 2012;34(10):1811–2.
32. Barker F, Jannetta P, Bissonette D, Larkins M, Jho H. The long-term outcome of microvascular decompression for trigeminal neuralgia. N Engl J Med. 1996;334(17):1077–84.
33. Gardella L, Viruega A, Rojas H, Nagel J. A case of a patient with SUNCT syndrome treated with Jannetta procedure. Cephalalgia. 2001;21(10):996–9.
34. Black D, Dodick D. Two cases of medically and surgically intractable Sunct: a reason for caution and an argument for a central mechanism. Cephalalgia. 2002;22(3):201–4.
35. Lagares A, Gómez P, Pérez-Nuñez A, Lobato R, Ramos A. Short-lasting unilateral neuralgiform headache with conjunctival injection and tearing syndrome treated with microvascular decompression of the trigeminal nerve: case report. Neurosurgery. 2005;56(2):E413.
36. Sprenger T, Valet M, Platzer S, Pfaffenrath V, Steude U, Tolle T. SUNCT: bilateral hypothalamic activation during headache attacks and resolving of symptoms after trigeminal decompression. Pain. 2005;113(3):422–6.
37. Guerreiro R, Casimiro M, Lopes D, Marques J, Fontoura P. Video NeuroImage: symptomatic SUNCT syndrome cured after trigeminal neurovascular contact surgical decompression. Neurology. 2009;72(7):e37.
38. Irimia P, González-Redondo R, Domínguez P, Díez-Valle R, Martínez-Vila E. Microvascular decompression may be effective for refractory SUNCT regardless of symptom duration. Cephalalgia. 2009;30(5):626–30.
39. Williams M, Bazina R, Tan L, Rice H, Broadley S. Microvascular decompression of the trigeminal nerve in the treatment of SUNCT and SUNA. J Neurol Neurosurg Psychiatry. 2010;81(9):992–6.
40. Lambru G, Shanahan P, Watkins L, Matharu MS. Occipital nerve stimulation in the treatment of medically intractable SUNCT and SUNA. Pain Physician. 2014;17(1):29–41.
41. Miller S, Watkins L, Matharu M. Long-term follow up of intractable chronic short lasting unilateral neuralgiform headache disorders treated with occipital nerve stimulation. Cephalalgia. 2017;38(5):933–42.
42. Leone M, Franzini A, D'Andrea G, Broggi G, Casucci G, Bussone G. Deep brain stimulation to relieve drug-resistant SUNCT. Ann Neurol. 2005;57(6):924–7.
43. Lyons M, Dodick D, Evidente V. Responsiveness of short-lasting unilateral neuralgiform headache with conjunctival injection and tearing to hypothalamic deep brain stimulation. J Neurosurg. 2009;110(2):279–81.
44. Bartsch T, Falk D, Knudsen K, Reese R, Raethjen J, Mehdorn H, et al. Deep brain stimulation of the posterior hypothalamic area in intractable short-lasting unilateral neuralgiform headache with conjunctival injection and tearing (SUNCT). Cephalalgia. 2011;31(13):1405–8.
45. Miller S, Akram H, Lagrata S, Hariz M, Zrinzo L, Matharu M. Ventral tegmental area deep brain stimulation in refractory short-lasting unilateral neuralgiform headache attacks. Brain. 2016;139(10):2631–40.
46. Palmisani S, Al-Kaisy A, Arcioni R, Smith T, Negro A, Lambru G, et al. A six year retrospective review of occipital nerve stimulation practice—controversies and challenges of an emerging technique for treating refractory headache syndromes. J Headache Pain. 2013;14(1):67.
47. Holle D, Naegel S, Krebs S, Katsarava Z, Diener H, Gaul C, et al. Clinical characteristics and therapeutic options in hypnic headache. Cephalalgia. 2010;30(12):1435–42.
48. Raskin N. The hypnic headache syndrome. Headache. 1988;28(8):534–6.
49. Lanteri-Minet M, Donnet A. Hypnic headache. Curr Pain Headache Rep. 2010;14(4):309–15.
50. Lanteri-Minet M. Hypnic headache. Headache. 2014;54(9):1556–9.
51. Bahra A, May A, Goadsby P. Cluster headache: a prospective clinical study with diagnostic implications. Neurology. 2002;58(3):354–61.
52. Cittadini E, Matharu M, Goadsby P. Paroxysmal hemicrania: a prospective clinical study of 31 cases. Brain. 2008;131(4):1142–55.
53. Holle D, Naegel S, Obermann M. Hypnic headache. Cephalalgia. 2013;33(16):1349–57.

54. Holle D, Wessendorf T, Zaremba S, Naegel S, Diener H, Katsarava Z, et al. Serial polysomnography in hypnic headache. Cephalalgia. 2010;31(3):286–90.
55. Pinessi L, Rainero I, Cicolin A, Zibetti M, Gentile S, Mutani R. Hypnic headache syndrome: association of the attacks with rem sleep. Cephalalgia. 2003;23(2):150–4.
56. Naegel S, Huhn J, Gaul C, Diener H, Obermann M, Holle D. No pattern alteration in single nocturnal melatonin secretion in patients with hypnic headache: a case-control study. Headache. 2016;57(4):648–53.
57. Cohen A, Kaube H. Rare nocturnal headaches. Curr Opin Neurol. 2004;17(3):295–9.
58. Holle D, Naegel S, Krebs S, Gaul C, Gizewski E, Diener H, et al. Hypothalamic gray matter volume loss in hypnic headache. Ann Neurol. 2010;69(3):533–9.
59. Denuelle M, Fabre N, Payoux P, Chollet F, Geraud G. Hypothalamic activation in spontaneous migraine attacks. Headache. 2007;47(10):1418–26.
60. Schulte L, Allers A, May A. Hypothalamus as a mediator of chronic migraine. Neurology. 2017;88(21):2011–6.
61. Cohen A. SUN: short-lasting unilateral neuralgiform headache attacks. Headache. 2017;57(6):1010–20.
62. Singh N, Sahota P. Sleep-related headache and its management. Curr Treat Options Neurol. 2013;15(6):704–22.
63. Diener H, Obermann M, Holle D. Hypnic headache: clinical course and treatment. Curr Treat Options Neurol. 2011;14(1):15–26.
64. Lisotto C, Rossi P, Tassorelli C, Ferrante E, Nappi G. Focus on therapy of hypnic headache. J Headache Pain. 2010;11(4):349–54.
65. Pareja J, Kruszewski P, Caminero A. SUNCT syndrome versus idiopathic stabbing headache (jabs and jolts syndrome). Cephalalgia. 1999;19(25_suppl):46–8.
66. Lane R, Davies P. Modified Valsalva test differentiates primary from secondary cough headache. J Headache Pain. 2013;14:31.
67. Sjaastad O, Bakketeig L. Exertional headache. I. Vågå study of headache epidemiology. Cephalalgia. 2002;22(10):784–90.
68. Sjaastad O, Bakketeig L. Exertional headache—II. Clinical features Vaga study of headache epidemiology. Cephalalgia. 2003;23(8):803–7.
69. Ran Y, Liu H, Zhang M, Dong Z, Yu S. Laugh-induced headache: clinical features and literature review. Headache. 2017;57(10):1498–506.

Chapter 19
Future Therapies for Trigeminal Autonomic Cephalalgias: Cluster Headache and Related Conditions

Peter J. Goadsby and Lars Edvinsson

The trigeminal autonomic cephalalgias (TACs) are a group of primary headache disorders linked by usually prominent cranial autonomic features [1] that when present are typically lateralized to the side of the pain [2]. The TACs are grouped under section 3 of the current International Classification of Headache Disorders-3 [3]. They consist of cluster headache [4], paroxysmal hemicrania [5], short-lasting unilateral neuralgiform headache attacks with conjunctival injection and tearing (SUNCT)/cranial autonomic feature (SUNA) [6] and hemicrania continua [7]. These are devastating problems with patients describing the pain of cluster headache as the worst they have ever experienced [8].

The current treatments for cluster headache are less than ideal, be it use limits and vascular issues with triptans [9] or efficacy and tolerability issues with medicines such as verapamil, lithium and topiramate [2]. Few, least of all patients, would argue that new therapies are not required. We review here treatments on the horizon, either just arrived or close by, which provide real optimism that we can manage patients with these disorders much better in the near future. We will address the developments by condition since the treatments for the disorders are one of the more important distinguishing features.

P. J. Goadsby (✉)
NIHR-Wellcome Trust King's Clinical Research Facility & SLaM Biomedical Research Centre, King's College London, London, UK
e-mail: peter.goadsby@kcl.ac.uk

L. Edvinsson
Department of Internal Medicine, University of Lund, Lund, Sweden

© Springer Nature Switzerland AG 2020
M. Leone, A. May (eds.), *Cluster Headache and other Trigeminal Autonomic Cephalgias*, Headache, https://doi.org/10.1007/978-3-030-12438-0_19

19.1   Cluster Headache

Broadly the treatment of cluster headache (CH) can be considered as either acute, i.e. treating the immediate attack, or preventive, the later short-term bridging or medium- to long-term prevention.

19.1.1   Acute Attack Treatment

All patients with CH require an acute therapy, or at least a discussion of options. Current widely used treatments include triptans; serotonin $5HT_{1B/1D}$ receptor agonists; sumatriptan 6 mg s/c, sumatriptan 20 mg IN or zolmitriptan 5 mg IN; or inhaled oxygen 100% 12–15 L/min [2]. When considering new approaches, one way to do this is by considering the limitations of the current therapies and how new approaches may help.

19.1.1.1   Can We Make Oxygen Delivery More Efficient?

The currently accepted approach to oxygen therapy in acute cluster headache is described as high flow, 12–15 L/min, and was established evidentially by a randomized placebo-controlled double-blind multi-attack crossover study as effective [10]. One approach that is being explored to improve the performance of oxygen is "ultra-high flow" delivered by a demand valve where inspiratory effort alone limits flow rate. There have been some reported advantages, including patient preference [11], although this method would be well served by a rigorous study.

19.1.1.2   How Do We Treat More Than Two Attacks a Day?

A common problem in practice is patients who have more than two attacks a day. If they have three and respond to zolmitriptan NS, this seems a reasonable solution [12]. However, if they do not, or have more attacks, there can be a problem. Oxygen can be used for any number of attacks although it does not always work and is certainly a cumbersome approach in many ways. Smaller doses per attack of sumatriptan s/c may be used [13]; this area deserves further consideration. One important new addition to acute cluster headache therapy is non-invasive vagal nerve stimulation (nVNS), using the gammaCore device. This delivers a proprietary electrical signal consisting of five 5000-Hz pulses repeated at a rate of 25 Hz. A typical dose is a 120 s of stimulation. There are now two randomized sham-controlled studies that demonstrate superiority at 15 min on the pain-free outcome [14, 15]. The device is well tolerated and there is no limit on daily dosing. Indeed repeated dosing may have some preventive effect [16]. Interestingly, the positive effect on acute attacks was only seen in episodic cluster headache not chronic cluster headache [17].

19.1.1.3 My Patient with Cluster Headache Has Significant Cardiovascular Disease; with What Do I Treat Acute Attacks?

In a clinical cohort of middle-aged, often cigarette smoking males, this is not an uncommon problem. Triptans may be relatively or absolutely contraindicated in such patients because of increased cardiovascular risk [9]. While oxygen is an obvious way forward, again it does not work for everyone and has important logistic limitations. Again for episodic cluster headache, acute attacks may be treated with non-invasive vagal nerve stimulation (nVNS) for which there is clear randomized controlled trial evidence [17]. Based on a study that demonstrated octreotide 100 mcg s/c to be more effective than placebo at 30 min [18], pasireotide [19] is currently being explored for the acute treatment of cluster headache (NCT02619617). Pasireotide has a different receptor binding pattern being high affinity for the somatostatin receptor (SSTR)-5 and less so for 1, 2 and 3, whereas octreotide binds mainly to SSTR-2 [20]. SSTR activation has no known or observed vascular effects so that, if effective, it would be a welcome addition to our options for treating acute cluster headache.

19.1.2 Preventive Treatments for Cluster Headache

Most patients will benefit from at least short-term preventive approaches in cluster headache, and some certainly require long-term prevention. For short-term prevention, typical choices are greater occipital nerve region injection (GONi) with local anaesthetic and a corticosteroid [21, 22] or oral corticosteroids [23]. The former is not universally effective, and the latter has the issue of potential osteonecrotic consequences [24]. Patients with chronic cluster headache need preventives in the longer term. Current approaches with verapamil, lithium, topiramate or melatonin have their many limitations [4].

19.1.2.1 What Can I Use for Short-Term Prevention in Cluster Headache?

In patients who have failed previous GONi or may be unsuitable, there were few realistic choices. Some have advocated short-term nocturnal ergotamine [25] or a more modern version, frovatriptan [26]. These have limitations, including either the issue of concomitant cardiovascular disease or the relative contraindication of concomitant triptans. It has been shown that either spontaneous [27] or nitroglycerin-triggered [28] acute cluster headache attacks are associated with elevated levels of calcitonin gene-related peptide (CGRP). Monoclonal antibodies to CGRP have been tested now extensively in migraine and are effective attack preventives [29]. Galcanezumab, a CGRP monoclonal antibody [30], was tested in a randomized placebo-controlled double-blind study in episodic and chronic cluster headache. It was administered s/c monthly for two doses; at the primary endpoint of weeks 1–3, 75% of galcanezumab patients had a ≥50% reduction in attacks compared to baseline [31]. The treatment was well tolerated with no new adverse events than injection site pain, as reported in controlled trials in migraine [30, 32–35]. Interestingly, there was no significant effect in chronic cluster headache [31]. Similarly, a press release reports that fremanezumab, a CGRP monoclonal antibody effective in migraine prevention [36, 37], in a study in chronic cluster headache (NCT02964338) has been stopped for futility; the episodic cluster headache study (NCT02945046) continues.

19.1.2.2   What Can I Do for Patients with Medically Refractory Chronic Cluster Headache?

There may be no more suffering a patient than those with medically refractory chronic cluster headache [38, 39]. When medicines have failed, clinicians have typically turned to invasive approaches. Radiofrequency lesions [40] or Gamma Knife [41] of the trigeminal ganglion has been used, either important side effects, such as anaesthesia dolorosa, or an outcome no better than natural history, respectively. The sphenopalatine ganglion has been ablated [42, 43] with modest outcomes. The trigeminal nerve root has been sectioned [44] with complications including death. These procedures have been sensibly abandoned. Deep brain stimulation of the region of the brain at the posterior most portion of the hypothalamus, which is active in cluster headache [45], have been reported as being useful [46, 47], although brain surgery has serious, albeit rare, morbidity [48]. Notably a randomized controlled trial was negative [49]. The advent of a less specific, yet safer approach, occipital nerve stimulation [50, 51], made it in turn the preferred option, although lead migration, infection [52] and longer-term battery replacement issues and reduced efficacy have been issues.

The sphenopalatine ganglion, which sits in the pterygopalatine fossa draped across the maxillary branch of the trigeminal nerve [53], is a logical target for the treatment of cluster headache. An important component of the pathophysiology of acute cluster headache attacks is activation of the trigeminal autonomic reflex [54], which accounts for the cranial autonomic features, such as lacrimation, conjunctival injection, nasal congestion, aural fullness and periorbital oedema. The outflow pathway for these symptoms traverses the facial, VIIth, cranial nerve and synapses in the sphenopalatine ganglion (SPG) [55]. Based on this anatomy and clinical experience that the SPG may be a therapeutic target [43, 56, 57], an SPG microstimulator has been developed. In a study, CH-1, comparing SPG stimulation to a sham with no stimulation and a sub-perception stimulus in a randomized crossover design in 32 subjects with chronic cluster headache, 67% of attacks have pain relief at 15 min compared to 7% for each of sham and sub-perception treatments [58]. Interestingly they also reported that 36% had a ≥50% reduction in attack frequency [58]. Most recently the CH-2 study compared SPG stimulation to a sham stimulation that produced a cutaneous TENS-like effect to preserve blinding in subjects with chronic cluster headache. SPG stimulation was more effective than sham at achieving pain relief at 15 min (odds ratio 2.62) and reduced weekly attack frequency by 50% in subjects on active treatment and 28% on sham stimulation [59]. There were no serious adverse events, save surgical events that all resolved. Long-term open-label experience demonstrates that most patients, attack responders or frequency responders, maintain benefit out to at least 24 months [60].

19.2 Indomethacin-Sensitive TACS: Paroxysmal Hemicrania and Hemicrania Continua

Of the TACs, paroxysmal hemicrania (PH) and hemicrania continua (HC) can be very rewarding to treat or remarkably frustrating. Patients respond to indomethacin, by definition. When indomethacin cannot be tolerated, one can use medicines such as topiramate or melatonin, although none are spectacular as indomethacin is.

19.2.1 What Can I Treat Indomethacin-Sensitive Headache Patients with when They Do Not Tolerate Indomethacin?

When patients with PH or HC cannot tolerate indomethacin, their quality of life reverses quickly to that prior to diagnosis and treatment. We have seen of nine patients with HC who could not tolerate indomethacin, seven reported a positive effect on pain with non-invasive vagal nerve stimulation (nVNS) [61]. Similarly, of six patients with PH, four reported significant benefit for nVNS [61]. It is a well-tolerated approach and offers much to patients with very limited treatment options.

19.3 Comments

The diversity in modes of treating TACs and their relatively low success rate point towards the need of rethinking the pathophysiology. The drugs and procedures listed above are by and large focusing on targets outside the CNS. The modulation of the cranial nerves suggests some common pathways. With that in mind future neuroanatomy and function studies will provide avenues for basic research that can help this group of subjects with severe and long-lasting pain syndromes.

References

1. Goadsby PJ, Lipton RB. A review of paroxysmal hemicranias, SUNCT syndrome and other short-lasting headaches with autonomic features, including new cases. Brain. 1997;120:193–209.
2. Nesbitt AD, Goadsby PJ. Cluster Headache. Br Med J. 2012;344:e2407.
3. Headache Classification Committee of the International Headache Society (IHS). The international classification of headache disorders, 3rd edition. Cepahalalgia. 2018;38:1–211.
4. Hoffmann J, May A. Diagnosis, pathophysiology, and management of cluster headache. Lancet Neurol. 2018;17(1):75–83.
5. Cittadini E, Matharu MS, Goadsby PJ. Paroxysmal hemicrania: a prospective clinical study of thirty-one cases. Brain. 2008;131:1142–55.
6. Cohen AS, Matharu MS, Goadsby PJ. Short-lasting Unilateral neuralgiform Headache Attacks with conjunctival injection and Tearing (SUNCT) or cranial Autonomic features (SUNA). A prospective clinical study of SUNCT and SUNA. Brain. 2006;129:2746–60.
7. Cittadini E, Goadsby PJ. Hemicrania continua: a clinical study of 39 patients with diagnostic implications. Brain. 2010;133:1973–86.
8. Schor LI. Cluster headache: investigating severity of pain, suicidality, personal burden, access to effective treatment, and demographics among a large International survey sample. Cephalalgia. 2017;37(1S):172.
9. Dodick D, Lipton RB, Martin V, Papademetriou V, Rosamond W, MaassenVanDenBrink A, et al. Consensus statement: cardiovascular safety profile of triptans (5-HT$_{1B/1D}$ agonists) in the acute treatment of migraine. Headache. 2004;44:414–25.
10. Cohen AS, Burns B, Goadsby PJ. High flow oxygen for treatment of cluster headache. A randomized trial. J Am Med Assoc. 2009;302:2451–7.
11. Petersen AS, Barloese MC, Lund NL, Jensen RH. Oxygen therapy for cluster headache. A mask comparison trial. A single-blinded, placebo-controlled, crossover study. Cephalalgia. 2017;37:214–24.
12. Dixon R, Gillotin C, Gibbens M, Posner J, Peck RW. The pharmacokinetics and effects on blood pressure of multiple doses of the novel antimigraine drug zolmitriptan (311C90) in healthy volunteers. Br J Clin Pharmacol. 1997;43:273–81.
13. Gregor N, Schlesiger C, Akova-Ozturk E, Kraemer C, Husstedt IW, Evers S. Treatment of cluster headache attacks with less than 6 mg subcutaneous sumatriptan. Headache. 2005;45(8):1069–72.
14. Silberstein SD, Mechtler LL, Kudrow DB, Calhoun AH, McClure C, Saper JR, et al. Non-invasive vagus nerve stimulation for the Acute treatment of cluster headache: findings from the randomized, double-blind, sham-controlled ACT1 study. Headache. 2016;56:1317–32.
15. Goadsby PJ, de Coo IF, Silver N, Tyagi A, Ahmed F, Gaul C, et al. Non-invasive vagus nerve stimulation for the acute treatment of episodic and chronic cluster headache: a randomized, double-blind, sham-controlled ACT2 study. Cephalalgia. 2018;38:959–69.
16. Nesbitt AD, Marin JCA, Tompkins E, Ruttledge MH, Goadsby PJ. Initial experience with a novel non-invasive vagus nerve stimulation device for the treatment of cluster headache. Neurology (Minneap). 2015;84:1–5.
17. de Coo IF, Marin J, Silberstein SD, Friedman DI, Gaul C, Tyagi A, et al. Non-invasive vagus nerve stimulation for acute treatment of episodic and chronic cluster headache: pooled analysis of data from two randomised, double-blind, sham-controlled clinical trials. Cephalalgia. 2017;37(1S):175–6.
18. Matharu MS, Levy MJ, Meeran K, Goadsby PJ. Subcutaneous octreotide in cluster headache-randomized placebo-controlled double-blind cross-over study. Ann Neurol. 2004;56:488–94.
19. McKeage K. Pasireotide in acromegaly: a review. Drugs. 2015;75(9):1039–48.
20. Lesche S, Lehmann D, Nagel F, Schmid HA, Schulz S. Differential effects of octreotide and pasireotide on somatostatin receptor internalization and trafficking in vitro. J Clin Endocrinol Metab. 2009;94(2):654–61.

21. Ambrosini A, Vandenheede M, Rossi P, Aloj F, Sauli E, Pierelli F, et al. Suboccipital injection with a mixture of rapid- and long-acting steroids in cluster headache: a double-blind placebo-controlled study. Pain. 2005;118:92–6.
22. Leroux E, Valade D, Taifas I, Vicaut E, Chagnon M, Roos C, et al. Suboccipital steroid injections for transitional treatment of patients with more than two cluster headache attacks per day: a randomised, double-blind, placebo-controlled trial. Lancet Neurol. 2011;10:891–7.
23. Jammes JL. The treatment of cluster headaches with prednisone. Dis Nerv Syst. 1975;36:375–6.
24. Mirzai R, Chang C, Greenspan A, Gershwin ME. The pathogenesis of osteonecrosis and the relationships to corticosteroids. J Asthma. 1999;36:77–95.
25. Symonds C. A particular variety of headache. Brain. 1956;79:217–32.
26. Gaul C, Jurgens T. Frovatriptan for prophylactic treatment of cluster headache. Headache. 2011;51:1008–9.
27. Goadsby PJ, Edvinsson L. Human *in vivo* evidence for trigeminovascular activation in cluster headache. Brain. 1994;117:427–34.
28. Fanciullacci M, Alessandri M, Figini M, Geppetti P, Michelacci S. Increase in plasma calcitonin gene-related peptide from extracerebral circulation during nitroglycerin-induced cluster headache attack. Pain. 1995;60:119–23.
29. Ong JJY, Wei DY, Goadsby PJ. Recent advances in pharmacotherapy for migraine prevention: from pathophysiology to new drugs. Drugs. 2018;78:411–37.
30. Oakes TMM, Skljarevski V, Zhang Q, Kielbasa W, Hodsdon ME, Detke HC, et al. Safety of galcanezumab in patients with episodic migraine: a randomized placebo-controlled dose-ranging Phase 2b study. Cephalalgia. 2018;38(6):1015–25.
31. Martinez JM, Goadsby PJ, Dodick DW, Bardos JN, Oakes TMM, Millen BA, et al. A placebo-controlled study of galcanezumab in patients with episodic cluster headache: from the 8-week double-blind treatment phase. Headache. 2018;58:1289–90.
32. Dodick DW, Goadsby PJ, Spierings ELH, Scherer JC, Sweeney SP, Grayzel DS. CGRP monoclonal antibody LY2951742 for the prevention of migraine: a phase 2, randomized, double-blind, placebo-controlled study. Lancet Neurol. 2014;13:885–92.
33. Skljarevski V, Matharu M, Millen BA, Ossipov MH, Kim BK, Yang JY. Efficacy and safety of galcanezumab for the prevention of episodic migraine: results of the EVOLVE-2 phase 3 randomized controlled clinical trial. Cephalalgia. 2018;38:1442–54. https://doi.org/10.1177/0333102418779543.
34. Skljarevski V, Oakes TM, Zhang Q, Ferguson MB, Martinez J, Camporeale A, et al. Galcanezumab for episodic migraine prevention: a randomized phase 2b placebo-controlled dose-ranging clinical trial. JAMA Neurol. 2018;75:187–93.
35. Stauffer VL, Dodick DW, Zhang Q, Carter JN, Ailani J, Conley RR. Evaluation of galcanezumab for the prevention of episodic migraine: The EVOLVE-1 Randomized Clinical Trial. JAMA Neurol. 2018;75:1080–8.
36. Dodick DW, Silberstein SD, Bigal ME, Yeung P, Goadsby PJ, Blankenbiller T, et al. Effect of fremanezumab compared with placebo on the prevention of episodic migraine: a randomized clinical trial. JAMA Neurol. 2018;319:1999–2008.
37. Silberstein SD, Aycardi E, Bigal ME, Blankenbiller T, Dodick DW, Goadsby PJ, et al. Fremanezumab for chonic migraine preventive treatment. N Engl J Med. 2017;377:2113–22.
38. Goadsby PJ, Schoenen J, Ferrari MD, Silberstein SD, Dodick D. Towards a definition of intractable headache for use in clinical practice and trials. Cephalalgia. 2006;26:1168–70.
39. Leone M, Franzini A, Broggi G, Dodick D, Rapoport A, Goadsby PJ, et al. Deep brain stimulation for intractable chronic cluster headache: proposals for patient selection. Cephalalgia. 2004;24:934–7.
40. Mathew NT, Hurt W. Percutaneous radiofrequency trigeminal gangliorhizolysis in intractable cluster headache. Headache. 1988;28:328–31.
41. Donnet A, Valade D, Regis J. Gamma knife treatment for refractory cluster headache: prospective open trial. J Neurol Neurosurg Psychiatry. 2005;76:218–21.

42. Filippini-De Moor GPG, Barendse GAM, van Kleef M, Troost J, de Lange S, Sluijter ME, et al. Retrospective analysis of radiofrequency lesions of the sphenopalatine ganglion in the treatment of 19 cluster headache patients. Pain Clin. 1999;11:285–91.

43. Narouze S, Kapural L, Casanova J, Mekhail N. Sphenopalatine ganglion radiofrequency ablation for the management of chronic cluster headache. Headache. 2009;49:571–7.

44. Jarrar RG, Black DF, Dodick DW, Davis DH. Outcome of trigeminal nerve section in the treatment of chronic cluster headache. Neurology. 2003;60:1360–2.

45. May A, Bahra A, Buchel C, Frackowiak RS, Goadsby PJ. Hypothalamic activation in cluster headache attacks. Lancet. 1998;352:275–8.

46. Leone M, Franzini A, Bussone G. Stereotatic stimulation of the posterior hypothalamic gray matter in a patient with intractable cluster headache. N Engl J Med. 2001;345:1428–9.

47. Leone M, Franzini A, Cecchini AP, Broggi G, Bussone G. Hypothalamic deep brain stimulation in the treatment of chronic cluster headache. Ther Adv Neurol Disord. 2010;3(3):187–95.

48. Schoenen J, Di Clemente L, Vandenheede M, Fumal A, De Pasqua V, Mouchamps M, et al. Hypothalamic stimulation in chronic cluster headache: a pilot study of efficacy and mode of action. Brain. 2005;128:940–7.

49. Fontaine D, Lazorthes Y, Mertens P, Blond S, Geraud G, Fabre N, et al. Safety and efficacy of deep brain stimulation in refractory cluster headache: a randomized placebo-controlled double-blind trial followed by a 1-year open extension. J Headache Pain. 2010;11:23–31.

50. Burns B, Watkins L, Goadsby PJ. Successful treatment of medically intractable cluster headache using occipital nerve stimulation (ONS). Lancet. 2007;369:1099–106.

51. Magis D, Allena M, Bolla M, De Pasqua V, Remacle JM, Schoenen J. Occipital nerve stimulation for drug-resistant chronic cluster headache: a prospective pilot study. Lancet Neurol. 2007;6:314–21.

52. Burns B, Watkins L, Goadsby PJ. Treatment of intractable chronic cluster headache by occipital nerve stimulation in 14 patients. Neurology. 2009;72:341–5.

53. Gray H. Anatomy of the human body. Philadelphia: Lea & Febiger; 1918.. www.bartleby.com/107/

54. May A, Goadsby PJ. The trigeminovascular system in humans: pathophysiological implications for primary headache syndromes of the neural influences on the cerebral circulation. J Cereb Blood Flow Metab. 1999;19:115–27.

55. Goadsby PJ, Lambert GA, Lance JW. The peripheral pathway for extracranial vasodilatation in the cat. J Auton Nerv Syst. 1984;10:145–55.

56. Sluder G. The role of the sphenopalatine (or Meckle's) ganglion in nasal headaches. NY Med J. 1908;87:989–90.

57. Ansarinia M, Rezai A, Tepper SJ, Steiner CP, Stump J, Stanton-Hicks M, et al. Electrical stimulation of sphenopalatine ganglion for acute treatment of cluster headaches. Headache. 2010;50(7):1164–74.

58. Schoenen J, Jensen RH, Lanteri-Minet M, Lainez JM, Gaul C, Goodman AM, et al. Stimulation of the sphenopalatine ganglion (SPG) for cluster headache treatment. Pathway CH-1: a randomized, sham-controlled study. Cephalalgia. 2013;33:816–30.

59. Goadsby PJ, Sahai-Srivastava S, Kezirian EJ, Calhoun AH, Matthews DC, McAllister PJ, et al. Sham-controlled study of sphenopalatine ganglion stimulation for chronic cluster headache. Headache. 2018;58:1316–7.

60. Jurgens TP, Barloese M, May A, Lainez JM, Schoenen J, Gaul C, et al. Long-term effectiveness of sphenopalatine ganglion stimulation for cluster headache. Cephalalgia. 2017;37:423–34.

61. Tso AR, Marin JCA, Goadsby PJ. Non-invasive vagus nerve stimulation for treatment of indomethacin-sensitive headaches. JAMA Neurol. 2017;74:1266–7.

.

The manufacturer's authorised representative in the EU is Springer
Nature Customer Service Centre GmbH, Europaplatz 3, 69115 Heidelberg,
Germany. If you have any concerns regarding our products, please
contact ProductSafety@springernature.com

Printed and bound by CPI Group (UK) Ltd, Croydon, CR0 4YY
29/04/2026
02099454-0004